REVERSING
ALZHEIMER'S

REVERSING ALZHEIMER'S

The New Toolkit to Improve Cognition and Protect Brain Health

Dr. Heather Sandison
with Kate Hanley

HARPER

An Imprint of HarperCollins*Publishers*

REVERSING ALZHEIMER'S. Copyright © 2024 by Heather Sandison, ND. All rights reserved. Printed in the United States of America. No part of this book may be used or reproduced in any manner whatsoever without written permission except in the case of brief quotations embodied in critical articles and reviews. For information, address HarperCollins Publishers, 195 Broadway, New York, NY 10007.

HarperCollins books may be purchased for educational, business, or sales promotional use. For information, please email the Special Markets Department at SPsales@harper collins.com.

FIRST EDITION

Designed by Bonni Leon-Berman

Library of Congress Cataloging-in-Publication Data has been applied for.

ISBN 978-0-06-333908-8

24 25 26 27 28 LBC 7 6 5 4 3

For Darlene, for showing me what is possible
so that I could support so many others.

Why is there an elephant on the cover of this book?

Elephants are known for their excellent memory, and of course the goal of this book is to help you and your loved ones preserve cognition. Also, oftentimes, memory loss is the elephant in the room—that topic that everyone knows needs attention, but can feel too scary to talk about. And finally, elephants are matriarchal. Since women are two-thirds of the dementia sufferers and two-thirds of the dementia caregivers, that elephant on the cover is a nod to how women can also lead the way in preventing and reversing this insidious disease.

— H.S.

CONTENTS

FOREWORD

Many who read the title of this book by Dr. Heather Sandison—*Reversing Alzheimer's*—will object, claiming that reversing Alzheimer's is simply not possible. At least, that is the claim of mainstream medicine. And yet, as Dr. Sandison has shown clearly in this book, and in her recent clinical trial, reversing the cognitive decline of Alzheimer's disease is not only possible but it is occurring repeatedly in patients at multiple sites. In her new book, Dr. Sandison delves deeply into how she and others are accomplishing this remarkable result, offering a road map for anyone who is at risk for cognitive decline or who has begun such decline. The patient outcomes she and her team have achieved are far superior to anything reported in a pharmaceutical clinical trial.

How have Dr. Sandison and her team accomplished what billions of dollars of pharmaceutical research and development have not? She chose not to focus on writing prescriptions for synthetic chemical band-aids for the chronic illnesses that are compromising the health of most of us, but rather to peer deeply into the underlying physiology to determine the root causes of illness in each patient. She then treated each patient with a personalized approach. By incorporating twenty-first-century medicine in its best practice, this approach has already led to improved outcomes in diseases from lupus to rheumatoid arthritis to cardiovascular disease to cancer.

In 2017, Dr. Sandison attended a course that my colleagues and I offered in which we translated our decades of basic research on neurodegeneration into a novel clinical approach to reverse cognitive decline. She recognized the potential of such a protocol immediately and has devoted her career to the treatment and prevention of cognitive decline. Inspired by a dire need for more humane assisted-living facilities—institutions that did not simply watch residents decline while managing their struggles with zombifying drugs—she founded Marama. Marama is the first assisted-living facility to actually improve cognition of their residents. The ramifications of Marama are difficult to overstate—this establishment will be the model for all assisted-living facilities in the coming decades, the first to witness residents' improvements to the point of regained independence.

When Dr. Sandison saw the positive results of the practices she devised for her patients, she raised support for and conducted a trial proving to the medical community the possibility of improving cognition in patients with cognitive decline. Her results were starkly in contrast to recent drug trials—which at best slow the decline, and modestly at that. Her study was published in the well-respected, peer-reviewed *Journal of Alzheimer's Disease*.

Next in her efforts to make a difference, she created an at-home solution for the many who either could not afford in-residence costs at an assisted-living facility, or who desired to care for their family members with cognitive decline at home. Reversing Alzheimer's at Home, a course that is improving at-home care for the many in need, has been enormously helpful to scale her approach for families with different needs.

And now, with this book, Dr. Sandison offers her experience, deep knowledge, and advice to address the practical aspects of achieving the reversal of cognitive decline. In its pages, you will find the rationale, the tools, and the recipes for best outcomes.

As you might well imagine, these fundamental advances have not come without pushback from the old guard: as several have reasoned, "If this were true—that the cognitive decline of Alzheimer's disease could be reversed—it would be on the front page of every newspaper in the world; since it's not, it must not be true." But that assumes that the key opinion leaders are objective, which is rarely the case, especially when there are billions of dollars, tenure, many government grants, and prestigious awards at stake. Others have claimed, "Well, of course my doctor is doing everything possible, so she'll know (or he'll know) what is best." Sadly, in this day and age of rapid doctor visits, business-controlled healthcare, and managed costs, much of medical practice is outdated and ineffective.

So not surprisingly, any paradigm-shifting claim such as reversing Alzheimer's will be met with its share of skepticism; but as Confucius said, those who claim that something cannot be done should not interfere with those who are doing it. Skepticism is one of the very few pastimes that requires no energy or expertise. If one has the sagacity to prove a hypothesis or conclusion correct or, alternatively, to refute it rationally, that is an important contribution. However, if one is unable to do either, but does not wish to appear thick, then he may proudly claim to be a "skeptic."

Thankfully, the work of Dr. Sandison is making Alzheimer's optional. As she has shown, the reversal of cognitive decline is no longer a fantasy or future goal, it is an ongoing process today. I challenge anyone who does not believe her claims to read this book. If you have concerns for yourself or a loved one about cognitive decline, I urge you to visit Marama, to meet with patients who have improved, to learn the protocol, and to see for yourself that the era of untreatable, unpreventable Alzheimer's disease is truly and thankfully over.

Dale E. Bredesen, MD
Singleton Endowed Chair in Neurology
Pacific Neuroscience Institute
Novato, California
October 14, 2023

Hope for Alzheimer's

Let me guess. You opened up this book because you are:

- scared of, or already developing dementia yourself,
- currently caring for a loved one with dementia, or
- a healthcare provider who wants to help your patients protect their cognition.

Statistically speaking, you're most likely to be in the first group. After all, a whopping 64 percent of all Americans say that their biggest fear about growing older is that they will suffer from dementia. That's over 212 million people.

But you're also in good company if you're a caregiver—according to the Alzheimer's Association, there are 11 million Americans providing unpaid care to people with dementia. And this number will only grow as the number of people with Alzheimer's increases. After all, aging is the biggest risk factor for Alzheimer's. So as the enormous baby boomer generation ages—currently, every day ten thousand Americans turn sixty-five—the number of people in the US with Alzheimer's is expected to reach 8.5 million by 2030, and 11.2 million by 2040.

You're least likely to be in the third group—a healthcare provider who wants to help your patients protect their cognition. The standard narrative around dementia—even among medical practitioners—is that it is a long, slow, torturous decline for which there is very little you can do to mitigate, much less treat. I hope this book will help to change that narrative. (And if you are in this third group, I'm so happy you're here.)

No matter which group you're in—you could even be in all three—I think you'll be delighted to learn that dementia can be prevented, and even reversed. In my work as the founder and medical director of Solcere Health Clinic, a San Diego–based brain optimization clinic, and Marama, the first residential memory-care facility to have the goal of returning its residents to independent living, I see it happen regularly.

The remarkable improvements in cognition that I have witnessed are thanks in large part to a complex systems medicine approach to Alzheimer's treatment that supports all aspects of brain health using a comprehensive and robust set of tools, including diet, exercise, sleep, the remediation of toxic exposures and infections, and stress reduction. It's a far cry from the typical treatment for Alzheimer's, which relies on pharmaceutical treatments that, despite having FDA approval as treatments for Alzheimer's, don't have a measurable beneficial impact on cognitive function and have concerning side effects (such as an increased risk for brain bleeds and swelling). And what I have seen time and time again is that this new Alzheimer's toolkit works.

My First Dementia Patient

I was skeptical at first that Alzheimer's could actually be reversed. In fact, I have a distinct memory of my neurology professor in naturopathic medical school saying that suggesting there was any way to treat Alzheimer's disease was false advertising. This was in 2012, two years before Dr. Dale Bredesen, a neurologist at the UCLA Mary S. Easton Center for Alzheimer's Disease Research and Care and the Buck Institute for Research on Aging, published his first paper, documenting the improvements in cognition three patients experienced after following a complex treatment protocol that serves as the foundation of the protocol that I outline in these pages. And it was five years before his groundbreaking book, *The End of Alzheimer's*, came out. There's a rule of thumb that it takes twenty years for medical research to trickle down into medical practice, and I am thankful for Dr. Bredesen doing as much as he has done to condense that time frame and get more medical practitioners trained and more patients educated in his thorough approach so that more patients can benefit from it.

Despite my beliefs that there was nothing you could do to treat Alzheimer's, I signed up for a training with Dr. Bredesen after hearing him speak at a medical conference, because for the first time, the complexity of the intervention seemed like it could possibly match the complexity of the disease process. I hoped it would work, but it felt like the kind of hope you get when you have nothing else to lose.

Then I saw my first dementia patient after my training.

Darlene's dementia had progressed to the point that she was only able to speak in one-word sentences. Her score on the Montreal Cognitive Assessment (MoCA)—a standard clinical tool used to evaluate cognitive function that gives people a score from 0, the worst, to 30, which is a perfect score—was a 2. Her husband was desperate, ready to try anything that might help, but he needed some guidance and a little hand-holding. That's where I came in.

Even though she couldn't add much to our conversation, Darlene's personality shone through her brightly patterned floral dress, her studded black leather backpack, and her vibrant pink lipstick. She had a huge smile and bright eyes that met yours and let you know that she was with you. She was a former schoolteacher, and you could easily see that Darlene was used to holding attention and interacting with those around her.

Working together, Darlene and her husband dove into the program headfirst. They had her mercury fillings replaced, moved out of their bedroom that had grown moldy following a roof leak, started eating a ketogenic diet, went on long walks every day, and got back to the ballroom dancing they had always enjoyed three times a week. Six weeks later, her MoCA score had increased to a 7. She was speaking in full sentences, participating in the conversation, even bickering with her husband about something that had happened the night before. It wasn't a cure, but it was significant progress in a short time—and a far cry from the torturous decline we've been told is the only path Alzheimer's can take. And it was enough for me to rethink everything I had been told about what was possible for those suffering with dementia. If these improvements were possible for Darlene, what was possible for everyone else?

Since those early days working with Darlene, I have seen firsthand that this evidence-based protocol helps people—people with severe cognitive impairment as well as people who have only mild memory loss—get better. I *know* now that there's hope. And after you read the stories of other patients that I'll include in this book, you will, too. You'll meet Nancy, a widow whose MoCA score went from a 23 (mild cognitive impairment) to a 30 and who decided she didn't need to move into the senior living complex she had already paid a deposit on, because she was having too much fun running her business, dating, and thrifting with friends. You'll also read about Dean, who remembered his grandkids' names and stopped being incontinent after just three months on the protocol. And so many others. You'll hear the stories of people who are in similar circumstances and stage of cognitive decline as your loved one is (or you are). And you'll see that it's possible to get back to where they (or you) were—and maybe even better than before.

Approaching brain health from multiple angles is common sense, but uncommon practice. Except at Marama, where it's what we do, day in and day out. We evaluated the effects of our approach in a 2023 study that was published in *The Journal of Alzheimer's Disease*. Of our twenty-three study participants, seventeen of them experienced cognitive improvement in just six months. While a nearly 75 percent rate of success is encouraging, indeed—especially when compared to the 0 percent expectation of improvement the traditional medical approach has to offer dementia patients—what I really find exciting is that these were people implementing the same program that I outline on these pages on their own, at home. They didn't do everything perfectly. Some participants never fully got into ketosis. No one took every supplement. And still, their cognition got significantly better.

And because the brain has a relationship to every other major system of the body, the benefits of following the protocol we use at Marama and evaluated in our clinical study extend beyond the brain:

- Enhanced insulin sensitivity, which then dramatically improves type 2 diabetes
- A reduction in high blood pressure that is protective of heart health (many of our patients both at Solcere and Marama reduce or eliminate their need for blood pressure medications)
- An improvement in mental health by lessening the experience of depression and anxiety and boosting mood
- A reduction of fall risk
- Improved gut health
- A lessening in symptoms and severity of autoimmune diseases
- An increase in sleep scores
- A boost in quality of life

As excited as I have been by the results of the study, I'm not surprised, because it matches what I see clinically—when patients are given the direction and have the willingness to take it, even imperfectly, the vast majority tend to improve.

Effective, and Doable, but Not Easy

While I *am* offering real, life-changing, global hope, I'm *not* saying it's easy to turn the tide on Alzheimer's and get cognitive changes to start going in a positive direction. I wish I could say that it was. I long to be able to tell patients and families that I have an easy pill or IV that will make their suffering stop and bring their loved one back. The reality is it takes energy, time, consistency, and resources. While this protocol works, it can feel overwhelming. This book is here to distill the protocol into a step-by-step process so that you—and your loved one, if you're a caregiver—can start reaping the benefits.

As dementia is a complex disease and the brain a complex organ within a complex system, the protocol is multifaceted. There are a lot of moving parts, including changing the foods you eat, getting more and different types of exercise, supporting your ability to get good sleep (which is when your brain takes out the trash and repairs itself), engaging in activities that challenge your brain, doing simple but powerful practices to counteract stress, and addressing your environment in order to reduce potential toxic exposures. You need more than just information in order to follow it—you need a little help with getting organized, staying motivated, and taking some of the stress out of caregiving. That's where my clinical experience comes in. Through my real-world functional medicine clinic, my residential-living facility (Marama), and my virtual group coaching program (Reversing Alzheimer's at Home), I've helped hundreds of people utilize the tools of the new Alzheimer's toolkit in their daily lives. I don't expect you to be able to do it all. But every little piece you can weave into your daily routines can provide benefit—that's why I include guidance on what to choose to do if you do only one thing throughout the book.

If you find yourself looking for additional support, we have created video summaries of each chapter and a workbook to guide you through the most actionable steps. Download it at ReversingAlzheimersBook.com.

I also know that the more tools you implement, the more significant those benefits will be. The potential gains these tools can create aren't limited to cognitive function—choosing to engage in the things that support your brain health can give you a new sense of meaning and purpose, and deepen your connection to others. This isn't just about ticking things off a list, but about reorienting your life in a way that supports all definitions of health—cognitive, physical, mental, emotional, and even spiritual.

While I can't promise an easy fix, I can promise hope—hope that our elders can stay sharp and vital, in community with their loved ones, and enjoying themselves while also sharing their wisdom and perspectives. And hope that if dementia runs in your family, you can stop fearing the worst and make a plan to maintain your dignity, joy, and yes, cognition, throughout your senior years.

As much as I am devoted to improving health and health span (the number of years we stay well), my ultimate goal is twofold: (1) making dementia a rare, yet reversible, occurrence, and (2) facilitating intergenerational wisdom transfer. The world is desperate for solutions, and we can't afford to lose the counsel and perspective of our elders. We need our wisest change-makers, and we need the people who are compassionate and devoted enough to care for our elders to have the bandwidth to participate in making the world a better place for the generations that follow.

Let's Get Started

We've already lost too many people and too much time spent in fear of developing Alzheimer's disease. By turning the page and embarking on your Reversing Alzheimer's journey, you are beginning to reclaim your focus, energy, and potentially even your loved ones from dementia.

Before you get going, I want to share a story about a 1979 plane expedition to Antarctica. This flight was adventure tourism, meant to be a scenic tour of the southernmost continent. The route was carefully calculated to depart from New Zealand, fly over the ice floes and penguin colonies, and then return to New Zealand eleven hours later. But there was an infinitesimal error in the mathematical calculations that guided the route, and the plane crashed into Mount Erebus, which the pilots couldn't see due to fog.

While this story doesn't have a happy ending, it shows the incredible power of even tiny changes. I've included hundreds of ideas in this book that will help you take better care of your own brain as well as the brain of the person you're caring for. You can't do them all, and certainly not all at once. Start with just a few and add on as you can. And know that every idea you implement and make a new habit can compound into profound benefits over time. Do what you can and be gentle with yourself about the rest. That way, you'll be more likely to continue, adding on to your Reversing Alzheimer's plan as you go, knowing that each incremental change can help you avoid the mountain as well as enjoy the ride along the way.

Understanding the Problem

CHAPTER 1

The Truth About Brain Health

At age seventy-five, Nancy came to see me because she was noticing some cognitive decline. Nancy and her partner had run a small business for years. Since her husband had died, she was having a hard time keeping up with the paperwork the business required. Preparing her taxes—something she'd always done easily—was giving her fits and sending her spiraling into overwhelm. While Nancy was ready to sell the business and officially retire, the age-in-place senior living community she planned to move into wouldn't accept her if she had measurable cognitive decline. With no children or living siblings, that facility was Nancy's best hope for spending her later years in community with others, and she was scared the door to that opportunity was closing.

Nancy needed to reverse any cognitive impairment she had already experienced, and she needed to do it quickly. You could see the effect of stress on her face—she had noticeable dark circles under her eyes. Her scalp was itchy and toenails were discolored. She had enrolled in an online class for brain games, but she was too overwhelmed to actually show up to the classes. Nancy was also very anxious, calling my office every day, leaving three or four voicemails every night. If you might describe someone as needing a little hand-holding, she needed both hands held, all day.

Once we evaluated her, we determined that she fit the definition of mild cognitive impairment according to the Montreal Cognitive Assessment (MoCA). Out of a possible 30 points (the highest score), Nancy scored a 23, just shy of the cutoff for normal age-related cognitive decline.

From a medical perspective, it's no wonder that Nancy's scalp and nails were bothering her—she had an overgrowth of yeast that had spread from her gut to her skin and nails. I prescribed her supplements to support her thyroid and adrenals—the stress had really taken its toll on these glands, which were overworked and struggling—and put her on bioidentical hormone therapy to send her brain signals that helped it stay sharp. Nancy also adopted a ketogenic diet, which helped with the yeast overgrowth, and started taking long walks every day and getting to a tai chi class a day or two each week. We also discussed her sleep hygiene and she started turning the TV off an hour before bed (she made it a point to stick to funny movies instead of twenty-four-hour news channels up until that time) and taking a magnesium glycinate supplement and a progesterone pill at night to help her body relax enough to sleep.

Within about three months, Nancy's MoCA score was up to 27, and she decided that she didn't actually need to move into the senior living community. She got caught up on her taxes, and was showing up for all her brain training classes. Nancy definitely didn't like that the ketogenic diet required as much cooking as it did, but she solved that problem by cooking extra for her neighbors—sharing food and helping other people energized her.

After six months, Nancy got back to a MoCA of 30, and her life blossomed. She started dating. Her new favorite pastime became thrifting with friends, and when she'd come into our office for her follow-up visits, she'd be wearing colorful outfits such as a bright purple dress with a big red belt. She was clearly having fun and loving life.

I share Nancy's story because it demonstrates so well how cognitive decline can actually move in reverse. When you give the brain the nutrients and the conditions it needs to be healthy—and remove the irritants and toxins that harm it—it can rewire and repair itself at any age.

A Complex Disease Requires a Complex Approach

It's impossible to separate brain health from whole-body health. Whatever is happening in your gut, in your cardiovascular system, in your sense organs (eyes, ears, nose, and skin), and in your musculoskeletal system is going to be felt in your brain. And whatever's happening in your brain is going to impact all your other systems, too.

The definition of health that I ascribe to is *homeodynamic balance within a complex system.* That means that imbalance is the opposite of health—in other words, chronic imbalance equals chronic disease. And that balance is ever changing—it's not set it and forget it.

A mentor and friend of mine, Daniel Schmachtenberger, defines imbalance as "too much, too little, in the wrong place, or at the wrong time." An example of too much is eating a carb- and sugar-heavy diet that leads to excessive levels of glucose, which then leads to glycation of your neurons (a process where a sugar molecule bonds with a brain cell and essentially caramelizes it, contributing to cognitive decline). Too little could mean not enough exercise so that the body doesn't get the signal to keep building its capacities. An example of "in the wrong place" is high levels of glucose and insulin in your bloodstream because your insulin receptors have burned out and no longer work (in what's known as insulin resistance). And "at the wrong time" is having high levels of cortisol, which naturally spikes in the morning and helps you have the energy to get up and move through the day, at night, when it's time to sleep.

But to really be able to address everything that is impacting your brain health, we have to zoom our lens out a little farther and consider the things that our brains are influenced by that happen beyond our physiology. This includes mental health, such as trauma, negative self-talk, and your own self-awareness. (After all, if you don't realize that your cognition is declining, you'll be a lot less incentivized to do anything about it.) In addition, the external stressors you experience in your life, and that come from just being alive in the world today, have a big impact on your health, and on your bandwidth for doing the things that take care of your health. Some stressors come from our society, such as all the "isms" (racism, sexism, ableism, and ageism, for starters), and the belief that working twenty-four/seven is the only way to be. Our relationships to other people, and how isolated or connected we feel to individuals and to society at large, also play an important role in our cognitive health.

According to the great wisdom traditions, medicine and healing operate in four dimensions:

- Inside (internal)
- Outside (external)
- Me (individual)
- We (collective)

To get well we will need to incorporate all four dimensions. If we leave any out, we will miss healing opportunities.

On the next page is an image that maps each of the influences on cognitive health—it's inspired by the work of Ken Wilber, an American philosopher who points us back to this truth of how we can categorize all life according to these four dimensions. Here, I've modified this concept to pertain specifically to brain health.

Many of the interventions we use at Solcere and that I outline in this book apply to the upper right quadrant of this graph—they apply directly to the brain and the body. By writing this book I am working in the lower left quadrant—working to shift our collective narrative around aging and the medical approach to managing dementia, and even changing the idea that there's "nothing you can do" about Alzheimer's until we find a magic cure. And by reading this book, you are addressing the upper left quadrant—your attitudes about aging, beliefs around what's possible for your brain health as you age, your awareness of your own cognitive health, and your confidence that you can positively impact your brain health. As you and other people read this book and start to share your stories and insights with more people, you are addressing the lower right quadrant.

I know, it's a lot. And yet, it's doable. In this book I will walk you through it step by step. Since dementia has many factors, and any approach to preventing or reversing dementia needs to take into account every one of those factors—that's how you don't overlook something crucial, and how you bring balance back to your being.

In this book I will walk you through each of the factors and give you the road

THE TRUTH ABOUT BRAIN HEALTH 7

Individual Internal	**Individual** External
My inside state	My brain and body
Self-awareness	Toxins
Self-talk	Nutrients
Attitudes	Hormones
Feelings	Infections
Beliefs	Structure

Social networks	The culture
Isolation	How society thinks about me:
Community	Ageism Sexism
Friendships	Racism Ableism
	Social structures:
	Health insurance policy
	Government safety nets

Collective Internal	**Collective** External

map, so you can be methodical and measured about discovering which factors are influencing you, and then take steps to remedy them. Some factors likely won't apply to you or your loved one at all—but you'll still have the confidence of knowing that you systematically considered everything you could potentially do to protect your current and future self from cognitive impairment.

Getting Started: Assessing the Physical Influences of Brain Health

One of my primary teachers is Dr. Dale Bredesen, whose integrative approach to treating dementia is the basis of much of my work. In my opinion he deserves a Nobel Prize for his work to change how we think about neurodegenerative disease against much resistance. He also deserves credit for some great analogies that I share regularly with my patients and throughout this book. One of my favorite analogies of his is how he describes the brain as a country—he calls it My Brain-i-stan.

Just like any sovereign country, you want your brain to have plenty of resources for building and maintaining infrastructure. The roads, bridges, planes, and trains that help citizens get around their country are the equivalent of the neurons, neuronal connections, and neuronal pathways in your brain. You also want a trash system that functions well so that the roads and sidewalks don't get blocked—in My Brain-i-stan, that's your systems of detoxification, including your lymphatic and glymphatic systems, which remove waste from cells throughout your body and in your brain, respectively. You don't want to be accepting trash from other countries that then overwhelm your own sanitation department; the same goes for your brain, in that you don't want to be ingesting a lot of toxins via your food, lawn care, traffic exhaust, mold, or heavy metals. And you don't want My Brain-i-stan to have to constantly be in defensive mode, warding off attacks and repairing damage from invaders. You want plenty of building blocks for that infrastructure, which for your brain means plenty of nutrients from food and, in some cases, supplements. And you want reliable information from the rest of the world to help My Brain-i-stan work with its neighbors—just as your brain needs plenty of input from your sense organs, your hormones, and neurotransmitters to function at its best.

You can assess the overall health of My Brain-i-stan by looking at the six integral components of a healthy brain:

- TOXINS, which can keep your body stuck in a defense mode (think inflammation) and divert resources away from creating new neurons and neuronal connections, as well as directly cause damage to your brain.
- NUTRIENTS from the foods you eat can either help or harm the brain. The brain needs specific nutrients (namely, amino acids, vitamins, minerals, and fats) to support its function. And too many carbs and sugar can damage the brain.

- STRESS is like Goldilocks—both too much and too little are detrimental to the brain. Too much makes your brain and nervous system hyperfocused on getting you out of that stressful situation, while too little means your brain has no reason to form new neuronal connections.
- STRUCTURE refers to your physical makeup and includes your genetics, chronic pain, and even the shape of your airways (which then impact how much sleep and oxygen you get and, thus, how much cleaning and repair your brain gets each night).
- INFECTIONS not only divert resources away from brain function and maintenance but, like toxins, can directly cause damage to the brain itself and send the brain into protection mode by stimulating inflammation.
- SIGNALING refers to all the chemical messengers in the body that interact with the brain, including reproductive hormones such as estrogen and testosterone, and proteins, such as peptides and brain-derived neurotrophic factor (BDNF).

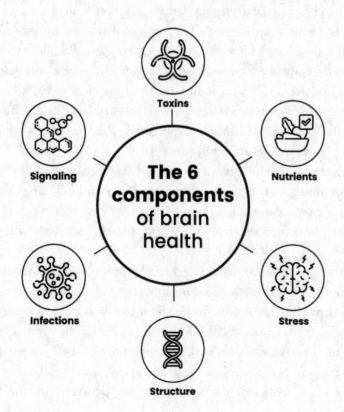

Let's take a deeper look at how each of these influences My Brain-i-stan. And just know that we will cover how to balance each of these areas in the chapters to come. But in case you are excited to start making changes already, I'm including the one thing you can do now that will start to turn the tide as you get the rest of your Reversing Alzheimer's program in place.

Toxins

Toxins are a fact of life. After all, every cell in your body needs to consume energy, a process that creates waste products, and those waste products can become harmful if they are allowed to build up. In addition, we live in a toxic world—with heavy metals in our dental fillings, fish, drinking water, and household dust; hormone-disrupting chemicals in our food containers and personal care products; neurotoxic compounds excreted by mold; pesticides and herbicides on our food and on our lawns and parks; and particulate matter from car exhaust and industrial processes in our air.

The good news is your body has multiple detoxification processes. In the brain, the glymphatic system takes out the trash each night while you sleep. In the body, the venous and lymphatic systems sweep away dead cells, viruses, bacteria, and waste products and delivers them to the liver, where anything the body no longer needs can be shunted into the digestive tract via the bile and excreted through your stool. The kidneys and skin help excrete toxins through urine and sweat.

The bad news: It's still easy to get "too much" (referring back to that definition of imbalance) on the toxin front, so that your body can't efficiently process and get rid of toxins. Then they store up in your tissues and wreak havoc on the complex system that is your overall health, including your brain health.

Toxins are a heavy burden on the brain, as processing them requires nutrients and energy. If you are continually dealing with new toxic exposures, your body will go into defense mode and divert nutrients and energy away from building memories and detracting from your cognitive processes.

The most prevalent toxins that show up in my patients are heavy metals (such as mercury, cadmium, lead, and arsenic), chemical toxins (from pesticides and herbicides, drinking water, and personal care and house-

hold products, such as glyphosate, parabens, and phthalates), and biological toxins (such as the mycotoxins released from mold spores).

If you do one thing to reduce your toxic exposures: Take your shoes off
at the door, and open your doors and/or windows for an hour every day. (I
realize this is technically two things! They're each so simple, I feel that I'm
not making too big of an ask.)

Taking your shoes off means you leave any pesticides on the grass or
sidewalk you walked across, particulate matter that's settled out of the air
(from traffic exhaust or pollen), or bacteria at your front door. Because it
never rains on your rugs or carpet, the pesticides and herbicides we track
into the house are often even higher than what they are outside.

Opening your doors and windows helps usher in outside air and flushes out
your indoor air, which tends to be considerably more polluted than outside air.

Poor Nutrition

Although your brain makes up only 2 percent of your total body weight,
it alone is responsible for consuming 20 percent of the calories your body
requires for daily functions.

Beyond needing energy to work, your brain also needs specific nutrients
in order to perform its many vital functions, including creating, storing,
and retrieving memories; coordinating functions throughout the body;
regulating emotions; and modulating various executive functions, such as
prioritizing and decision-making. Your brain function is orchestrated by
neurotransmitters—chemical messengers such as serotonin, dopamine, and
melatonin. It takes energy and building blocks to form neurotransmitters,
as well as to bind those neurotransmitters to receptor sites where they can
transmit their messages, and then to metabolize them once their message is
sent. The basic categories of nutrients your brain requires are:

- AMINO ACIDS, which are found in protein and which are used to manufacture neurotransmitters and signaling peptides.
- VITAMINS AND MINERALS, such as B vitamins, vitamin C, zinc, and
  magnesium, which help the brain utilize and metabolize the neurotransmitters.

- FATS, which the body can metabolize into fatty acids known as ketones. Ketones are the preferred source of fuel for the brain—in the rare instances when both glucose and ketones are available, the brain will use up ketones first before turning to glucose to meet its energy needs. In addition, the brain itself is largely made of fat, and the myelin sheaths, which encase and protect nerves and neurons in the brain, are comprised of fat—without enough fat, your brain won't have the building blocks it needs to maintain its tissues.

Without enough of these nutrients, your brain health can become impaired.

There are four major parts of the process of feeding yourself. They are intake, digestion, absorption, and then elimination of anything the body doesn't need. What you eat (your intake) is dictated by your choices and tastes, but also by your economic reality, where you live, and your culture. Everything else—your ability to digest, absorb, and eliminate—is largely ruled by:

- STRESS. Your autonomic nervous system, the branch of the central nervous system that rules the functions of the body that happen without your conscious awareness, is divided into two parts: the sympathetic, which rules the fight, flight, or freeze functions, and the parasympathetic, which is responsible for the rest, digest, and heal roles of the body. When you are stressed, your sympathetic nervous system is activated, which means that digestion is down-regulated. Because your body is prepped to run away from a threat or defend itself, it won't have the bandwidth to create the digestive enzymes necessary to break down your food, or to send blood flow to your digestive organs to help with metabolizing and circulating the nutrients in your food. Your brain won't get a chance to send signals to the pancreas and GI tract to release the hormones that calibrate hunger and the feeling of being full. If you are too stressed to sit down and chew your food, you don't start the process of digestion where it should start, which is with enzymes in your saliva that help break down your food and trigger acidity in the stomach and the release of digestive enzymes that further that work.
- YOUR GUT LINING. Your body's ability to absorb nutrients is dictated by the integrity of your gut wall. If it's healthy, the gut lining is selective

and lets in only properly digested nutrients, which can then be distributed throughout the body. But if it's overly porous—or you have what's known as leaky gut—it will let all kinds of unhelpful things both into and out of the digestive tract and into the bloodstream, such as undigested food, toxins, viruses, and bad bacteria. This permeability can trigger the body to release defender immune signals, such as cytokines, that trigger inflammation in an attempt to fight off the perceived invaders, moving your body away from growth and repair and toward defense and attack.

- ELIMINATION. If you're having less than one bowel movement per day, two things are happening—there's less surface area of the intestines available to absorb nutrients from the food you eat, and toxic waste products aren't leaving your body and thus can be reabsorbed as your stool sits in your GI tract. That leads to an accumulation of toxicity, which is the exact opposite of what we want to happen.

- MICROBIOME. The bacteria that live in your gut play a huge role in your whole-body health, particularly brain health. Good gut bacteria influences many of your neurotransmitters—in fact, there are more neurotransmitters in your gut than in your brain. They also play a big role in digesting your food and liberating the nutrients your brain needs to function. Yet another reason why sugar and excess carbs are detrimental is that they feed bad bacteria, which then grow in number and crowd out friendly gut bugs. It's like your gut is a neighborhood—do you want your neighbors to be taking care of their homes, watering their lawns, and keeping their exteriors painted, or do you want neighbors who leave their trash in the yard and let their home fall into disrepair?

If you do one thing to take better care of your brain through diet, start seeking out lower-carb alternatives to some of the foods you eat most regularly. If you love crackers, try almond flour or flaxseed-based crackers. If your go-to carb of choice is rice, try cauliflower rice or quinoa. If it's pasta, try some of the bean-based pastas out there. If it's candy or other sweet treats, try one of the chocolate bars that use an allulose, monk fruit, or sugar alcohol (which don't impact your blood sugar), instead of regular sweetener, such as Lily's, or the Brownie Fat Bomb recipe on page 293. If you love cereal, switch to a grain-free granola (it will often say "keto" on the label). Without diving into a full-on ketogenic diet, which I will invite you to do and guide you through in Chapter 7, you can start to retrain your palate to appreciate new, better-for-you foods.

Stress

Study after study shows that high stress is connected to poor memory and poor cognition. A major player in this connection is elevated levels of the stress hormone cortisol, which is associated with poor cognitive function and impairments in spatial memory, executive function, language, processing speed, and social cognition (the ability to interact with other people).

When we're under significant stress, all our resources are directed toward warding off the threat, and there's little energy or attention left over for thinking clearly, especially about complex situations. Think of being on-stage and performing in front of others, and your mind goes blank—that's a classic example of stress's effect on the brain. We need to be in a restful state in order to become more creative and less reactive.

Social isolation is one of the most identifiable—and preventable—sources of stress associated with dementia. If you have had your driver's license taken away, or you live in a secluded spot, or it's hard to leave the house due to a disability, or you can't hear as well as you used to, or maybe you experience shame about your declining cognition, you are more likely not to spend regular time with others. However, we are social creatures, and we need social connection to live a healthy life as we age.

When you experience stress, your adrenal glands start churning out cortisol. Cortisol on its own—and in the right amounts, at the right time—is a helpful hormone. It typically rises naturally in the morning and helps us get out of bed and get going. Throughout the afternoon and evening, cortisol is supposed to drop as melatonin—which primes us for sleep—rises. It's only when cortisol is high all day and night that its negative cognitive effects are compounded. High levels of cortisol that are sustained over time have neurotoxic effects on the hippocampus (the area of the brain associated with memory) and are connected to an overload of beta amyloid, which causes neuron dysfunction via multiple mechanisms, including oxidative stress, membrane changes, and neurotransmitter receptor changes.

I'll talk more about reproductive hormones in the "signaling" section of this chapter, but when you are stressed, the protein sex hormone-binding globulin (SHBG) rises, which then goes on to bind with testosterone and estrogen, reducing circulating amounts of those reproductive hormones, which means your brain gets less of their message to keep itself and the body systems vital and youthful. It's an example of the cascading effects of one input. (Don't forget that stress impairs digestion, too.) From an evolutionary perspective, if we're stressed, we should not be focused on procreating, because we need to focus exclusively on survival.

Even though stress is typically something we experience too much of, there are negative effects of having too little stress, too. Sometimes, getting older can mean that your stress is limited, because you spend a lot of time at home (perhaps because you can't drive, or to minimize fall risks), and you watch a lot of TV. I'm not here to judge anyone's life choices, but, if you don't give your brain and body reasons to stay strong and resilient, they will atrophy. I know we've had a collective idea that retirement is a time to take it easy, but if you take it *too* easy, it will get harder and harder to move and think as you might like to.

If you do one thing to reduce stress: Prioritize social time, whether it's catching up with friends or loved ones on the phone or in person, getting to a regular class of some sort (yoga, dancing, language), volunteering, or stopping to chat with a neighbor instead of hurrying past because you feel you don't have time. We are social animals. We *need* connection to others. We get stressed when we're isolated. It doesn't matter if your connection is with one or two people or a large group, it only matters that you spend time relating to others.

Structure

Structure refers to your physical makeup, from the macro level—the alignment of your bones, the health of your organs and tissues—to the micro level—your genetic makeup.

There are five different aspects of structure that have a specific relationship to brain health.

- **SLEEP APNEA.** One of the biggest and most common structural issues that has a negative impact on cognitive health is sleep apnea—when your airways get obstructed during sleep, reducing or even completely stopping the flow of air multiple times throughout the night. All your organs require oxygen to function, especially your brain. Without treatment, sleep apnea is essentially repeated micro brain damage each night.
- **CHRONIC PAIN.** Structural issues and chronic pain often go hand in hand, as a nerve that is being pinched by misaligned bones or discs or tight muscles and connective tissues can lead to distraction, or impair blood flow to your brain, which then deprives it of nutrients and leads to waste materials building up and potentially triggering inflammation.

  Living in chronic pain is also physically draining and emotionally stressful. It can directly affect your stress hormones and mental health. In addition, narcotics sometimes prescribed to make pain more manageable dull cognitive function. If you're in chronic pain, you're stuck in defend and attack, not focused on infrastructure building—but there is hope.

  The resource I recommend most frequently to patients in chronic pain is the book *Pain Free* by Pete Egoscue, who focuses on whole-body alignment and with whom I was lucky to work early in my career. In my time at his clinic, I watched people with debilitating pain resolve their pain and eliminate their need for surgical interventions. (To find an Egoscue-trained therapist near you, check the Resources section.) The program I outline in this book also helps to address chronic pain by helping you practice more mindfulness, get more exercise (which produces natural pain-relieving chemicals), enjoy better sleep, and nourish yourself with an anti-inflammatory ketogenic diet.
- **HISTORY OF BRAIN INJURY.** Repeated traumatic injury to your brain can cause structure-related dementia, something that's seen in football players, other athletes, and victims of domestic violence or motor vehicle accidents.
- **YOUR GENETICS.** The gene known as APOE (which codes for apolipoprotein E, a protein involved in the metabolism of fats) is linked to both dementia and cardiovascular disease—to be clear, this gene doesn't cause dementia or Alzheimer's, but it does impact your risk of developing it. Because this chapter is already jam-packed, I'll cover the genetics of dementia in Chapter 2.

If you do one thing to support your structures, determine if you have sleep apnea, and if you do have it, follow the treatments for it. I recommend this regardless of how much you weigh or snore. You can ask your doctor for a sleep study, or there are many wearable devices that will track your oxygen levels as you sleep. If you see that your oxygen levels are dropping repeatedly throughout the night, treat it immediately and aggressively, because even mild sleep apnea equates to mild brain damage every night. There are multiple ways to treat sleep apnea—refer to Chapter 5 for an overview of options.

Infections

When you experience an infection from bacteria, fungus, parasite, or virus, your body goes into attack mode, and in that war you'll get collateral damage in the brain, primarily via inflammation. If these microorganisms reach the brain, they can trigger microglial cells (the brain's immune cells) to wage an attack, leading to inflammation and even neuronal cell death. Inflammation also decreases blood flow and contributes to a leaky blood-brain barrier and perpetuates the likelihood that more infectious microorganisms will further affect the brain.

In lab studies, scientists see that some infections are associated with the development of amyloid plaques in the brain. Amyloid is likely part of your brain's attempt to protect and defend itself against infection. However, it can be too much of a good thing and lead to brain cell dysfunction over time.

What we understand from the science and what I have seen in my clinical experience is that the infections that have the most bearing on brain health are herpes (oral or genital), the oral bacteria *P. gingivalis*, Lyme, and Covid. Let's look at these briefly one by one.

- HERPES can occur in the mouth (showing up as cold sores) or in the genitals and sometimes other unexpected places. Once you contract herpes, it lives in your nervous system where it can be dormant for a long time, only to reemerge after a stressor. Having frequent herpes outbreaks (which includes even a yearly cold sore) is associated with a threefold risk of dementia. The good news is that managing outbreaks with antiviral medications such as acyclovir and valacyclovir has been shown to reduce dementia risk—if you know you have the herpes virus, speak to your doctor about having these medications on hand so that you can take them at the very first sign that a sore may be developing. If you are prone to outbreaks, also consider taking 500 mg of lysine twice daily.

- P. GINGIVALIS. There is a direct link between oral health and whole-body health—including brain health—and much of it has to do with bacteria. Oral health is associated with life span, in that the number of teeth you have is significantly correlated with longevity.

  You may know that if you have heart problems or artificial joints, you need to take antibiotics before you go to the dentist; that's because there is bacteria in your mouth that can get into your bloodstream when you have deep cleanings, create inflammation in your blood vessels, and even potentially cause blood clots and strokes. It can also trigger inflammation in your brain.

  The oral bacteria *P. gingivalis* has been found in the brains of Alzheimer's patients, and it is correlated with inflammation, as well as the plaques and tangles that are often found in the brain of those with dementia. If every time you brush and floss you see even trace amounts of blood, you are potentially introducing *P. gingivalis* bacteria into your bloodstream, which then increases your risk of both cardiovascular disease and dementia. If you have the variant of APOE4 that is associated with greater risk of developing dementia, these infections are more likely to trigger inflammation and lead to misfolded amyloid proteins.

- LYME DISEASE, which is a bacterial infection carried by ticks, is becoming increasingly common. With Lyme, many people resolve the infection with the standard treatment, which is two to three weeks on the antibiotic known as doxycycline. But for others, either the antibiotic doesn't help them, or they don't realize they were infected in the first place. Then some stressor comes along—moving, losing sleep, getting sick, or just living through a challenging time—and throws off their immune system. Then they can develop chronic Lyme. Testing for the presence of the bacteria is highly variable, and the infections themselves have complex life cycles—you may test at a time when the bacteria is dormant and hiding.

The way we usually test for these infections is through a blood test that looks for antibodies the immune system creates in response. But the Lyme bug Borrelia, and common co-infections with Lyme—including Babesia, Bartonella, Ehrlichia, and other vector-borne bugs—suppress your immune system, making it easy to get a false negative on testing. This means you could actually have the infection but the lab results tell you, you don't, as the virus can hide without creating a measurable immune response.

One of the most common symptoms chronic Lyme causes is brain fog and cognitive decline. We don't know that it causes Alzheimer's, but it's clearly negatively affecting the brain. Doing all the things in this book will help your immune system come online and meet the infection in an effective way, and function as optimally as possible and get you primed to work with a Lyme-literate doctor (see the Resources section for guidance on finding one near you) to fight the infection and any co-infections.

- COVID-19 popularized the concept of the cytokine storm, when a helpful molecule known as a cytokine is released in levels that are so high that they become dangerous. If you already have a baseline level of elevated inflammation for whatever reason—nutrient imbalance, brain injury, chronic pain, toxin load, a lot of stress, poor sleep—and then add Covid to that, it triggers more inflammation. If you're already predisposed to a reduction in cognitive function, Covid has the potential to nudge you farther down the path to cognitive impairment by adding inflammation to an already inflamed system. Studies are showing that long Covid is accompanied by memory issues and brain fog, even in young people and people with no other conditions. A study published in *JAMA*, the *Journal of the American Medical Association*, found that even a nonsevere Covid infection is associated with an elevated risk of early onset cognitive decline.

If you do one thing to address your infectious load: Brush and floss twice daily, no exceptions. If you see any blood, it doesn't mean you should stop brushing or flossing in that spot—it means that area needs even more cleaning, as it may be harboring a potential infection. Go see a biological dentist, who appreciates the whole-body effects of all dental interventions and who can help assess and address oral infections.

Signaling

A big reason that the many different parts of your body—its organs and systems—work synergistically as a whole is because of the many signaling molecules that are continually sending messages that tell your various parts what to do, when to do it, and how much to do it. These include hormones, proteins, and peptides. And in order for your brain to be at its best, you need your signaling molecules to be in balance. Let's take a quick look at these, one by one:

- SEX HORMONES. Of course, estrogen, testosterone, progesterone, follicle-stimulating hormone, and luteinizing hormone are involved in fertility and libido. But you may not realize that there is a very well-established link between reproductive hormones and cognitive health. They support the flow of neurotransmitters that is critical to the cognitive process, helping your brain learn new things and maintain executive function. Knowing this, it's no wonder that one of the many symptoms of perimenopause is brain fog and memory impairment. After all, think back to when you were in your late teens and twenties—that's when you were building skills and refining your ability to think clearly and critically, and also when your reproductive hormones were at their peak.

  As we age, our levels of reproductive hormones decline. There are ways to replenish your levels—and some are definitely better than others. Up until about 2002, it was standard practice to give peri- and postmenopausal women synthetic estrogen and progestin (a synthetic form of progesterone) to relieve menopausal symptoms and protect bone health. The practice fell out of favor after research revealed the medication increased the risk of heart disease and breast cancer. I still continue to prescribe bioidentical hormone therapy, as it appears to be safe for women under age sixty or within ten years of menopause, in topical instead of oral forms, and to patients who don't have a family history of heart disease and breast cancer.

  There are natural estrogens (estrone, estradiol, and estriol), phytoestrogens (dong quai, black cohosh, soy, hops, maca), and xenoestrogens (synthetic chemicals that attach to estrogen receptor sites in the body, making it harder for natural estrogen to work). When a natural or phytoestrogen binds with an estrogen receptor site, it turns on the faucet to a predictable cascade of downstream effects. I think of it like a beautiful tropical waterfall. When a xenoestrogen docks on a receptor site, it not only blocks that predictable waterfall from happening, it kicks off its own domino effect that paves the way for hormonal imbalance, inflammation, and even cancer. Remember, balance is about the right thing in the right place in the right amounts at the right time. Xenoestrogens are the wrong thing, in the wrong place, in the wrong amounts—and something for which it's always the wrong time. Even with bioidentical hormones, my aim as a doctor is to get my patients just enough, not too much.

Reducing your toxic load will also typically reduce your xenoestrogen exposure, as they are found in chemicals such as parabens and phthalates in conventional personal care products, plastics, and food storage products.

I'm definitely not saying that taking bioidentical hormones return you, cognitively or otherwise, to your twenties again. But they can bring some of your cognitive function back online—as well as provide protection for your bone health.

I admit, I came to bioidentical hormone therapy skeptically, but what I've seen over and over again with my patients is that it is a helpful piece of the puzzle in terms of promoting cognitive function.

There is one risk to taking bioidentical hormones, and that is that if you currently have a form of cancer that is sensitive to estrogen or progesterone—be it breast, ovarian, or uterine—it can augment that cancer's growth, which is definitely not what we want. However, if you don't have cancer, and cancer doesn't run in your family but dementia does, I think the risk of potentially furthering cancer is far outweighed by reduction of your greater risk of cognitive decline. Hormone therapy does not increase your risk of developing cancer—it increases the growth of cancer if you have it. To mitigate any risk, before I prescribe bioidentical hormones to any patients, we do lots of screening—mammograms, or MRIs, and potentially ultrasounds, as appropriate—and we do it repeatedly to keep an eye on things.

If you are interested in exploring whether bioidentical hormone therapy makes sense for you, see the Resources section for guidance on finding an accredited healthcare provider to help.

- PEPTIDES are amino acids, which come primarily from protein sources, that are broken down into smaller components. If peptides are like pearls on a string, an amino acid is a single pearl. Peptides send signals that tell cells how to behave. The most famous peptide is insulin, which tells cells to take up glucose from the blood into the cells where it is then turned into ATP, the fuel our cells run on.

  Our understanding and use of peptides is still in its early days. But there are a handful of peptides that are specifically supportive of cognitive function and are very safe for us—that's the good news. The less-good news is that they aren't easy to come by, and they can be expensive. I'll cover peptide use for treatment and prevention of cognitive decline more in depth in Chapter 12.

- BRAIN-DERIVED NEUROTROPHIC FACTOR (BDNF) is a protein pre-cursor (also known as a propeptide) that is generated by muscle tissue. It promotes the survival of developing neurons and helps them specialize in whatever function the brain needs at that time. As such, it's related to learning and memory, and it helps with neuroplasticity. In other words, BDNF is an elixir of youth for your brain. And you don't need expensive treatments to get more of it—you make more every time you exercise.

  Research shows that the amount of BDNF you have is directly cor-related to the size of your hippocampus—the brain region associated with memory. The more BDNF a person has, the bigger their hippocampus tends to be, and the better people tend to perform on tests of learning, memory, and spatial memory.

If you do one thing for better signaling: exercise. The key is to do more than whatever you have been doing. Pushing yourself, just a little bit, will trigger the release of BDNF, which has direct benefits on your brain, memory, and cognitive performance. If you already get plenty of exercise, mix it up and do something different. Play a different sport or engage in a new routine. If you run, take a new route.

Some of the things on this list you can't control. Maybe you live near a power plant or a highway or a waste treatment plant that exposes you to a higher concentration of pollutants, and it's not feasible for you to move. Or maybe your loved one is the one experiencing cognitive decline and is really resistant to any form of exercise, despite your best efforts to get them moving. The good part of having such a long list of influencing factors is that there will always be something else on the list—another tool that you have to effect positive change. So focus on the things you *can* control.

The Brain May Be Complex, but the Way Forward Is Simple

If you are concerned about your or your care partner's cognitive function—maybe it's memory lapses, or general sense of fogginess or confusion, or a string of little things that you fear might be adding up to a dementia diagnosis—you probably start with an appointment with a primary care physician. You want to be proactive. You might be feeling scared. But you also want to do anything you can to slow or reverse the disease process.

You'll probably get a referral to a neurologist. Who will probably recommend a neuropsych assessment that takes hours to complete, is stressful, and doesn't change your course of treatment. A neurologist *might* tell you to eat blueberries, as there is research that says you can benefit cognition by eating one-half cup a day. They might order an MRI or other imaging to rule out things like a brain bleed or tumor, which is helpful. They also might take away your driver's license. And then they'll probably say, "I want to see you again in six to twelve months." Typically, the only hope you'll be left with is that a new medication will be available, or that there might be a new clinical trial you could be recruited for.

Most people walk away from that neurologist's appointment with nothing new, and maybe no more driver's license, with no real answer to that burning question, "What can I do?"

And the reason the conventional medicine approach has so little to offer is because it's been looking for one root cause that it can treat with one medication—a search that has left billions of dollars spent, decades of time allocated, and four hundred unsuccessful clinical trials in its wake—and no real hope on the horizon. When the truth is, the brain is a complex organ, and dementia is a complex disease that requires a multifaceted approach.

With so many factors at play, I understand that it may sound overwhelming to address all the things that can negatively impact your cognitive function. But it's really a back-to-basics approach—eat better, move more, get more sleep, do more things that challenge you, and spend more time with people you love. As we showed in our study, there's so much you can do. And those things bring with them a nearly 75 percent chance that you will see some measurable benefit—and maybe a whole lot of benefit—in a manageable time frame.

There's a big difference between the Bredesen approach that I use with success with the residents at Marama and the patients in my clinic and the conventional approach. It makes you wonder, why? If this is so successful, why don't more doctors recommend it, or even seem to know about it? That's what we'll cover in Chapter 2.

CHAPTER 2

How Have We
Gotten It So Wrong?

Something I hear again and again from people who learn of our successes in improving cognitive function in patients with Alzheimer's is, "If this works, why haven't I heard of it?" And it's a great question.

The short answer is two-pronged:

- It has been difficult to conduct the research on an intervention that has multiple components (such as diet, exercise, stress reduction, medications, and supplements) until fairly recently.
- For decades the research we have been able to conduct has been focused mostly on a single thing that isn't the full picture of why people develop Alzheimer's.

Put simply, our research paradigm hasn't matched the complexity of the disease.

Let's take a closer look at these two factors.

The Realities of the Research World

First, the medical research community has until very recently been devoted to experiments that test one intervention at a time. Studies that seek to evaluate the effectiveness of multimodal interventions were rarely given the green light by internal review boards (IRBs). As a result, the vast majority of dementia research has focused on testing the effects of one particular molecule (typically, a pharmaceutical) on one particular measure of health (the plaques and tangles that are seen in high amounts in patients with Alzheimer's). This is despite the fact that—as we covered in Chapter 1—the brain is a complex organ, and dementia is a complex disease with multiple aspects.

IRBs are hugely important. They were established to protect human research subjects in the aftermath of unethical studies, such as those conducted on Black men in Tuskegee, Alabama, in the 1930s, where they were infected with syphilis without their consent or knowledge and denied known treatments. It's only been since the mid-2010s that IRBs have begun to approve studies that evaluate multifactorial interventions. Even still, the process of getting that green light is arduous—even in the early 2020s, it took my team eighteen months to get IRB approval on our pilot study.

As a result, the science that evaluates multipronged approaches to dementia is in its infancy. Research is lagging because it takes time to build a body of scientific evidence, and we've only recently been able to get through the gatekeepers. So to dismiss the early studies that have been done outright (such as the studies that Dr. Dale Bredesen and his team have published, and that I and my team have completed) because they're not big enough is like wanting to skip over childhood and adolescence and go straight to adulthood. It might sound nice to zoom past some of the more frustrating years of development, but those are where we learn formative lessons that shape the adults we become.

To be clear, I'm not criticizing IRBs. They are a vital piece of the research process, especially when study subjects have dementia—we need to make sure that vulnerable human subjects aren't being taken advantage of and are receiving excellent care. IRBs *should* be gatekeeping. And they should also—and they are beginning to—ensure that studies are testing potential remedies that actually improve patient outcomes and experience and not just reduce plaques and tangles.

An Oversimplification of the Problem

That leads me to the second, even bigger, reason why more people don't know about the hope offered by the protocol I outline in this book to improve cognition and reverse Alzheimer's. The medical community has had a single focus on reducing beta-amyloid plaques and tau tangles—the diseased structures found in the brains of many Alzheimer's patients during autopsy. Despite the fact that dementia is a complex disease with many factors, we've been training our sights on the neuropathology of the disease. Basically, we've been hoping for a silver bullet—some drug that would improve outcomes and, of course, make millions or even billions of dollars while it also improved millions or even billions of lives.

And as you'll learn, the decades of science we've conducted haven't even shown that plaques and tangles are a true cause of Alzheimer's, nor shown that when you reduce them, cognitive function improves. Rather, we've discovered that only 2 percent of people—from newborn all the way up to old age—*don't* have any plaques or tangles. Even though they are widely prevalent, the presence of plaques and tangles sometimes have no effect on cognition. In fact, a full 30 percent of people over age sixty-five have enough plaques and tangles to meet the criteria for Alzheimer's, yet only 10 percent of people sixty-five and older experience measurable cognitive impairments. That's right—the majority of the time plaques are present, there is no accompanying dementia. It's the same way some people can be bone-on-bone in their joints, or have a massively herniated disc, but experience no pain whatsoever, while someone with only mild cartilage or disc damage can be immobilized with pain. Pathology does not always equal disease.

So how did it come to pass that we've spent decades and untold billions of dollars on researching dementia, yet still don't have a scientifically validated approach to treating it, or even a full understanding of how it develops? Unfortunately, our scientific investigations into the true causes of chronic and degenerative cognitive impairment have been flawed from the beginning.

We've Been Focused on the Wrong
Thing from the Start

There have been three main missteps in our scientific investigations of the causes of severe dementia that have had far-reaching effects, or what Karl Herrup, Ph.D., professor of neurobiology and an investigator at the Alzheimer's Disease Research Center at the University of Pittsburgh School of Medicine, calls in his book *How Not to Study a Disease* "the three inflations." The first one occurred shortly after the very first recorded instance of what we now think of Alzheimer's disease, and it shows how we have been one-sidedly focused on plaques and tangles since the very beginning.

The First Inflation

The first patient to be identified with what is now termed early-onset Alzheimer's disease was a German woman named Auguste Deter, who began exhibiting symptoms of dementia in her fifties, and who died from the disease at the age of sixty-six in 1906. She was a patient of Dr. Alois Alzheimer, a young doctor who was mentored by the author of a neurology textbook, Emil Kraepelin. After Deter's death, Alzheimer and Kraepelin performed an autopsy and saw abnormal formations in her brain. Kraepelin wrote it up as a case study in 1906 and then, in 1910, included the case study in a new neurology textbook he was putting together. It was, after all, a sensational story, complete with gory physical details about a patient's brain, and including it would help sell more textbooks. The problem is that a single case study doesn't mean much—it's literally the story of one unusual case, and it was inappropriate to include in a textbook one case study that wasn't part of an established pattern. Nonetheless, it happened, and the link between early-onset dementia and plaques and tangles was born. Notice that I said "early onset," which is a distinct and rare form of dementia—not the much more common form of the disease that manifests after age sixty-five that we now call Alzheimer's. (See box at right for more information on the distinction between the two).

THE TWO TYPES OF ALZHEIMER'S

There are two distinct types of Alzheimer's disease—one is very rare, and caused primarily by genetics, while the other is much more common and influenced by a range of factors.

Early-onset Alzheimer's disease (also known as familial or presenile Alzheimer's)

Many people will use the term "early-onset Alzheimer's" to describe the beginning symptoms of dementia—such as having a hard time finding the word you want to say, or forgetting why you walked into a room—when the term really defines severe cognitive impairment that begins in someone who is in their forties or fifties and progresses quickly.

Early-onset Alzheimer's is also called familial Alzheimer's because it has a strong genetic component, and different gene variants are associated with it than with late-onset Alzheimer's. For early-onset, the genes in play are APP (which codes for the amyloid precursor protein) and PSEN (which codes for a protein known as presenilin). The specific mutations for APP occur on chromosome 21, for PSEN 1 on chromosome 14, and for PSEN 2 on chromosome 1. These genetic mutations are believed to contribute to the formation of amyloid plaques and, thus, are called "deterministic" genes. They are also extremely rare—only 1 percent of the population has them. Interestingly, most of the research on Alzheimer's disease has looked at this familial type.

Late-onset Alzheimer's disease (also known as sporadic Alzheimer's)

This is the more common form of Alzheimer's disease, which typically starts to develop after age sixty-five. While there is a genetic component to this disease, it is believed only to increase risk, not directly contribute to the formation of the disease.

The gene involved in this form of Alzheimer's is known as APOE, as it codes for apolipoprotein E, a protein involved in the metabolism of fats and the distribution of cholesterol via the bloodstream. There are three variants of APOE, aptly named APOE2, APOE3, and APOE4, and we get one allele from each of our parents. APOE2 is the least common and may actually be protective against developing Alzheimer's. APOE3 is the most common allele, and is believed to neither increase nor decrease risk. APOE4 has been associated with an increased risk of developing Alzheimer's, and if you have two of the APOE4 alleles, that risk is greatest. About 25 percent of people have one APOE4, only 2 to 3 percent have two. Getting genetic testing to see which variants of APOE you have can give you an indicator of how strong your predisposition toward dementia is.

APOE genotype	Percentage of population with this genotype	Lifetime risk of dementia
APOE3/APOE3	60 percent	9 percent
APOE3/APOE4	20–30 percent	30 percent
APOE4/APOE4	2–3 percent	Greater than 50 percent

In order to assess your genetic risk, 23andMe offers a direct-to-consumer Genetic Health Risk test that uses a saliva sample, or your doctor or healthcare provider may work with a lab that uses either a blood sample or cheek swab. (We use Lab Corp or Quest at Solcere.) It's important to know that simply having the APOE4 allele, or even two of them, doesn't mean you will develop Alzheimer's, or that if you don't, you won't. It's a good idea to consult with a genetic counselor who can help you sort through the implications—health, emotional, and otherwise. You can find a genetic counselor through the National Society of Genetic Counselors (nsgc.org).

If testing determines that you have two APOE4 alleles, there is good news: According to research by Yale gerontologist Dr. Becca Levy, people with this combination can reduce their additional risk by developing a positive attitude about aging—which following the protocol in this book can help you do (even if you are fearful about developing dementia), because it provides two crucial things—a road map and hope.

The Second Inflation

The second time the theory that elevated levels of plaques and tangles were the cause of dementia happened in the mid-1970s. After World War II ended, the US federal government began coalescing the beginnings of the agency that we now recognize as the National Institutes of Health (NIH). Over time, nearly thirty institutes were established to fund research in specific areas of health, including the National Cancer Institute (NCI), the National Institute of Neurological Disorders and Stroke (NINDS), and the National Institute of Mental Health (NIMH). In 1974, the National Institute of Aging (NIA) became the eleventh institute of the NIH. The leaders of the NIA had to vie with all the other institutes to secure funding from Congress, and arguing that the study of aging, which is unavoidable, deserves to draw funds away from research on something like cancer, which is treatable, was a hard sell. So the leaders of the fledgling NIA developed a strategy to find a disease that was an accepted part of the aging process—one that the public was afraid of. Alzheimer's disease was a perfect fit. The only problem? Alzheimer's disease at that time was defined, thanks to the research of Alzheimer and Kraepelin, as a relatively rare disease that began in one's fifties or sixties. Otherwise, the cognitive losses that occurred in older age were viewed as benign senile dementia. In order for this strategy to work, Alzheimer's would have to be viewed as much more common, and much more sinister.

A two-page editorial published in the *Archives of Neurology* in 1976 furthered the cause perfectly. Titled "Editorial: The Prevalence and Malignancy of Alzheimer Disease: A Major Killer," the article argued that the plaques and tangles that were a hallmark of the relatively rare early-onset Alzheimer's were widely common and contributing to the much more common senile dementia. The NIA leaders had their smoking gun, which they took to Congress to lobby for ever-bigger budgets. It worked. The NIA began receiving more and more funding, to the point that today, it has a $2.6 billion budget—two-thirds of which is spent on Alzheimer's disease research. While we want to be spending plenty of money on finding treatments to this devastating and costly disease, the problem is that most of those dollars have been focused on reducing plaques and tangles—and not on exploring other causes or treatments that focus on improving cognitive function.

It's worth pointing out that not only do perfectly healthy people have plaques and tangles in their brain (I have them; my four-year-old daughter likely does, too), but also that amyloid plaques are prominent in the brains of people with Parkinson's disease, Huntington's disease, traumatic brain injury, and epilepsy. Yet, Alzheimer's is the only disease to be defined by their presence. Even as far back as 1968, we had research that showed that only about half of cases with senile dementia actually have a significant presence of plaques and tangles. Years later, one examination by a prominent neurological pathology researcher, Heiko Braak, MD, looked at 2,332 autopsied brains of people from one to one hundred years old and found only ten that had absolutely no plaques or tangles. Yes, plaques and tangles are an important factor in Alzheimer's disease, but they are by no means the only one. Yet we weren't finished with our dogged determination to make them enemy number one.

The Third Inflation

The third major inflation occurred in 2010, when the NIA convened three working groups to do a comprehensive review of what we knew about Alzheimer's thus far and update its definition. This was a chance to at least scrutinize our reliance on the idea that plaques and tangles were causative factors in late-onset Alzheimer's. One of the papers produced by these working groups expanded the diagnostic criteria for dementia to include a preclinical phase where there are no symptoms but plaques are forming. This shift makes a certain amount of sense, as we know there are slow-building changes happening in healthy people who will go on to develop Alzheimer's. Yet it doubled down on the idea that it's the presence of plaques that is a defining feature of Alzheimer's. Now people over sixty-five who do have plaques and tangles but no impairment in cognitive function were no longer considered healthy—they were, as Herrup termed it, "sick people without symptoms."

By saying that people with plaques but no symptoms had preclinical Alzheimer's, the working group essentially tripled the prevalence of Alzheimer's with the stroke of a pen. Naturally, this finding made the race to find a drug to reduce the presence of these biomarkers even more frenzied. And it created an opening for drugs to target this preclinical phase where there are no symptoms, only plaques. Since this shift, millions of dollars have been funneled toward searching for a drug that will reduce plaques and tangles before symptoms present. Despite our best efforts and hopes, 99.6 percent of the research on pharmaceutical interventions for Alzheimer's has failed—meaning, they have not provided a statistically significant improvement in outcomes such as cognition and function when compared with placebo.

We need to be more open to other approaches to preventing and reversing Alzheimer's, not just because the disease is rising in prevalence and stealing too many minds, and not only because of our long history of having tunnel vision when it comes to researching possible treatments, but also because it has recently come to light just how misguided and wrong our approach to seeking an effective pharmaceutical treatment has been. Basically, we've been snookered.

Manipulated Images Further Degrade the Case for Focusing on Amyloid Plaques

It would be bad enough if we had mistakenly pursued only one potential treatment for Alzheimer's because we hadn't followed the scientific method correctly or had made the disease sound more prevalent than it is in an effort to secure more funding dollars. But it's looking like there was some outright deception thrown in the mix, too.

A July 2022 article in *Science* detailed how the images used in some seminal Alzheimer's research appears to have been falsified. One particular 2006 study that was published in the journal *Nature* seemed to find that beta-amyloid plaques cause dementia in rats. The study has since been cited more than twenty-six hundred times and played a major role in dictating the direction that Alzheimer's research has taken ever since—seeking a drug to reduce the formation of plaques, rather than searching for something that actually improves cognitive scores and quality of life for Alzheimer's patients. As an example, in 2021 alone, $1.6 billion went toward researching drugs that prevent or repair beta-amyloid plaques. If these allegations of falsified images are true, it sadly means that much of this research was justified with junk science.

It wasn't just the images in one study that have been called into question.

A follow-up article in *Science* published in November 2022 identified one particular researcher involved in the paper in question. This researcher has published over the course of two decades, and when all his papers were analyzed by a former student (now a neuroscientist at Vanderbilt University), a microbiologist and forensic image analyst, and another "image sleuth," they found "suspect images" of brain tissue in thirty-three papers. Many of these studies have been or are in the process of being reviewed and even retracted. But the damage has been done.

No wonder none of the drugs that have been developed since 2006 that target beta-amyloid plaques have been found to meaningfully improve cognition—they're based on junk science.

Where Has All This Research Gotten Us?

Surely, in the decades since the second inflation and all the dollars spent on research in the past five decades, there must have been some promising developments, right? Let's take a look at the first drug to be approved for the treatment of Alzheimer's in twenty years—the monoclonal antibody treatment known as aducanumab that received FDA approval in 2021. Administered via IV, a year's worth of aducanumab costs $56,000. In one study it did slow the progression of cognitive decline—yet the majority of data collected showed there was no benefit at all. In fact, eight out of ten members of the Federal Drug Administration advisory board voted not to approve aducanumab. It received approval anyway because it was the only drug in two decades found to have some efficacy, and the medical establishment felt desperate to say there is some new treatment available. Once it was approved, three members of the independent advisory committee to the FDA resigned in protest, with Harvard professor of medicine Dr. Aaron Kesselheim calling it "probably the worst drug approval decision in recent US history." It's hard to call aducanumab a treatment since it doesn't make anyone better—it only potentially helps them get worse more slowly, making the already drawn-out, torturous process of Alzheimer's take longer. On top of that, the drug's side effects include an increased risk of brain bleeds and brain swelling, both of which require MRIs and doctor's visits to manage. For $56,000 per year, how much value does that add to society? (Turns out, none: Biogen halted production of aducanumab in 2024.)

In 2023, the FDA approved lecanemab, a second similar monoclonal antibody drug that also targets plaques and tangles with less risk and less cost than aducanumab. It was hailed as a big deal, yet it still hasn't been shown to improve cognitive function or quality of life. Donanemab is a similar medication in Phase III trials but not yet FDA approved, with the same side effects of brain bleeds and brain swelling. With all these drugs, the positive outcome is a slower disease process, not significant improvement.

The most commonly prescribed medications for dementia are memantine and donepezil. Although some patients report a slight improvement in cognition initially, analysis of ten studies including over twenty-seven hundred patients showed that using these very common medications that are meant to help people with dementia actually makes cognition worse. *Do not* stop these medications if you or a loved one is on them. Stopping them can often make things get worse fast, and the decline can be next to impossible to recover from. If you haven't started them, I don't recommend it. If you already have, just keep the dose stable and put this new Alzheimer's toolkit to work.

There are a few other pharmaceutical drugs that are prescribed for dementia. In the table on the following page, I walk you through the current drug options as of this writing. As you'll see, none provide much hope.

When I look at this list and think of the injustice of the decades of time and the millions upon millions of dollars we've spent, only to pin all our hopes on a couple of exorbitantly priced pharmaceuticals that create more problems than they solve, it really lights a fire under me. As tempting as it is to get upset and point fingers, it's important to remember that the people who study Alzheimer's care so much, and we all have the same goal of helping people and reducing suffering. It's not time to cast blame, but it is time to pivot. We need to devote our time, energy, resources, and research dollars toward finding an approach that offers a real solution, even if it doesn't fit the pharmaceutical paradigm.

We have to work even harder to make up for lost time, and to change our thinking around how to treat this disease. We don't have time to wait. Thankfully, there are some bright spots in our evolving understanding of Alzheimer's disease.

DRUG NAME	BRAND NAME	COST	GOAL	RISKS
Aducanumab (since discontinued)	Aduhelm	$56,000 per year	A monoclonal antibody treatment that attacks beta-amyloid proteins and reduces plaques, yet has not been shown to improve cognitive function or quality of life; IV administration	Brain swelling, brain bleeds—two risks that require regular MRIs to monitor
Lecanemab	Leqembi	$26,000 per year	A monoclonal antibody treatment that attacks beta-amyloid proteins and reduces plaques, yet has not been shown to improve cognitive function or quality of life; IV administration	Brain swelling and brain bleeds—but with a lower risk than aducanumab
Memantine	Namenda	Can cost up to $8 per 5 mg pill—and prescription can be for as high as 20 mg/day. Those costs come down with generics and using an online subscription service.	Believed to improve memory by targeting N-methyl-D-aspartate (NMDA) receptors and blocking the action of glutamate, a stimulating neurotransmitter that is associated with Alzheimer's symptoms. It also blocks excess calcium from entering and damaging brain cells.	Relatively mild side effects, including dizziness, headache, confusion, constipation, diarrhea. The biggest risk is that you need to wean off of it; the brain can get dependent on it and then cognition can suffer if you stop too quickly.
Donepezil hydrochloride	Aricept	About $50/month	This cholinesterase inhibitor increases the amount of acetyl choline—a neurotransmitter that has been linked to memory problems when it is deficient—by stopping it from breaking down.	Benefits are typically temporary. Coming off of it creates withdrawal in the brain. I prefer to increase choline by eating choline-rich foods, such as eggs, liver, salmon, chicken breasts, red meat, cauliflower, and broccoli—all parts of the ketogenic diet. They taste great, and no withdrawals!
Sildenafil	Viagra	$70/pill for Viagra; $8.50 for the generic sildenafil, a cost that can come down to as low as $2 per pill with an online subscription	Relaxes the smooth muscles of the vascular system, increasing circulation (which then delivers more oxygen and nutrients and flushes away more waste products throughout the body—although exercise provides this same benefit); research is mixed on whether regular use is associated with lower rates of dementia—some studies say yes, others say no.	Sudden loss of vision or hearing; low blood pressure; can exacerbate risks of cardiovascular events. Because it is so frequently prescribed for erectile dysfunction, nearly all the research has been conducted on men.

Science Is Just Beginning to Get on Board with the Many Risk Factors

Most of the research world has been so focused on finding a pharmaceutical treatment for amyloid plaques and tau tangles that they haven't acknowledged other risk factors, although this has recently begun to change. In 2017, *The Lancet*, one of the oldest and most influential peer-reviewed medical journals, published a commission report examining the evidence for modifiable risk factors of dementia and Alzheimer's. The keyword here is modifiable— meaning these are contributors to dementia that can be changed or avoided. Of course, it makes sense that there are things you are exposed to or choose to do (such as smoking) or not do (such as exercise) that have a long-term impact on your cognitive health. Yet despite how logical this assumption is, we haven't been having a collective conversation around preventing dementia. Instead, we've been furthering the idea that there's nothing to be done except wait for the drug. And yet, here is *The Lancet* saying that there is lots of great evidence that suggests that you can reduce, prevent, or delay the onset of dementia. In this first report, they listed nine modifiable risk factors. In 2020, they issued an updated report that brought that total up to twelve modifiable risk factors, which, the authors said, "account for around 40 percent of worldwide dementias, which consequently could theoretically be prevented or delayed."

The twelve modifiable risk factors listed by *The Lancet* 2020 report include:

- LESS EDUCATION. In general, the more education you have, the less likely you are to develop dementia. There are two sides to this: getting a primary and secondary education as a young person, when neuroplasticity is highest, is believed to expand cognitive reserves. On the other side, staying cognitively active throughout life helps keep the brain sharp—some studies even find that later retirement age is associated with decreased dementia risk.
- HEARING LOSS. The information gathered by your senses stimulates your brain, so it makes sense that a decline in hearing—even hearing loss at subclinical levels—is significantly associated with an increased risk of dementia. If you already have hearing loss, get fitted for and regularly use your hearing aids. And if you don't, take preventive measures to protect

your hearing by wearing ear protection when exposed to loud noises, such as concerts, and keeping the volume on your earbuds at a moderate level.

• TRAUMATIC BRAIN INJURY (TBI). Even mild brain injuries—such as a concussion without a loss of consciousness—is associated with an increased risk of dementia. The more severely, and the more times the brain is injured, the more the risk goes up. The takeaway—wear a helmet when biking, skiing, and riding a scooter or motorcycle, and wear a seat belt every time you're in a car (including a taxi or ride share).

• HYPERTENSION. High blood pressure at midlife (at any time over forty) seems to pave the way for dementia. In fact, the authors of *The Lancet* article concluded, "antihypertensive treatment for hypertension is the only known effective preventive medication for dementia." Hypertension is defined as systolic blood pressure of 130 mm Hg and above. It's important to note that blood pressure can lower with dementia, so if you are sixty-five or older with low blood pressure, it could indicate the presence of dementia, and not an absence of risk.

• WEIGHT. Although there is a foundational shift happening in our culture at large and within the medical community away from focusing on obesity as a cause of disease, there are still numerous studies that have found that clinical obesity and a higher body mass are associated with an increased risk of developing dementia, and that losing even a small amount of weight (4.4 pounds, or 2 kilograms) at midlife in people with a body mass index (BMI) of 25 or higher is linked to a significant improvement in attention and memory. While not intended as a weight-loss plan, the eating plan in this book can help with weight loss if you or your loved one has extra weight to lose.

• EXCESSIVE ALCOHOL CONSUMPTION. While there is conflicting evidence on whether light drinking offers some protection against developing dementia, the research is clear that having more than twenty-one alcoholic drinks per week significantly increases risk; even drinking fourteen drinks per week was associated with a smaller hippocampus (a part of the brain heavily involved in learning and memory). One French study found that a full 56.6 percent of people in the study with early-onset Alzheimer's had an alcohol use disorder listed in their medical records. Alcohol is a neurotoxin, after all.

- PHYSICAL INACTIVITY. As you'll learn much more about in Chapter 6, moving your body improves circulation everywhere, including to your brain, and that means more nutrients and oxygen delivered and more waste products flushed away. In several long-term studies that evaluated dementia risk, people with the lowest levels of physical activity experienced the highest risk.

- DEPRESSION. Depression in mid-late life tends to increase dementia risk, although dementia can also be a cause of depression. Evidence suggests that depressive episodes in the first half of life are associated with greater incidence of dementia. While there isn't clear evidence to suggest that taking antidepressants reduces this increased risk, the takeaway is that you do want to take good care of your mental health—something that regular exercise, staying socially active, and pursuing hobbies can help with.

- TYPE 2 DIABETES. The link between type 2 diabetes and dementia is so strong that Alzheimer's is known as type 3 diabetes. The good news is that type 2 diabetes can be reversed, and the eating plan I outline in this book can help you get there.

- SMOKING. Just as smoking damages your heart and lungs, it also negatively impacts your brain. This is true even if the smoke is secondhand. There is hope, though—quitting, even later in life, can substantially reduce dementia risk.

- AIR POLLUTION. Exposure to monoxide, nitrogen dioxide, and particulate matter from traffic and wood-burning are associated with increased dementia risk. This risk factor speaks to environmental justice—often, poorer communities are more exposed to air pollution from car traffic, power plants, and trash-burning facilities. It's not always as easy as moving somewhere with cleaner air, but you can take advantage of air purifiers (local energy companies often subsidize these purchases).

- SOCIAL ISOLATION. Interacting with other people helps keep you on your toes, mentally, and is believed to both build cognitive reserves and to encourage other healthy behaviors, such as engaging in exercise and having an outlet for your emotions. According to multiple long-term studies, the more social contact you have, the lower your dementia risk and better your cognitive function later in life.

- SLEEP DISTURBANCES. Although not included in the official list of twelve modifiable risk factors, the 2020 report does address the negative consequences on cognition of poor sleep, so I'm listing it here. Regular sleep disturbance (such as insomnia, restless sleep, or sleep apnea) is linked to chronic inflammation, lack of oxygen, and increased amyloid plaques and tau proteins (which form tangles)—all of which are associated with an increased risk in dementia and clinically diagnosed Alzheimer's. Although more sleep isn't necessarily better—research has found increased risk in getting less than five hours as well as more than ten hours of sleep per night. The use of hypnotic sleep aids (benzodiazepines like Ambien or Xanax) is also associated with greater risk of dementia. A better approach is to build better habits around sleep hygiene, get more movement (which tires you out), reduce stress, treat sleep apnea, and try some nonhypnotic sleep supplements—all of which the program I outline on these pages does.

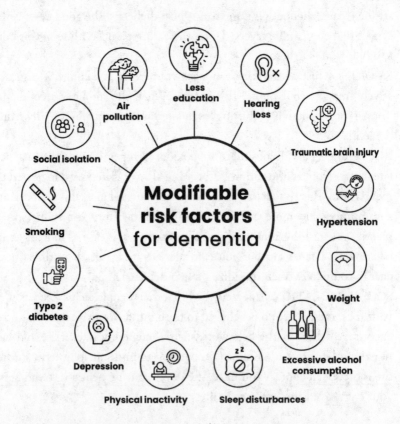

One risk factor that was not included in either report that is *somewhat* modifiable is caring for a loved one with dementia, as caregivers have a risk of developing dementia that is 250 to 600 percent greater than the general population. While you may not be able to avoid taking care of your loved one with dementia—nor would you want to, even though it is an undeniably challenging role—you can learn to care for yourself in ways that reduce that risk as well.

Essentially, this book is about mitigating these modifiable risk factors, both those that have been outlined by *The Lancet*, and those that are more commonsense, such as stress, toxic exposure, and ultra-processed foods (I wouldn't be surprised if these are included in *The Lancet*'s next update).

As helpful as this information is and as exciting as the paradigm shift it points to is, why did it take until 2017 to be introduced? And how are we not talking about it more?

If you bring up any of these twelve risk factors with your neurologist and ask for guidance on changing your relationship to them, your doctor may roll their eyes at you. If you or your loved one are already experiencing some cognitive impairment, your doctor will likely suggest Aricept—with a caveat that it may not work, or if it does help you, it won't work for long— and suggest a follow-up appointment in six to twelve months to measure the decline. It's maddening, but now you know why: there's a bunch of controversy in the medical and research establishment when it comes to Alzheimer's, and it wasn't until the late 2010s that reputable journals were acknowledging that there are modifiable risk factors that we can treat.

By 2025, there will likely be another version of this report that has still more modifiable risk factors, but why wait? Let's use common sense now. Especially since so many of the suggested actions to reduce risk are so low-risk, with pleasant side effects—such as better mood, better sleep, and better connection to people who love you.

A Protocol That Works

As I mentioned in the introduction, I was drawn to the work of Dr. Dale Bredesen and his approach to treating Alzheimer's because he took a multifactorial approach—the complexity of his protocol seemed to match the complexity of the disease. And since my very first patient after taking that training, I have seen the proof that it works. But to be fair, Dr. Bredesen's work has garnered its fair share of criticism. Since we're talking about the messiness of the scientific process and the controversy that surrounds Alzheimer's research, I want to address the criticisms of Dr. Bredesen's work, too.

One of his most outspoken critics is Dr. Joanna Hellmuth of the Memory and Aging Center at the University of California, San Francisco, who published her grievances in *The Lancet: Neurology* in 2020.

Among Hellmuth's points are that Bredesen didn't declare any conflicts of interest. There are few people whose interest feels clearer to me than Dr. Dale Bredesen's. My every experience of him is that he is passionate and committed to getting helpful, hopeful, effective information about preventing and reversing neurodegenerative diseases out to as many people as possible as fast as possible. He has done this by committing himself to the science at some of the most prestigious institutions in the country, writing a book, and supporting businesses that support those suffering with dementia as an adviser. He does all this in the face of public criticism from colleagues. Hellmuth also points out that Bredesen didn't include enough information about his methods and how he selected his participants so that other researchers could try to replicate his results; however, his 2017 book *The End of Alzheimer's* describes what was done at length. I also struggled to describe how I treated patients in my clinical trial since it is more appropriate to describe them in a book of the length of the one you are reading than in a short article. Hellmuth also calls out Bredesen for publishing in journals that are known to be predatory—meaning, they may require payment in order to be considered for publishing, have little editorial oversight, and/or make unfounded claims to their potential authors about the legitimacy of the journal. Bredesen's findings would have been better accepted if they had been published in reputable journals, and yet his research is destabilizing to academic experts, big pharma business, and bureaucratic government agencies, and there is a huge amount of interest in marginalizing changes to the paradigm. But the most recent studies—and my clinical experiences—show his approach works.

The number one criticism of the Bredesen protocol—from more voices than Hellmuth's—is that there's not enough research. And this point is absolutely true. We *do* need more research. As recently as 2017, when Dr. Bredesen first published *The End of Alzheimer's*, he was still getting turned down by IRBs when proposing a multimodal intervention instead of a single variable like a drug.

In his work, and in my own, we are following the process that gets us to the point where we can do a big randomized controlled trial—a process that takes years and millions of dollars, yet it has already been started. We're not just twiddling our thumbs waiting for things to change. And the body of evidence that we are building along the way is highly compelling. I hope as the results become clearer and the paradigm shifts, we can all do more collaborating and less criticizing, working together to focus our time, money, and energy on solutions.

Here's a basic timeline of how our thinking on the causes and treatments for dementia have changed over the last decade:

- In 2011, Bredesen's proposal for a multimodal ReCODE trial + tropisetron is rejected by the IRB and with it his funding for the trial is revoked.
- In 2014, Bredesen published a case series, reporting on the successful experiences of ten patients who followed his protocol, nine of whom improved.
- In 2016, Bredesen and team published another case series including extensive objective data on ten participants.
- In 2017, *The Lancet* published its first report on nine modifiable risk factors of dementia based on the analysis of many other peer-reviewed research articles.
- In 2018, Bredesen published another case series of one hundred dementia patients.
- In 2020, *The Lancet* released a follow-up report with twelve modifiable risk factors.
- In 2022, Dr. Kat Toups, Bredesen, and other researchers published an observational trial with twenty-five participants showing 84 percent of twenty-five participants with MoCA scores 19 and above had an improvement in cognition following a nine-month intervention.
- In August 2023, my team and I published the results of our feasibility study in the *Journal of Alzheimer's Disease*. It showed that 73.9 percent

of participants (17 of 23) with starting MoCA scores from 12 to 23 had improvement in cognition following a six-month intervention.

- Currently, Dr. Bredesen's team is recruiting for a seventy-participant randomized, multisite, controlled trial that has been IRB-approved. I cannot wait to see and share their results.

- We are in the midst of an industry-wide paradigm shift and a scientific paradigm shift to be more inclusive of study designs that are multimodal with multiple interventions, and that include lifestyle-related interventions. The science *is* progressing.

The Way Forward

If we want to protect brain health well into our eighth, ninth, and tenth decade of life, we have to let go of the idea that there will be one pill that will save us and we won't have to change anything else. We have to approach brain health from multiple angles, not just one. This is common sense, but uncommon practice.

I understand that we as a country as well as individual researchers have poured so much time, energy, and hope into the theory that amyloid plaques cause Alzheimer's disease that it's hard to consider we may have gotten it wrong. We have to stay open to other theories, and not automatically shut down alternative hypotheses. That's how the scientific process works—we question interpretations of the data and consider other possibilities. It's time to look at other approaches.

In my years of clinical experience I have seen too many people get better not to share the steps we've taken to achieve those improvements. Although the science is evolving, it's moving too slowly for the people who are already suffering or who are at high risk. I fully relate to Dr. Bredesen in that I cannot in good conscience wait for there to be enough science to satisfy someone else's standard. I feel compelled to tell people now that there is hope and a path.

I do hold out hope for a pharmaceutical drug that gets rid of the plaques and tangles and some of the pathophysiological changes that happen in the brain without the side effects of brain inflammation and brain bleeds. That way, theoretically, we could still remove the triggers of dementia and do any necessary cleanup of previous damage with pharmaceuticals. It's an exciting possibility, yet even with these drugs, we still need to prevent damage from happening in the first place.

It's time to admit that we've gotten Alzheimer's research wrong since the beginning. We need to shift our focus away from reducing plaques and tangles and toward the things that actually improve cognition and patient experience. We need to treat the brain like the complex system that it is. We need a new Alzheimer's toolkit.

SECTION 2

Getting Started

CHAPTER 3

Unpack the New Alzheimer's Toolkit

Pinning the vast majority of our scientific attention on combatting amyloid plaques isn't the only misguided assumption we've been operating under, and not the only way we've been getting the prevention and treatment of dementia wrong.

We've also been fed a lot of ideas that are quite harmful to the brain. We've been told that you should eat eight to ten servings of grains every day and avoid fat—which is exactly the opposite of what your brain needs. Your brain is made out of fat, and its neurons are sheathed in it. It prefers to use fat for fuel over carbohydrates. In addition, when we have more glucose lying around than we can truly use, that excess sugar can bond with our brain cells and essentially caramelize them in a process known as glycation.

In addition, we've been forced into a lifestyle where we are expected to spend eight hours sitting at a desk and—if you're not one of the employees who are now allowed to work remotely—maybe even driving an hour each way to get to your desk. We don't move enough to circulate nutrients to and waste products away from the brain; our lack of exercise means we also don't create the signaling molecules that tell our brain to stay active and form new connections. And we're told that we can sleep when we're dead, meaning that we miss out on hours of cleaning and repairing that keep all our organs, especially our brains, functioning well.

To top it all off, we've been socialized to think that if we have a health issue, we should go to the doctor to get a pill or have surgery, and the issue will go away. That's just not how the body works.

If we want to protect brain health well into our eighth, ninth, and tenth decade of life, we have to let go of the idea that there will be one pill that will save us and we won't have to change anything else. We have to approach brain health from multiple angles, not just one.

After all, as we've covered, the brain is a complex system. And while that makes it highly unlikely that any one drug is going to protect the brain from dementia, it is also great news—because it means that there is a broad array of strategies that support brain health. And when you layer these strategies together, you can significantly improve cognitive function.

It's time to open up the lens on what we can do to protect our brains and see that we have multiple tools—eight, to be precise—that, taken together, comprise a new Alzheimer's toolkit.

Better yet, these tools aren't terribly sophisticated or costly, and they have very few risks. They are things that you are likely already familiar with, so the learning curve isn't very steep. In fact, you're probably already doing a couple of them to some extent. But when you prioritize and optimize these tools, and bring the ones that you haven't been using into the mix, the benefits you create ripple out far beyond the brain, to your gut health, mental health, heart health, and more.

What are these eight practical yet magical tools?

- A nutrient-dense, high-fat, and low-carb ketogenic **diet** that gives your brain plenty of fuel and reduces harmful by-products of burning glucose
- **Exercise**, which cues all parts of your body, including your brain, to grow stronger and more resilient
- Brain-stimulating **activities** to maintain existing neuronal connections and trigger the formation of new neural pathways
- A supportive daily **routine** that reduces stress and makes doing the things that promote brain health more doable

- A serene and nontoxic **environment** that promotes being present and nourishes—rather than compromises—brain health
- Restorative **sleep** to help your brain clean and heal itself
- Loving **communication** between you and your care partner to reduce stress and foster connection
- **Care for the caregiver**—meaning, you, so that you can model healthy behavior for your loved ones, reduce your own risk of developing dementia, avoid burnout, and provide the best possible care

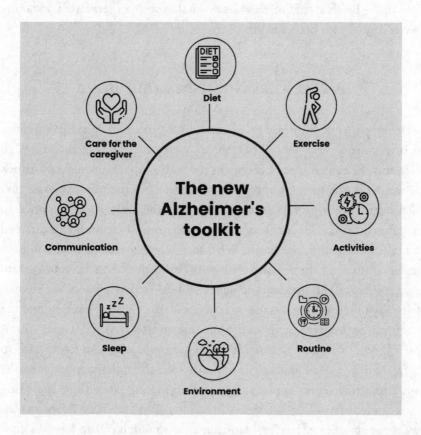

As you can see, nothing here is revolutionary. Yet taken together, these eight tools compose a holistic brain care plan because not only do they give the brain what it needs to thrive, they also address the root causes of brain dysfunction that we covered in Chapter 1.

A key premise of the power of this toolkit is that the choices you make

every day—about what to eat, how much to move, when to go to sleep, what kinds of activities you do, etc.—have the biggest influence on your health. When you optimize those choices, you can go an awfully long way toward giving the brain what it needs to function well—even to regain function it has already lost. No matter where you're starting from, it's never too early or too late to start taking better care of your brain.

In this chapter I'll give you a brief introduction to all eight tools, including one thing you can start doing differently in these areas right away—even before you've finished reading this book—so that you can get started on taking better care of your brain health.

A Diet That Nourishes Your Brain

Remember, while the brain makes up only 2 percent of your body weight, it is responsible for over 20 percent of energy expenditure each day. In fact, it is the biggest user of energy in the body—approximately two-thirds of the ATP (the form of energy manufactured in the mitochondria that fuel nearly every process in the body) that the brain uses is applied to firing neurons, while a full one-third goes toward cleaning, repair, and maintenance within the brain. With such a high need for fuel, you have to be consuming things that feed your brain, not harm it. You want to give the brain the nutrients it needs to heal, repair your brain tissues, fight toxins, create neurotransmitters, and maintain your neurons and the connections between your neurons. That means nutrient-dense, lower-carb foods. Nutrients to provide the building blocks, and lower carb to help stabilize your blood sugar and even out the roller coaster of spikes and drops that create so many cognition-impairing side effects, including lightheadedness, anxiety, fatigue, irritability, and a decrease in focus. You want the stability of having blood sugar in the high 60s to low 80s consistently, instead of zooming up to 150 or higher after a carb-heavy meal and then dropping to 71 after your body has cranked out a bunch of insulin to counteract the resulting glucose spike. When your blood sugar is in a steadier state, you're more predictable, regardless of where you are on the dementia spectrum.

A healthy diet also fosters the gut microbiome, which then benefits the brain via the gut-brain connection. (Your healthy gut bacteria are responsible for aiding digestion, providing a first line of defense for the immune system, and even manufacturing some nutrients and neurotransmitters that the brain needs to function.) And it helps you have a bowel movement every day, which is important for detoxification, digestive health, colon health, and preventing colon cancer. (If you're not currently having a daily bowel movement, see the troubleshooting section of Chapter 6 for some suggestions that can help make regular bowel movements a reality.)

More specifically, research shows that ketones—the fatty acids that the body creates when using fat, and not glucose, for fuel—are the brain's preferred form of food, and that they help the brain perform better. While no one, not even people with severe dementia, need to continually be in ketosis for the rest of their lives, spending three to six months on a ketogenic diet will jump-start the brain's healing in someone who already has cognitive decline. (I will outline in detail what foods to eat to get into ketosis in Chapter 7.) And if you're in prevention mode, spending about a quarter of the year in ketosis—whether that's one week a month, one month a quarter, or two to three days per week—can help elongate your brain span (how many years your brain stays healthy and functional).

Remember the story of that flight to Antarctica that I shared at the end of the introduction? The choices you make every day, even the small ones, are what determine your health over the course of your life. If you can decide, *I am no longer someone who eats a standard American diet with its high amount of ultra-processed, sugary foods*, it will change the trajectory of your health. Or even, *I am no longer someone who drinks soda*, this can have a profound impact on your health over time.

What I see clinically is that the higher the level of ketones in your blood, the more your cognitive function comes online. While a ketogenic diet was a key part of what helped our study participants achieve their significant gains in cognitive function, that doesn't mean it's ketosis or bust—simply eating fewer ultra-processed foods and more of the foods on the Phase 1, 2, and 3 lists in the back of this book will often still net you improvements in cognition. That basically means eating more things that don't come in a package, or if the foods do come in a box or a bag, that packaging doesn't contain words in the ingredients list that you can't pronounce (an easy way to tell if a food is ultra-processed or not).

If you do one thing to improve your diet: Hopefully, you've already started raising your carb-consciousness and begun to swap out some of the carb-heavy foods you eat most often for lower-carb alternatives (the guidance I offered in Chapter 1 in the "Poor Nutrition" section). To build on this new awareness, start aiming to keep your daily carb consumption under 100 grams. That could look like having one piece of avocado toast for breakfast instead of a whole bagel or cereal, having soup and salad instead of a sandwich and chips for lunch, swapping your side dish of potatoes or rice for quinoa or cauliflower rice at dinner, and having berries with a little whipped cream or a few squares of dark chocolate instead of ice cream for dessert. I don't really like to get too hung up on counting every gram of carbs you consume, because it can be stressful and overwhelming (which is the opposite of what we want!). But many times my patients don't realize how many carbs they've been eating. Becoming aware of how many carbohydrates you're eating in a day will help you eat less of them—after all, you can't change a habit you don't know you have. Just this one change would do a ton of good—including bringing down glucose and insulin levels (and therefore reducing inflammation), and upping consumption of the nutrients that support brain health (protein, vitamins and minerals from vegetables, and fats).

Exercise to Make Your Brain More Resilient

Honestly, exercise is so powerful a health intervention that if we could just bottle it, we could probably get rid of chronic disease. Exercise does take time and effort, but making this one activity a regular part of your life addresses so many causal factors of dementia that it can profoundly reduce your risk.

The overarching reason that exercise is such a powerful health protector is that it is what's known as *hormetic*, or a beneficial stressor. Basically, when you put your body through its paces, the body is forced to use up resources, and your tissues can even be broken down a bit (that's what happens when you lift weights: your muscles tear a tiny bit). In that sense, you're introducing stress to your system, but that stress is a force for good because it triggers your body to get more efficient at using its resources and your tissues to grow back even stronger. In other words, exercise makes your body—including your brain—more resilient.

Exercise benefits several of the root causes of neurological disease:

It improves *structure* by increasing your cardiovascular capacity and boosting circulation, which delivers oxygen and nutrients to the brain.

It reduces *stress* in multiple ways—by giving you an outlet to blow off steam, by producing feel-good hormones such as endorphins and lowering the stress hormone cortisol, and, depending on what kind of exercise you choose, getting you outside and into nature, which is a well-known stress reliever. It can also be social, and a great way to spend time with friends or even meet new people, which helps address the loneliness and social isolation that *The Lancet* lists as one of the modifiable risk factors for Alzheimer's disease.

It improves *sleep* by tiring you out.

It strengthens immune function, which reduces the risk and effects of *infection*—all those muscular contractions and moving against gravity improves the flow of lymphatic fluid, which delivers immune cells and flushes away invader cells. A 2019 review found that moderate exercise mobilizes immune stem cells, helping the body defend itself against pathogens, reduces systemic inflammation, and protects against the typical age-related decline in immunity known as immunosenescence.

It promotes *detox*, both through increased circulation and through sweating.

It improves *signaling*, as challenging and strengthening your muscles triggers the release of multiple signaling molecules, known as exerkines, that have demonstrated neuroprotective functions.

There are four types of exercise that are particularly valuable for boosting brain health, which I'll cover in depth in Chapter 6. For now, you only need to know that whatever type of exercise you do, when you can push the intensity (not necessarily the duration, but the amount of energy required to complete a workout) and get into the sweet spot of being outside your comfort zone without overdoing it, you trigger a cascade of signaling molecules that protect and repair the brain. This is a key point about the value of exercise as a tool for improving brain health—you have to do more than you're typically used to doing. In other words, walking is great, but if that's been your go-to exercise for a while now, it's not enough to protect brain health.

When your form of movement is something new to you, such as ballroom dance, tai chi, or golf, or something that is continually different, like a Zumba class with new routines, exercise is also cognitively stimulating as it keeps you in learning mode, creating new neuronal connections.

If you do only one thing: Change up your current exercise routine in a way that challenges your brain and amps up the intensity. If you are a devoted walker, find a new route that includes hills or stairs. If you're open to trying something different, check out a new exercise class that you've been meaning to try.

Challenge Your Brain—and Have Fun—with Activities

When it comes to cognitive function, it is definitely use it or lose it. That means it's on each of us to do things that stimulate our brains (or, if you're the caregiver to someone with dementia, to keep them engaged). Activities are how we keep our brains sharp, and luckily there are so many ways to enhance neuroplasticity and keep new neuronal connections and pathways forming so that cognitive function stays strong or improves. While they can include crosswords and sudoku (depending on your current cognitive score), the key to keeping your cognition strong is continually challenging your brain to either learn something new or to dig deep in order to remember something you may have forgotten.

We know from the articles in *The Lancet* about the modifiable risk factors for Alzheimer's, the more educated you are earlier in life, the more cognitive reserve you have. Although that's not to say that if you don't have a lot of formal education you're doomed. Everyone's brain can benefit from stimulation, which means that adopting the attitude of being a lifelong learner is key for brain health. Pursuing activities and topics that you're interested in, staying curious, and actively seeking to continue learning new things helps extend your brain span. Just as importantly, it helps you stay engaged in life, approach things with curiosity, and pursue things that you enjoy.

Creating new routines; shopping, cooking, and eating in a different way; learning new disciplines like meditation; and pursuing new physical practices like dancing or playing pickleball all engage your brain. Even following the guidelines that I outline in this book—and reading this book and learning more about the way the brain works!—help you create those new pathways. Whenever you can make the activities you do social—going dancing with a friend, taking a class with others—it will have even more benefit, because you will also be remedying any isolation or loneliness that we know can be a risk factor for dementia.

If you do only one thing: If you're in prevention mode, use this as your motivation to start learning that hobby or skill you've been meaning to check out but haven't gotten around to. That could mean learning a new language (by signing up for a class or using an app), a new musical instrument, or a new sport. If you're already noticing that your cognitive function isn't what it once was, expand on something you already know how to do—start cooking a new cuisine or using new culinary techniques, learn some new songs on the instrument you already know how to play (or refresh yourself on how to play the song you performed at your eighth-grade recital), or challenge yourself to use the language you studied in school. And if you are caring for a loved one with dementia, engage them in a sing-along to music they once knew well and loved, or encourage them to remember facts they once knew (such as asking someone who was once an avid gardener to name the plants in the garden). Bonus points for choosing activities you can do with other people— like salsa dancing, playing a sport, or forming a knitting bee.

If the thought of doing one more activity adds to your stress, lean into learning practical things that will help you maintain your independence as you age—when there's a problem with your dishwasher, look for a how-to video on YouTube that can guide you through fixing it yourself, for example. Or, always calculate the tip when you go out to dinner, keep seeking to discover new ways to drive to the places you go most frequently, or just try to figure out whatever problems you encounter in your daily life before calling in someone else to help.

Reduce Your Daily Stress with Routine

Establishing a rhythm to your and your care partner's day serves two important purposes: (1) it helps you find a time for all the pieces of your program so that you don't feel pressure to be doing all the things all the time. And (2) it provides a comforting structure for you and your care partner that reduces stress, rushing, and worry. In Chapter 5, I'll guide you on how to create your own daily routine that helps you feel calm and confident that you are doing what you can.

A grounding and supportive daily schedule focuses primarily on the morning (taking supplements, interacting with nature, and doing some sort of centering practice), midday (a time for activities, appointments, exercise) and evening (a time for oral care and rituals for healthy sleep).

Routine does more than provide a container for all the tools in your new Alzheimer's toolkit—it's also comforting to know what happens when. It makes it easy to plan out your days and weeks so that you can stress less about making sure you get things done.

I've said it before, and I'll say it again: the decisions you make every day—what to eat, what to do next, what time you get into bed, how often you floss your teeth, whether you turn on the TV or do a stimulating and satisfying activity—comprise the biggest, most powerful lever you have for positively impacting your health. Yet these healthy choices aren't always easy to make. Each choice can require a lot of willpower—a finite resource that can be quickly depleted. An effective way to keep making those healthy choices and lean on this lever as hard as you can with the least amount of effort is to make them part of your routine. That's how you get to make fewer decisions and make your daily healthy actions more automatic.

Honestly, helping you get into a routine that makes it easy to choose to do the healthy thing is the overarching goal of this whole book. There's so much information out there on *what* to do to be healthier; I want to focus more on *how* you do it, so that you can pull that lever as hard as you can.

Also, as someone progresses through dementia, routine becomes even more important. They may not remember what they did at the table where you do your activities the day before, but they know they're supposed to be sitting at that table after lunch every day. All humans want a balance between predictability and surprise. Varying your activities within the framework of a routine is how you find that balance. When new residents join us at Marama and they aren't yet familiar with our daily rhythms, they're agitated, on edge. When they have experienced the consistency of our schedule for a while (it takes some people a few days; for others, it's more like a few weeks), they're noticeably less anxious. Predictability creates that space to be more present and engaged in whatever activity you're doing.

If you do one thing: Pick one aspect of your day to "routine-ize": it could be your morning, lunch break, or evening. Make a bulleted list with everything you do during this time nearly every day, and hang that list somewhere in view. As you read through the rest of the book and learn more things you could be doing to care for your brain, think about what you can weave into your existing routine—and update your list. Giving a new task a home in your daily routine will make it easier for that new habit to stick.

An Environment That Supports You

Setting up your environment makes it easier for you to stick to your daily routine. For example, having exercise equipment on hand and a dedicated space for using it makes it much easier to actually work out. (And making sure there aren't cookies sitting out on the counter will also make it a lot easier to choose something healthier.)

In addition, reducing clutter in your space minimizes distractions and gives the brain more space to function. It doesn't mean you have to adopt a minimalist lifestyle (although, if you're so inspired, don't let me stop you!). Simply getting things off your countertops, moving bags out of the entryway, and clearing things out of your visual field is great for reducing stress. That's because the brain reads clutter as a to-do list, meaning you never get a chance to rest in the feeling of being caught up.

Another important piece of setting up your environment for better cognitive health is reducing your exposure to toxins. Our bodies are wise and elegantly equipped to detoxify, but if we're constantly pouring more toxins in, it's hard for cells to keep up, and they can get locked in constant defense mode. That means nutrients and energy get devoted to detoxing, and then you have less on hand to create brain infrastructure—new neurons, and new connections between those neurons. In Chapter 9, I'll walk you through the easy steps you can take to make your environment relatively free of toxins from things like mold, volatile organic compounds (such as those found in household paint and cleaning products, nonstick pans, and plastic products), and other common contaminants.

And the final piece of the environment puzzle is bringing in more natural elements—such as daylight, plants, and even art that features the natural world—a step that helps lower stress and boost immune function.

Ultimately, you want to set up your home in a way that helps you feel like you are on retreat when you are home, so you can get into a rest, digest, and heal state.

While setting up your home environment can be a big project, maintaining it after that initial push takes only a few minutes a day and pays off by helping both the caregiver and the care partner feel more relaxed.

If you do one thing: Declutter as many areas as you can. You'll be setting the stage for your brain to be less distracted and more present, and for you to be able to truly rest and recharge when you are home. Start with one room where you spend a lot of time. The good feeling you'll get from being in that newly pared down room will inspire you to move on to another area once you're done.

Refresh and Restore with Sleep

Getting restful sleep at night is a crucial piece of protecting brain health, primarily because sleep is when the brain takes out the trash. Just like the rest of the body has the lymphatic system—a series of channels that use fluid to deliver immune cells and wash away waste materials, the brain has the glymphatic system—a network of glial cells that pulses while we sleep and flushes out toxic waste products. Without good sleep, those toxins can build up—just as you need to wash your dishes every day or else your sink will overflow, your brain needs a chance to cleanse what accumulates during the day.

Sleep appears to have a direct relationship to beta-amyloid proteins, too. Incredibly, research has found that even people in their thirties and forties have more amyloid plaques after just one night of sleep deprivation. Over the course of years or decades, those are going to build up. Even though we haven't established that amyloid plaques *cause* dementia, we know they are related and at least a sign of Alzheimer's; if simply getting more sleep helps keep them at bay, then let's do it!

Beyond the glymphatic system, sleep is when the hippocampus consolidates memories and the amygdala does a lot of the work of processing emotions.

Although it's appearing well down the list of tools, sleep is a great place to start because it kicks off a virtuous cycle. The more rested you are, the more energy you have to exercise and do activities, and the more willpower you'll have to avoid sugar and the more motivation you'll have to choose keto-friendly foods instead. It's also hard to heal and get stronger without regular, restful sleep.

If you do one thing to improve your sleep—put a bubble around the three hours before you go to bed. During these final three hours of your day, don't eat (because digestion can distract your body from going into repair and restore mode while you sleep), minimize your screen time, since the blue light from screens and a gripping storyline in whatever you're watching can be stimulating, and try not to exercise too intensely (although an easy walk after dinner is a nice way to boost digestion) because it raises cortisol and your core body temperature, both of which need to fall in order for you to sleep soundly. Instead, these hours can be time for you to do the things that are hard to make time for during the day—things like meditating, taking a relaxing bath, or connecting with loved ones and friends whether in person or on a phone call.

Prioritize Connection over Correction

Your relationship with your care partner is the foundation for everything you do with and for them, and communication is how you keep that relationship strong and positive. Because the person you're caring for is more than a list of to-dos—they have feelings, wants, and fears, just as you do—in every chapter of this book, I'll focus on how you can improve your communication so that your bond gets stronger and you each experience less resistance to making needed changes.

When your communication is in a good place, caregiving—while still stressful—can become a positive experience, because it can bring you closer to your care partner and help you express thoughts and feelings in a constructive way so that they don't fester and add to your stress.

A lot of times I hear from patients' families things like, "You don't understand, she's not willing to do that," or "He will spit in my face if I don't let him have a cookie after dinner." If you have challenges in getting your care partner to try the things in the new Alzheimer's toolkit, know that you are by no means alone. It can be made even more challenging because of your relationship dynamics with this person—it's easy to take a loved one's comments personally. Loving communication can help you rewire those dynamics and bring your relationship in to the present, so that you can engage them and help them in a way that's relevant to where they are and what they're capable of doing and understanding today. My refrain is "connection over correction"—it is much more valuable to connect with your loved one than to correct them when they aren't doing something "right." Throughout the book, I'll offer language to help you with certain scenarios and achieve that connection.

Regardless of our MoCA score, we all long for connection—communication is a big piece of how we can feel that connectedness. In addition, loving communication is quite practical—it's much more likely that your care partner will eat their meal and engage in activities if you can talk to them about it in a loving way. If you've been frustrated by trying to feel that connection with your care partner, it's completely understandable, and likely caused at least in part because you didn't know that there's another way to communicate and you fell back into old patterns that maybe weren't that healthy to begin with—and are even less relevant now that cognitive decline is in the picture. I've seen it happen again and again that once a caregiver learns a more loving way to communicate, it makes things a lot easier for everyone.

Loving communication ultimately reduces the caregiver's stress as well.

because you can de-escalate situations that could otherwise throw you and your whole day off.

If you do one thing to improve communication: Adopt the improv principle of "yes, and." Meaning, if your care partner has trouble remembering something, or says something that doesn't make sense, don't challenge them, or reject what they're saying. Rather, acknowledge what they said and then add on to it—the same way that improv scene partners will do in order to come up with a sketch on the fly. It does require a little creativity, but mostly, all it takes is a willingness to see life through your care partner's eyes. If they can't remember someone's name, don't say, "You really don't remember?" Try saying, "It's hard when you can't think of someone's name. You're thinking of Jean—or as I like to call her, Jeanie with the light brown hair." Or if they insist they had breakfast with their mom that morning, instead of saying, "No, your mom died twenty years ago," say, "Oh! What did you and mom have for breakfast?" (There's an excellent book from 2003 on this very topic called *Learning to Speak Alzheimer's*, by Joanne Koenig Coste—I include it in a list of recommended resources in the back of this book.)

Care for the Caregiver (Meaning You)

It's absolutely vital that you take care of yourself now, too. Why? If you are caring for someone with dementia, your act of love comes with a cost of a significantly increased risk of developing dementia yourself. After all, caregiving is extremely stressful, and it disrupts sleep, diet, and exercise— all the lifestyle things we're talking about that are so important to brain health. That's likely why science reflects that caregivers have a 250 to 600 percent increased risk of developing dementia. You don't want to end up being the patient.

Because caregiving is stressful, it's vital that you direct some of your caring efforts toward yourself, both so you can be there for your care partner and so you can grow during this experience and minimize your risk of needing care in the future.

In my experience, although caregiving comes with a host of logistical challenges that can increase your stress and make you feel like you don't have the time to get the exercise, sleep, healthy foods, and other tools in the toolkit that can so effectively reduce the risk of dementia, the biggest challenge to a caregiver's health is guilt. It's hard to feel like you're doing enough, or doing things correctly, and this worry conflicts with your desire to provide your loved one with the best care possible. I understand why you feel that way, but it doesn't serve you or the person you're caring for.

Here's the thing—because you are on the front lines, you know the suffering firsthand. Hopefully that front-row seat also means that your motivation is that much higher to put the new Alzheimer's toolkit to work in your own life. Just because you're not the person with the diagnosis doesn't mean you shouldn't also eat the brain-healthy diet, or do the brain-stimulating activities, or get the brain-boosting exercise—it actually means you should! And just as importantly, you need to find ways to develop compassion for yourself, let yourself off the hook, and figure out how to be kind to yourself. It is possible—and I look forward to diving in to the many strategies and resources you have to make it even more doable. But don't wait until you get to Chapter 10 to start. Please!

If you do one thing to take better care of yourself—enlist someone in helping you, whether you have to hire this person, reach out to a resource in your community (such as an adult day care class or a network of neighbors who provide rides and other simple tasks), or simply ask a friend or family member to help out. (You can also turn to page 70 for a list of caregiving resources.) As much as you may wish you could, it's not realistic to expect that you can do all the caregiving yourself. It would only set you up for burnout—and then you won't be able to take good care of your loved one. Caring for someone with dementia is not a one-person job.

You can't do this alone, so for everyone's sake, stop trying. Since you're reading this book I already know you're doing the best you can.

A Different Approach for Better Outcomes

I'm sharing this bird's-eye view of the tools we use at Marama—which our study participants followed, and which the rest of this book will break down in detail—so that you can get the lay of the land and see how the tools in the toolkit form a synergistic whole that can nourish your brain health, and so many other facets of your life. Using the toolkit also offers a richer, more rewarding daily experience, as well as a reduction in risk factors for the other prevalent chronic diseases of our time, such as heart disease, cancer, diabetes, and autoimmune diseases, because what's good for your brain is also good for your heart, your immune system, and your metabolic health.

As someone who uses each of these tools in her personal life, as well as seeing the power they have to benefit my patients at my clinic and Marama, I understand that they can be very different from the standard way of doing things for most people. But think about it—the standard way of doing things is what's gotten us into the crisis of 6.5 million Americans living with dementia (not to mention the myriad chronic diseases that are eroding too many people's quality of life for too many years).

That's why this new Alzheimer's toolkit offers a different approach to daily living—because we want different results.

While all these tools in the new Alzheimer's toolkit are based on common sense, they are uncommon practices. I know it's a big ask to adopt them all—or as many of them as you can manage at any given time. The number one rule of changing your life for the better is that it can't stress you out too much. Don't let the perfect be the enemy of the good.

But adopting any number of these tools will help, and the more you can weave into your daily life, the more benefit you'll receive: the latest science shows us that the more healthy habits we stack on top of one another, the better the outcomes we can achieve over time. I've outlined an approach that can help you prepare to make these changes in a way that increases your commitment and helps remove any mental or physical obstacles to putting in the work. Let's start setting the stage for applying these tools in the way that makes the most sense for your life, goals, and bandwidth.

To watch a summary video of this chapter and download the Reversing Alzheimer's workbook go to ReversingAlzheimersBook.com.

CHAPTER 4

Set the Stage with a Doable Plan

As powerful as each tool in the new Alzheimer's toolkit is on its own, their benefits increase when you stack them on top of one another. Excitingly, we are starting to have science that shows how taking good care of multiple areas of health over the long-term has the power to reduce the risk of developing dementia.

A US study that presented its initial findings at the 2023 annual meeting of the American Academy of Neurology tracked nearly fourteen thousand women age fifty-four and up for twenty years, giving them a score of either zero (for poor or intermediate health) or one (for ideal health) in seven categories: getting movement, eating a healthy diet, maintaining a healthy weight, not smoking, and avoiding high blood pressure, cholesterol, and blood sugar. While the perfect score was 7, the average score was 4.3. The researchers found that for every score increase of one point (which means bringing one additional aspect of health into an ideal range), the risk of developing dementia fell by 6 percent.

And a 2022 Chinese study followed more than twenty-nine thousand people age sixty or older for ten years. The researchers wanted to evaluate the impact of six healthy behaviors: eating nutritious food, getting regular exercise, not smoking, doing at least two social activities and two cognitively challenging activities per week, not smoking, and not drinking. Participants who performed at least four of these activities had significantly slower cognitive decline over the course of ten years than those who did only one or none of those behaviors. This was true even for the participants who carried an APOE4 gene.

While this means that the more tools you make part of your daily life, the more you stand to gain, but it can also open the door to overwhelm if you try to add a bunch of new habits at once. In this chapter, we'll cover the mindset, tools, and strategies that will help you implement new habits—or strengthen those healthy behaviors you already do regularly—in a way that makes them both more doable and longer lasting.

Managing Your Own Expectations

Every week, I meet with several patients—or family members of patients—who confess to me that they want to do everything they can to protect their or their family member's brain health. They want to go all in, but they are paralyzed by all the changes they could be making. I get it. It's natural to struggle with feeling that you have to address all the things you *could* be doing to protect brain health, especially when the stakes can feel so high.

So please hear me when I say: you cannot do everything. That means, any perfectionist tendencies you may have cannot drive the train. Remember, in my clinical trial, nearly 75 percent of people experienced measurable and significant improvements in cognition, and none of those people followed the protocol 100 percent. You don't have to incorporate every single tool in the toolkit to get meaningful results.

Of course, I want you to dive in and embrace as much as you can of what I've outlined on these pages, but making change is a process. It doesn't have to be perfect. That's why I've included so many suggestions of "if you do only one thing" up until this point—anything that you incorporate into your life will provide benefit. While adding more tools will provide additional benefit, some is always better than none.

As you read through the rest of the book, remember that you are the expert on you and your life. While I know that you might surprise yourself by how many changes you are able to make over time, you also know how much you are realistically able to take on in this moment.

Beyond managing your own expectations about how much you'll be able to do right away, the most important thing you can do at this point, before we launch into the whole program, is to create a thoughtful, doable plan. To that end, you need to get clear on your goals, acknowledge your obstacles, and think through some logistics. That's what this chapter will help you do.

Prepping Your Mind for Change

Because change is an emotional as well as a logistical process, some of the things I'll guide you through in this chapter address some of the fears and unhelpful thought processes that may be lurking in your mind. Behavior change isn't easy—otherwise, everyone would already be doing many of the things in this book, and we wouldn't be facing a dramatic uptick in the prevalence of dementia. Making different choices a new way of life requires your mind, body, and spirit to be on board.

To that end, my first suggestion for you in this chapter is to dedicate a notebook, journal, or document on your computer or note on your phone to your Reversing Alzheimer's journey. This is a place to capture your answers to reflection questions that I'll include throughout the rest of the book. It's also a place to log every step you take, write down your questions, capture your successes, and jot down notes about things you want to be sure to remember. Much more than a perfunctory exercise, this notebook can be a tangible record of the steps you took, the love and care you felt, and the progress you made. It can also help you troubleshoot later—if you start struggling with sleep at some point in the future, you can look back at your notes to see exactly what you did this time around to make improvements to your sleep. It can also inform your visits with your care provider, by keeping a log of your questions and also a record of the changes you've made so that your provider or coach can tailor their recommendations based on what you've been doing.

Once you have your notebook, here is your first assignment: set your intentions for the changes you are about to implement.

Take a few minutes to think ahead to the results you want to create by following the advice laid out in this book. Think ahead to six months from now, and answer these questions.

Reflection questions:
• What do you want to be different in six months? (Do you want to see an improvement in your or your loved one's MoCA score? Do you want to be exercising regularly? Do you want to have spent a significant part of that time in ketosis?)
• How do you want to feel in six months? (Do you want to be more clear-headed, energized, patient, optimistic, empowered?)

Write your answers down in the present tense, as if they have already happened. For example, "I am feeling well rested and energized. I have become addicted to my new exercise habits because they are so much fun and make me feel so good. And my bloodwork shows that I am no longer prediabetic."

There will be ups and downs through this process and times in the coming weeks and months when you will wonder whether the changes you're making are worth the effort. Having these intentions written down will help you reconnect with your desires and goals and help motivate you to keep going.

Get Support

No matter how much you may wish this weren't true, the fact is, you can't be the only person to care for your loved one. Even if you're reading this book because you are in prevention mode for yourself, and not actively caring for someone with cognitive decline, lasting change doesn't happen in isolation.

Even if you think everything is fine now, look for support before you need it so that when you do need it, you already have it lined up. I've talked to so many families in a state of desperation because they really need some help, but now they feel too overwhelmed to find it. Also keep in mind that when you are stretched thin, your loved one with dementia will be less safe, simply because you don't have the bandwidth to give them all the care they require on your own. You're so much less likely to get to that point if you start the process now.

An obvious place to consider looking for support is your closest relationships—your spouse, a sibling, an adult child or grandchild or other family member, a close friend (of yours, or of your care partner).

From here, I'll divide my guidance for possible resources for support into two categories: for caregivers, and for people in prevention mode.

For caregivers:

- FRIENDS AND FAMILY MEMBERS. Maybe they can run errands for you or spend a day with your loved one so that you can get a full day off (a vital piece of your care plan that I'll talk more about in Chapter 10). If you need ideas, some helpful asks for this person are to set up automatic grocery deliveries, schedule appointments, get bills on auto pay—any way to use technology to make things a little easier going forward. Typically, these things take the most time to set up and then need only occasional troubleshooting.
- HOME CARE SERVICES OR HOME HEALTHCARE SERVICES. Home care services can match you with a paid caregiver who can help with daily tasks like dressing, cooking, and cleaning for your loved one. If your loved one isn't sleeping, you might need a night caregiver. Home healthcare givers are medically trained professionals who can administer meds, help with toileting, and make sure the environment is safe. The Family Caregiver Alliance is a nonprofit devoted to helping people caring for a member find the information and resources they need. Their website, caregiver.org, is a great place to start.
- YOUR CHURCH OR OTHER EXTENDED NETWORK. You can ask for recommendations for trustworthy caregivers whom others have used, or perhaps even find someone looking for work. You may also be able to connect with others in a similar position who would be interested in forming a support group—or discover that one already exists that you can join.
- SOCIAL SERVICES. The US Administration on Aging has created a comprehensive website called the Eldercare Locator (eldercare.acl.gov) to help you connect with local resources for caregiving, transportation, housing, day care, navigating insurance benefits, and more.

- YOUR LOCAL SENIOR CENTER. They may have a daytime program that your loved one would enjoy and that would give you some relief. They may also have resources such as transportation to help you get your care partner to and from the doctor, physical therapy, and exercise appointments.
- ADULT DAY SERVICES. The National Adult Day Services Association (www.nadsa.org) can connect you with local adult day service centers that can help fill in gaps for care during the day as well as activities, exercise classes, and all-important opportunities to connect and be social. Many of the centers are covered by Medicare and Medicaid.
- CHEFS FOR SENIORS. This service offers chefs matched with seniors to come to their home and cook for them at regular intervals to reduce the burden of shopping and preparing meals. You can give them recipes to help them help you get into ketosis. (chefsforseniors.com)

If you're in prevention mode:
- FRIENDS AND FAMILY: Is there someone who might commit to exercising or signing up for some lessons to learn a new skill with you so that you have accountability and you also both get the benefit of socializing? Would someone be interested in changing their diet along with you? Has someone you know followed the ketogenic diet before and might be able to share some pointers and some favorite recipes? Is your partner willing and able to help you optimize your sleep?
- PROFESSIONALS: If you have room in your budget, Bredesen-trained doctors, nutritionists, health coaches, and other professionals can help you create a customized plan. (See Resources for guidance in finding one.)
- CLASSES: Joining in a group for your activities, exercise, or meditation is a great way to hold yourself accountable for doing them and for meeting people. Check out local yoga studios, gyms, churches, small businesses, and even your community library or hospital for classes.

Reflection questions:
- What parts of making changes to your diet and lifestyle are the hardest for you? Is it grocery shopping, or cooking? Is it getting motivated to exercise?

Finding the time to meditate? Having time to yourself (because you're a parent, or because you're spending a lot of time with your care partner, or even both)? Being clear about where you struggle will help you get just the support you need.

- Who are the people already in your life whom you could ask for support?
- What, specifically, could you ask them to do?
- What other resources do you want to investigate? When can you devote an hour or two in the next week to researching and making calls?

Figure Out the Best Place to Start

A journey of one thousand miles begins with a single step—so how do you know which step should be the first? My recommendation is to look for either the low-hanging fruit—the things that would be fairly easy to incorporate—or what's going to make the most difference. For example, if your diet is currently sugar- and carb-heavy; or if you have—or suspect you have—sleep apnea; or if you or your care partner are currently getting very little movement, tending to that area will likely have a big benefit.

In general, the areas that tend to need the most attention are diet, exercise, and sleep. So if you aren't sure where to start, pick one of these options—either the one you feel most drawn to, the one you feel you'll have the most success with, the one with the most room for improvement, or the one that you've already made some progress on but just need to take a few more steps to really get it dialed in.

When any one of these areas improve, you'll create a virtuous cycle. If you start with diet, you'll have more energy for exercise. If you start with exercise, you'll naturally sleep better and improve your blood sugar. If you start with sleep, you'll have clearer thinking to help you figure out ways to make changes to diet or exercise more doable. It's really just a matter of getting started.

If you aren't sure where you want to start, try this exercise that comes from the coaching world—it's called the wheel of life, and it helps you objectively assess how you are doing in eight different areas of your life. When I share this exercise in my Reversing Alzheimer's at Home online course or with my patients, people find it very thought-provoking. Because it's easy to have tunnel vision and focus on only one or two areas of life—namely work and family. The wheel of life guides you through stepping back and looking at the full picture.

To do it, look at the image below and give yourself a score from 1 to 10 based on what's been happening over the last month for each segment. Don't overthink it, and be honest. The goal isn't necessarily a 10 in each category. The goal is to identify what might be out of balance, either too low and neglected in your life or maybe even overemphasized. The question is, "Where is there room for more balance in my life?" If you are caring for someone, fill out a second wheel for them, talking through it if possible. (To download a companion workbook that includes a printable version of the wheel of life exercise, visit ReversingAlzheimersBook.com.)

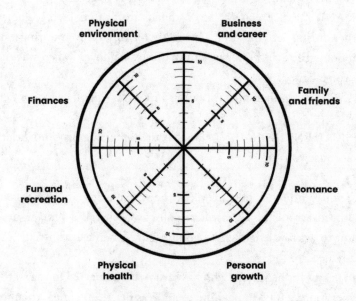

Wheel of Life

Let's take a quick tour through these categories, starting from the top of the circle:

- BUSINESS AND CAREER: This may not be applicable if your loved one or you aren't working now, but if you are, how do you feel about where you are, work-wise? If you are not currently working, this could refer to your contribution as a volunteer or mentor.
- FAMILY AND FRIENDS: Are you or your care partner interacting with people and feeling that foundational sense of connection? Do you have opportunities to socialize regularly (even introverts need this!)?
- ROMANCE: Do you feel loved, valued, and appreciated, and are you enjoying each other's company and a sense of connection and support?
- PERSONAL GROWTH: Are you staying open to new experiences and ideas, and either allowing or pushing yourself to evolve and change? Are you building skills?
- PHYSICAL HEALTH: How is your energy, your diet, your sleep? Are you getting regular checkups or are you behind on doctor and dental visits? Are you prioritizing or neglecting your physical body?
- FUN AND RECREATION: How much are you enjoying yourself—whether during activities that are strictly for fun, or even during work or when doing life tasks? Are you doing things you love? When was the last time you laughed?
- FINANCES: Is your money situation in a pretty good place, or causing you stress?
- PHYSICAL ENVIRONMENT: Does your home support your health, or does it cause you stress?

Once you're finished, take a look at the whole thing and, first, congratulate yourself for all the areas where you gave yourself a 7 or higher. (It's important to acknowledge what's going right!) Then ask yourself, "Where do I really need to focus?"

Donna cares for her mom, who has severe Alzheimer's. Donna started by getting her mom a CPAP machine to address her sleep apnea, then moved into adopting a ketogenic diet. Although Donna's mom has made some progress, it's felt really overwhelming for Donna, who's been burning the candle at both ends as a mom with a full-time job and now the additional role of caregiver.

Doing the wheel of life exercise showed Donna that she's not been feeling connected to her husband, and she hasn't had very much fun or recreation—she gave herself a 3 in both of these sections. In all other areas, she was doing pretty well. When Donna looked at her completed wheel of life, it was a forehead-smacking moment: *I need a date night with my husband and maybe we should plan a weekend away!* She hadn't fully realized just how much this area of her life needed attention.

It wasn't a surprise to me, as nearly all the people who have shared their completed wheel of life with me have given themselves low scores in fun and recreation. Seeing that low number in such a vital part of life typically leads to the question, "How can I make this more playful and fun?" Otherwise, what's the point? After all, laughing, enjoying yourself, and having fun are so important for mental well-being and feeling like a human being—not just a human doing.

It's vital to remember that taking care of yourself isn't just about you. It allows you to show up for your loved one with dementia and everyone else in your life. Plus, it's easy to skimp out on your own sleep, exercise, nutrition, stress relief, and play when you're caring for someone else. You can't serve from an empty vessel, so we need to make sure your cup is full. I'll talk more specifically about how to tend to all areas of your own wheel of life in Chapter 10, but it's still a good idea to go ahead and fill one out for yourself now so that you can identify where you need the most support and stand to receive the most benefit, even as you walk your care partner through the toolkit.

As you're doing the wheel of life exercise, keep in mind that this is a judgment- and criticism-free zone. You're not trying to fix; you're trying to take stock. Also, there are no right or wrong answers—just the ones that are true.

Reflection questions:
- When you look at your completed wheel of life, what truths emerge?
- What is something you can easily do that would start to improve the lowest score(s)?
- What is something you can do that would make the biggest difference?

Find the Time

A crucial early step to making the diet and lifestyle changes that can extend your brain span is to pause and think through your current schedule so that you can see where you might be able to do less of something so that you have more time for something new.

If this approach to brain health requires anything up-front, it's time. It also takes commitment and a little bit of extra effort. A big part of being able to make it happen is just getting organized and finding that time in your week.

Although it may not feel like it at first, the space *is* there if you allow yourself to think differently. Granted, this step does require an open mind and a willingness to get a little bit uncomfortable. But the investment of time and energy you put toward making a few changes will provide tremendous rewards.

I'm not asking you to figure out how to add even more things to your plate—you're not a superhero who can defy the laws of time, and you don't need to become a multitasking tornado. My goal for you is to realize that when you reshuffle and reprioritize some things, you do actually have enough time to do your brain-nourishing activities, and prepare more brain-friendly foods, and get your brain-boosting exercise. When you create space in your schedule so that you don't feel like you have to rush through or cram things into your already jam-packed days, these new pursuits can simply become part of a new, fulfilling, fun lifestyle. Remember how everything you can add has the power to amplify the benefits of any other intervention you're already doing, thanks to the compounding effect of stacking your interventions.

Before you start scheduling in anything new, it's best to take a look at how you're currently spending your time. That means it's time to open your calendar or planner, if you have one, and look at just the next week—if you don't have a planner, get out your notebook and jot down what you anticipate you'll be doing over the next seven days. If you don't use a calendar or organizer, this is a great opportunity to start using one; I absolutely live by mine, and the residents at Marama love being able to see each day's schedule posted on a whiteboard so that they know what to expect.

During this first pass, you're just trying to get a baseline for everything that happens in your typical week. You're simply evaluating what is. This will help you identify places where you can make space for the things you'll be incorporating from the new Alzheimer's toolkit.

As you look at your typical week, ask yourself what you might be able to eliminate—perhaps some TV watching or scrolling social media time, or a volunteer commitment that's no longer filling your cup, or maybe it's time to get the kids to start making their own breakfasts. The simple truth is that you're going to have to give something up so that you can devote some time and energy to this change in lifestyle. Be thoughtful. Allow yourself to think differently about what you "have" to do on a daily basis so that you can recognize the possibilities that are hiding in plain sight there on your calendar.

Once you've freed up some space for yourself—and I understand that this may take a little time—you want to embrace the power of structure to reduce stress and increase productivity. How do you do this? You plan your days in advance.

Let's start by imagining an ideal week. So, taking all the constraints out of the picture for a moment—whether those constraints are financial, logistical, or emotional—what would an ideal week look like for you?

If you're a caregiver, be sure to include an entire day off from caregiving so that you have time to take care of yourself and enjoy some regular downtime. Even if you aren't caregiving on a daily basis—perhaps you live far away and do more coordinating of care from a distance—you need a day a week during which any emergency calls go to someone else so that you can relax and recharge without that nagging feeling that the phone could ring at any time. When we dive into Chapter 5, you'll learn more about the power of routine, but at this point, envision starting your days with a morning routine that includes some time for taking meds and supplements, reflection, meditating, and/or interacting with nature. Sketch out an evening routine that includes time for stretching and decompressing in some way, with plenty of time for restful sleep. You also need time for activities, exercise, as well as shopping for, preparing, and eating meals. Are there weekly appointments you need to work in, like therapy or physical therapy? Know that as you go along, you will get better at stacking these things so that you're meeting multiple needs in one go. You can also find other people to help with making sure that your care partner gets taken to their appointments, etc.

Of course, there will be things that come up and take precedence over this ideal schedule; for now, keep your mind focused on what would be ideal. It will take time to get to a place where this ideal week resembles a typical week for you. So over the next few weeks, your goal is to start looking for areas of flexibility—places where you could potentially do less—as well as opportunities for you to get support—such as helping with grocery shopping or providing care for your loved one on your personal day.

For inspiration, I've included the schedule of a typical day at Marama at the back of this book. Keep in mind that implementing this schedule requires fourteen full-time staff, but this is the direction you want to head in. If you have the luxury of time and resources and a loved one who has already traveled down the path of cognitive decline, by all means, make this your life. Otherwise, don't expect to get here, but use it as a suggestion of what you might start adding in.

I've also included a sample Progress Tracker on page 318 at the back of this book to help you keep a simple record of the things you're doing on a daily basis to care for your cognition. While you may not be able to check all the boxes right away, it will help you celebrate your wins and stay present to other elements you can weave in as you have more bandwidth.

Now, setting the ideal week aside, go back to your actual plan for next week and see what you can realistically start to shift. Approach this with a big dose of self-compassion. Don't worry if you don't get it perfectly right today or tomorrow or next week, you can always start over. With any change, you're not going to get there overnight. It's a process.

Maybe there are things you're currently committed to that you can't just immediately stop. Or maybe it's something seasonal, like getting your taxes done, or you're about to go on a trip. Honor those things that need to be done, but then once they are complete, move toward that ideal week as much as you can.

Remember, you don't have to do everything all at once. Do what you can and appreciate any small step you're able to make. Also, though, it's possible that this exercise of looking at a real week of your life and imagining an ideal week may show you that you're not ready yet, and that's okay. I encourage you to keep reading the book so that the ideas and suggestions can start to percolate in your mind, but you may need to wait until your sister moves closer, or you've lined up some caregivers, or you've had a chance to reorganize your life a little bit so that you have more time. I want to give you a framework so that you can see how you can fit in brain-healthy activities and pursuits, not paralyze you. The goal of this exercise is to help you start to see what ways exist for you to start doing more of these things that make such common sense but are such uncommon practice. I want to make incorporating tools from the toolkit into your life less theoretical, and more practical, so that eventually many of them will become habit.

By having a plan and a schedule, you stack the cards in your favor and increase your chances. Planning is how you blaze a mental trail that you only have to follow, and then you don't have to weed whack your way through the day.

I know for me, personally, if I don't schedule things, they don't happen. If I don't have a yoga or Pilates class on my calendar, I'll get caught up in emails or running an errand and I'll miss it—simply because I didn't write it down on my schedule. Focus on what you can do and not what doesn't feel workable at this moment. The more you do, the more confidence you will have, but for now, you just want to get started.

A way to reframe the common thought "I don't have time for that" is to instead think "That's not a priority for me." Just listening to and possibly changing the way you talk to yourself might help you to understand how important something is to you and to help you reset your priorities or at least to understand what they are. Creating awareness around how you spend your time can help you shift your behavior.

Reflection questions:
- What are all the things you do in a typical week?
- Of these things, what are a couple of things you could potentially stop doing?
- What is a feasible morning routine?
- What is a doable evening routine?

- What does your ideal week look like—one that leaves plenty of space for the things that move the needle in a positive direction on brain health?
- What are three things you can do to make that ideal week start coming to life?

Prep Your Environment

Your home environment plays a big role in your daily habits. While there are a host of adjustments you can make to your or your care partner's home to make it more supportive of brain health, at this point, there are just a couple of things to do to help your environment be supportive in these early stages of your journey.

1. SAFETY. Look around the environment where your care partner lives and identify potential hazards—do you need to childproof the knobs on the stove? Do you need to hide or make inaccessible the knives? Are there cords, rugs, wastebaskets, or other items that need to be removed so that they don't contribute to falls? A lot of times as you go down the path of dementia, your eyes don't work as well—you can use this to your advantage by putting a dark rug in front of a door you don't want them to go out of, as they may see it as a hole and naturally avoid it. On the flip side, if there's a white toilet against a white wall, it can be hard to see, so consider painting the wall behind the toilet a darker color to provide contrast and make the toilet stand out. Would a baby gate be helpful to prevent your loved one from trying to go up or down stairs unassisted?
2. SUPPORTIVE OF HEALTHY CHOICES. Take an hour or two to make the things you want accessible, and the things you don't want inaccessible. That means getting out your card games, books, coloring, and engaging activities and leaving them either on the coffee table, or in a basket near the coffee table. Either move the TV or find a new, hidden place for the remote. If you've already cleared away clutter in one small area, per the "if you do only one thing" recommendation in Chapter 3, tackle a second spot. Know that you are literally making space for new habits and a new

way of being. And if you haven't yet done any streamlining of physical clutter, pick one well-used area to tackle now. Finally, hide any cookies or any ultra-processed foods and put a few keto-friendly snacks in clear containers right at the front of your fridge and/or cupboards—such as olives, fat bombs, guacamole and cucumber chips, nuts, seeds, and beef jerky.

3. ORGANIZED. Set up a whiteboard and/or calendar with your agenda for the day, or for each day of the week. (A monthlong calendar is likely too much information for your care partner to process.) This is how you and your care partner know what's happening next, and how you know that you've got time for everything.

Talk to Your Loved Ones to Get Their Buy-in (or Not)

I am not going to lie: the tools in the new Alzheimer's toolkit require some financial investment. Which means that money often comes up in family dynamics when following this approach. There are going to be those moments when you're comparing two options, as Susan was with her mom, of going to a biological dentist versus a regular dentist, and wondering, Do I really need to spend this money? In Susan's case, she wanted to make the investment in a biological dentist for her mom, but Susan's sister did not agree, and it was straining their relationship. (This strain was showing up on Susan's wheel of life—she rated her relationships a 6.)

Think of it this way: whatever you can invest in up-front now has the very real potential to prevent things that get very, very expensive. For example, it costs $15,000 per month to live at Marama. While not every memory-care facility costs this much, and some are covered by Medicare or Medicaid, long-term care comes with a high price tag, even if your loved one is living at home. In my own family, it was costing between $15,000 and $20,000 a month to have my grandma stay home, with all the caregivers, and buying the hospital bed and other supplies—and that was back in 2012. When I asked my dad to confirm my memory on this phase of care for his mother, his notable comment was "We sure were lucky. I don't think we could even find that care anymore." The longer you can maintain independence and delay a need for more hands-on care, it will save you so much later—not just in money, but also in quality of life. Viewed this way, it makes so much financial sense to spend $1 or $2 more for organic blueberries, or to get the dental work instead of putting it off, or to buy the air purifier.

Try to view every additional expense as an investment in your and your loved one's current health, future health, and quality of life.

That being said, not everyone in your family will agree every time that this is a worthy investment. Communicating your views can require a delicate balance of blunt honesty and acknowledging the other person's point of view and fear. There is often one sibling who is ready and willing to do everything they possibly can from a logistical and financial standpoint, while another sibling will say, essentially, *There's nothing we can do for Alzheimer's and this money you want to spend is money that I need for my kid's college education.* And often times, extra money to spend on supplements, providers, lab tests, and treatments just isn't there. The good news is that there are plenty of things you can do to protect cognition that are free, and this book outlines them. If money is tight, focus on what you can do at little to no cost, such as meditate, exercise, stay hydrated, and cut down on sugar and carbs. These daily choices can add up to big gains. (And for a deeper look at the cost of this protocol compared to the potential costs of doing nothing, refer to Chapter 11.)

If you reach an impasse with a family member—you really want to get your mom on a ketogenic diet, but your siblings and dad are resistant—I don't recommend fighting with your family and creating more stress, because that's not good for anyone—you, them, or your loved one. This is a radically different way of living. It won't be for everyone. Pick the tools you can easily implement without a lot of drama, but it's not worth blowing up relationships or knocking yourself out to do it perfectly.

If you're wondering what you might say to a loved one to get them on board, here's a sample script you might use to talk about the possibilities you're learning about in this book:

I know we all want the best for Mom. This approach has some good science behind it to show that people with Alzheimer's or cognitive impairment can get better. It is possible for us to create a lifestyle for Mom that supports brain function. There are inspiring stories in this book of people regaining their cognitive function that are incredible, and better yet, they are re-creatable. It can be challenging to incorporate every tool that's covered in the book, but everything that we can manage to implement has the potential to help Mom—and although it can be an investment, the longer we prevent her needing round-the-clock care, the more we will save in the future, and the more we'll be able to rest easy knowing we did our best for her.

Some other approaches you can try include:

- SHARING THE SCIENCE. The news that cognitive decline can be reversed hasn't reached the majority of people. You can share this book with them, invite them to attend one of my free webinars or online summits (see the Resources section for information on how to do that), or share the research papers that my team and Dr. Bredesen's team have published. Once someone has a basic understanding of what's possible, you can have a conversation about applying that science to your care partner's situation.
- HAVING A FAMILY MEETING. Create space for everyone to feel heard, and it can lower the likelihood that someone feels they had no say and no choice about making a plan for your loved one.
- WORKING WITH A PROFESSIONAL. It can be well worth the cost and energy of meeting with a therapist, religious leader, or other mentor to foster a thoughtful conversation about how to approach caring for your loved one.

Reflection questions:
- Who in your family is likely to be the most resistant to making these changes?
- What is their point of view?
- What might you be able to share with them that will address their fears?
- How much family tension are you willing to face?
- What can you do for your loved one without having everyone else's buy-in?
- What can you do to protect your own brain health?

Take the time that you need to work through the tools in this chapter—the stronger your foundation, the easier it will be to implement bigger changes in the chapters to come.

To watch a summary video of this chapter and download the Reversing Alzheimer's workbook go to ReversingAlzheimersBook.com.

Implementing
the Protocol

CHAPTER 5

Get Organized with Daily Routines

As I've mentioned, this protocol takes money, effort, and time. While there are ways to customize the protocol to your budget, and as you make the interventions a habit, they will feel less effortful, the one piece that stays consistent throughout is time. You may very well be feeling like extra hours are the one thing you just don't have—especially if you're already experiencing cognitive decline, or caring for someone who is. This feeling is so pervasive that it has an official name—time poverty, or the feeling that there's never enough time to do all the things you need and want to do. Yet time is perhaps the most essential ingredient in the Reversing Alzheimer's recipe. In this chapter, my goal is to help you shift from a sense of time poverty to time abundance. Because I know that once you create the space to start weaving into your days the pieces of this protocol, you will quickly start enjoying returns on that time investment—in more energy, more rest, and more confidence. And the way you do that is to embrace the power of routine.

Whether you realize it or not, you already have a daily routine. Every morning, I'm guessing you wake up, brush your teeth, get dressed, maybe drink a cup of coffee or tea, and check your email. And every night, you brush your teeth, change into what you wear to sleep, and get into bed. You already have the infrastructure in place—now we'll simply be adding to those founda- tions the tools of the new Alzheimer's toolkit and refining what already exists.

When you create a reliable rhythm of doing the things that protect your brain span, you no longer have to think about them. They become automatic. If you're going to reverse or prevent dementia, you need to use those brain- boosting tools regularly, not every once in a while. Consistency is the gas that fuels the Reversing Alzheimer's bus, because the choices you make every day impact you the most.

Routines are beneficial for everyone in prevention mode, but if you're a caregiver or someone who is already experiencing cognitive decline, they are even more vital.

If you're a caregiver, having a routine is paramount for managing your stress and protecting yourself from the increased risk of dementia that care- giving brings. You *need* time to yourself every day, even if it's only fifteen minutes, because caregiving can be draining on multiple levels. This alone time typically comes before your care partner wakes up, or after they go to sleep, making your morning and evening routines the perfect time to restore and nourish yourself. I know how tempting it is to use these quiet times for getting the dishes done, catching up on emails, or doing some- thing else on your to-do list, but taking the time to get present and reflect on your day pays back so much in return. Maybe you can get in a quick workout or meditation session, and it will help you maintain your mental health during this stressful yet meaningful and rewarding phase of life.

For dementia patients, the predictability of a routine is comforting. It makes it easier to transition from one activity to the next, which makes it less effortful to check off a lot of the boxes of the Reversing Alzheimer's protocol each day. At Marama, we post the daily schedule on a whiteboard, and our residents check it regularly. It gives them a sense of predictability that staves off anxiety and agitation.

The easiest parts of your day to "routine-ize" are typically the hour or so after you wake up, and the hour or so before you go to bed. I think of your morning and bedtime routines as the bookends to your day—they give your days a supportive structure. Your evening routine helps you get more restful sleep, and what you do in the morning sets the tone for the rest of the day.

If you can get your mornings and evenings in a good rhythm, it will make the middle of your day less of a roller coaster and more productive. Once you have more capacity, you can turn your attention to giving the middle section of your day a more consistent rhythm.

Evening Routine

I'm starting with the evening routine because when I ask patients, coaching clients, and webinar attendees I've just started working with what they're currently struggling with the most, their answer is almost always sleep. Any steps you take to invite more restful sleep into your life can pay off in ways you may feel as early as the next day—and can deliver long-term dividends, too. If you read this book and all that happens is you wake up feeling rested on a consistent basis, that alone can be life-changing.

I always advocate making changes that either will make the biggest difference or are the easiest to address. Sleep is one area where impact and ease intersect. While lasting change requires sustained effort, and your particular sleep challenges may require a few different interventions that take a few weeks or even months to really dial in, I do have hope that the things I outline in this section can help you sleep at least a little bit better starting tonight.

Contrary to what you might assume, a nourishing bedtime routine actually starts after dinner. That doesn't mean you have to start getting into your jammies at seven o'clock—but you can use those evening hours to take good care of your brain in an enjoyable way that also helps you be in a more receptive state for sleep when bedtime comes.

After-Dinner Activities

It's such a tempting time to settle down in front of the TV or computer screen, but the evening hours are a rich opportunity for connecting with other people or doing something that engages and/or soothes your brain. Here are some possibilities to consider that will help you make a gentle descent into bedtime:

- Playing games that suit you or your care partner's cognitive abilities, such as Uno, Bananagrams, Scrabble, chess, other board games, card games, or doing a puzzle
- Engaging with music, whether that's simply listening, singing along, or even playing an instrument
- Doing a spiritual practice, such as reading a text, meditating, or praying
- Pursuing something creative, such as drawing, coloring, or doing a Zentangle
- Doing something physical, such as going for a walk, doing some gentle yoga or stretching, or playing a game—like bocce, catch, or badminton—in the yard
- Connecting with others, whether by writing a letter, making a phone call, or sitting and visiting
- Tending to easy household chores, like folding laundry, watering plants, dusting, or tidying up after the day, that give you a sense of accomplishment and completion
- Self-care, such as using a red light or sauna bag (see Chapter 8 for more on these options)

Luckily, single activities can tick boxes in multiple categories.

Activity	Connection	Brain-engagement	Physical activity	Relaxation	Purpose and meaning	Creativity	Nature	Health promotion	Fun
Playing games	X	X			X	X			X
Music	X	X		X		X			X
Spiritual practice		X		X	X				
Creative pursuit	X	X		X	X	X			X
Something physical	X		X	X			X	X	
Social engagement	X	X		X	X			X	
Chores			X	X					
Self-care				X			X	X	X

Many find it a pleasant surprise to discover how nourishing your after-dinner time can be if you don't automatically reach for the remote. This is typically a quieter time of day—work emails lessen, there are no appointments to get to, or errands to run. The average American spends two and a half hours a day watching TV—getting out of the habit can be how you magically find the time to do the things that feel impossible to weave into a busy day.

All that being said, everyone needs a break now and then. If you feel like you're fighting with your care partner all day about everything else, maybe this is the moment you let go and decide to watch something. Working a break into your daily routine is not a bad thing. There are just two things to consider if you're going to watch after dinner: (1) Watch something light-hearted, funny, or uplifting, and avoid anything that could get your stress levels up, like the news, a crime procedural, or any kind of thriller that gets your heart racing; (2) make it a point to get up off the couch before you are already dozing off and leave yourself some time for a pre-bedtime ritual.

Pre-Bedtime Ritual

These are the activities you do at the very end of the day that help you care for yourself and that cue your body that bedtime is imminent. You likely already have a pre-bedtime ritual, such as brushing your teeth and getting into pajamas—now it's time to bring a little more awareness to this sequence of activities and build on them to make them a little more robust and more beneficial.

An important thing to keep in mind when it comes to pre-bedtime rituals is that you want to start earlier than you may think you need to—maybe eight or eight thirty during the winter months when it gets dark earlier, and nine or nine thirty in the summer when sunset is later. That's because when your bedtime is in sync with when it gets dark, your circadian rhythms tend to be more balanced, which means your body will be primed for sleep not too long after sunset. Also, we get more efficient and deep sleep in the earlier hours of the night. If you're wondering how efficient your sleep is, the most important predictor is how rested you feel in the morning. If you regularly wake up feeling tired, you stand to benefit greatly from a consistent pre-bedtime ritual.

I have a colleague who uses the analogy of sleep being like a bus—if you're sitting at the bus stop and the sleepy bus comes by, you want to go ahead and get on it because you're not sure when the second one will come around. If you're yawning at eight, start getting ready for bed. If you stay on the computer, checking email and going down the Facebook rabbit hole, and you may be up for several more hours, missing that opportunity for deep sleep and the brain rinsing it provides.

The foundation of an effective presleep routine is having a consistent bedtime that is as close to the time it gets dark as you can manage. It's true that some people are natural night owls—if this describes you, you can go a long way toward improving the quality of your sleep by sticking to a bedtime that is within a thirty-minute window each night. This will help your body predict when sleep is happening, making it easier to drift off and your sleep cycles more efficient, meaning your sleep will become more restful, even if it's happening several hours after the sun went down.

Possible components of a pre-bedtime ritual:

- Bathing. Taking a warm bath or shower before bed will temporarily raise your core body temperature, which will then cue your body's cooling processes and end up lowering that temp—and a cooler core temp is an important physiological condition for restful sleep.
- Reflecting on the day. Think about or write down things that happened earlier in the day that you're grateful for, make a list of the things you want to do tomorrow so that you don't have to remember them overnight.
- Read. Some people feel their eyelids get heavy after just a page or two, because they've been so regular with reading in bed that their body knows that sleep is coming. Use a clip-on amber booklight so that the light you need to read doesn't contribute to wakefulness.
- Prayer or meditation. If you didn't do a spiritual practice after dinner, doing a quick version now can help foster the relaxation you need to be able to drift off to sleep.
- Dental hygiene. Brushing, flossing, oil pulling, and water picking could all be part of an evening ritual with brushing and flossing being the min-

imum that you do. As the science tells us, good brain health is linked to good oral health.

Sleep Hygiene

Your body sleeps better under certain environmental conditions—I cover the adjustments you can make to your bedroom or sleeping space for optimal rest in Chapter 9. Here, I'm covering the practices you can do as part of your wind-down routine; these work even better when you combine them with the environmental tweaks I suggest in Chapter 9.

- Regulate the light: Because blue light is stimulating, you want to make it part of your ritual to turn off screens at least one hour before bed (longer if possible), close the blinds against any outside light (even moonlight, which is reflected sunlight, can make it more challenging to sleep), dim your bedroom and bathroom lights, and maybe switch to using an amber-colored night-light or reading light, and perhaps even put on a sleep mask to keep all possible rays away from your retinas.
- Set the temperature: Most people sleep best when the room temperature is in the sixties, so adjust your thermostat or fans accordingly.
- Muffle the sounds: Many types of noises can disrupt your sleep. Make turning on a white noise machine or fan, or maybe even putting in earplugs, part of your routine.
- Tend to your oral health: Be sure brushing and flossing are a regular, can't-miss, never-fail part of your nighttime routine. You may also need to insert an oral device, put on your CPAP machine, or put on mouth tape and/or nasal strips to help keep your airways open while you sleep.

A Note on Sleep, Snoring, and Cognition

If you are experiencing any level of cognitive decline, ask your doctor to order a sleep study to determine if your breathing—and thus, oxygen levels—are impaired during the night. You may be able to avoid spending the night in a sleep lab—with new technology you can wear a device while sleeping in your own bed that will track your oxygen levels and send a report to your doctor to interpret. It's simply too important that your brain has access to a steady supply of oxygen throughout the night to put off finding out if you have sleep apnea. There are potential alternatives to the CPAP machine, including:

- Raising the head of your bed a little bit by resting the legs on wooden yoga blocks.
- Investing in a memory foam pillow that will help keep your head in a position where your airways are open (a chiropractor can help you choose the right pillow).
- Working with a specialized dentist to get a mouth guard that repositions your lower jaw at night so that your airways stay open.

If your snoring is mild, mouth tape can retrain you to breathe through your nose instead of your mouth, which is the most effective way to oxygenate your blood. Somnifix mouth tape has a little slit in the middle so that you can inhale and exhale through your mouth if your nasal passages are blocked. Breathe Right Nasal Strips can also help increase airflow through your nose.

Sleep Supplements

There are many options for supplements and herbs you can take to help promote more restful sleep. I'm listing them here in the basic order of their potential for risk, from safest to riskiest. Although many of these are safe to try, I recommend working with your doctor to determine which might be best for you individually.

- AMINO ACID SUPPORT. Amino acids are helpful for producing restful sleep because your body uses certain amino acids to create calming neurotransmitters. You can either take the amino acids directly or take the nutrients that your body uses to manufacture the amino acids. Which route you take is influenced by whether you need help falling asleep, or staying asleep. For falling asleep, melatonin helps us get to sleep, and serotonin often helps us stay asleep.

If you struggle with settling down enough to fall asleep, the amino acids taurine, glycine, and theanine are all great to take the edge off and make it easier to drift off in the evenings. You can take them separately or in a blend (see the Resources section for the blend of amino acids and magnesium that I recommend to my patients.)

If your issue is staying asleep, 5-HTP is the building block your body uses to make the neurotransmitter serotonin, which helps prevent the rumination that can keep you up in the middle of the night. I recommend taking 100 to 200 mg before bed to help you stay asleep all night.

Other options if your issue is waking up in the middle of the night and having a hard time getting back to sleep, thanks to your racing thoughts:

- THEANINE, an amino acid that blocks the excitatory neurotransmitter glutamate and supports the production of relaxing neurotransmitter GABA. Doses range from 100 mg to 400 mg; I typically recommend patients start with 200 mg.
- GABA. You can also take the water-soluble form of GABA itself, which I've had patients describe to me as making them feel as if they've had one alcoholic beverage—nothing is as big a deal as it seemed just a few minutes ago, you're relaxed, and your mood tends to improve. Those relaxed feelings can help with getting to sleep. A typical dosage is 300 mg at bedtime.
- VITAMIN B6 AND ZINC. These two nutrients help convert glutamate into GABA. B6 also helps you make your own melatonin. I typically start with 25 mg of zinc and 50 mg of B6 as pyridoxal 5 phosphate (P5P) before bed. It is possible to get too much B6 and zinc, so work with a provider to measure your nutrient levels and stop B6 if you experience any numbness or tingling in your extremities.
- PHOSPHATIDYLSERINE helps break down cortisol, the stress hormone that can keep you up at night if it's high. I have patients who take anywhere between 100 mg and 2,000 mg each night. You'll have to experiment to see what works best for you.
- MAGNESIUM is a mineral that acts as a relaxant and supports the formation of calming neurotransmitters. The form of magnesium I recommend is magnesium threonate because it crosses the blood-brain barrier. I generally recommend about 1 gm of magnesium threonate after dinner

as powder in water or in capsule form. Magnesium citrate or oxide acts as a smooth muscle relaxant that helps alleviate constipation, making it easier to get the daily bowel movement that's so important for reducing toxicity.

- INOSITOL is sometimes referred to as vitamin B8; however, it is a form of sugar that can reduce blood glucose levels, improve insulin resistance, and support restful sleep. A form of inositol known as scyllo-inositol has been found to coat the surface of beta-amyloid proteins in the brain, preventing them from stacking on top of one another and forming plaques. A trial in Israel showed that high doses of inositol at 6 grams per day significantly improved language and orientation in Alzheimer's patients.

- MELATONIN is the antioxidant and neurotransmitter-like substance that cues sleepiness when it rises; if your issue is with falling asleep, melatonin may help. Although melatonin supplements line the shelves of every drugstore, I don't recommend it as a first intervention because (1) supplements generally contain much more melatonin than is necessary to help you drift off, and this dosage can make many people feel groggy the next morning (when our goal is to wake up feeling refreshed) and (2) when you continuously take melatonin as a supplement, your body will have less of a reason to make it, which means you'll potentially need more and more for it to remain effective. Your body makes about .3 mg of melatonin each night—to follow its lead, I recommend taking a dose of less than a milligram. Look for melatonin supplements for kids to find one with a low dosage—most adult supplements are either 2, 5, or even 10 milligrams. Use the smallest dosage that works for you.

- HERBS including valerian, chamomile, poppy, passionflower, lavender, and lemon balm are relaxants. I love taking herbs as a supplement, but on rare occasions some people have a paradoxical drug reaction and are up all night long. The best way I find to take sleep-promoting herbs is to brew them as a tea and enjoy that as part of your wind-down ritual.

- PROGESTERONE, the reproductive hormone, can induce sleepiness and relaxation; if you and your healthcare provider decide to try hormonal therapy (more on this in Chapter 11), take your oral progesterone at 100 to 200 mg before bed.

- CANNABIS. Now that recreational marijuana is legal in so many states, many of us have the option of taking a cannabis product that has been formulated to produce sleepiness. If taking a product that contains THC, CBD, or a blend of the two helps you get to sleep and you wake up feeling clearheaded, then by all means, take the minimum dose that works for you. Cannabis could also be helpful for treating symptoms of dementia, such as irritability, disinhibition, agitation, and difficulty sleeping—particularly if your care partner's doctor is suggesting an antipsychotic medication, cannabis might be a preferable option. But whether you're simply looking for better sleep or to mitigate dementia symptoms, you have to ask yourself, do you want to be encouraging a foggy mental state, or clearheadedness?

  I put cannabis in a similar category of riskiness as benzodiazepine medications (see below) when it comes to cognition. Although cannabis is not as addictive as benzodiazapines, our goal is to optimize mental function. And just because it's natural doesn't mean it's not without risk. Proceed with caution—start with the smallest dose, avoid smoking and vaping (stick to tinctures and edibles to avoid harming the lungs, with a careful eye on how much is in each dose), and try the sleep hygiene, wind-down rituals, amino acids, and herbs first.

- BENZODIAZEPINE MEDICATIONS, include Valium, Xanax, Halcion, Ativan, and Klonopin. I recommend avoiding these medicines as much as possible because they are highly addictive. Additionally, they don't improve sleep that much. They are amnesic (meaning, they impair memory, yet another reason to avoid them), so you forget you didn't sleep well. Worst of all, for our purposes, they are associated with cognitive decline. Although not technically considered benzodiazepines, similar medications with similar risks include Ambien and Lunesta.

- ANTIHISTAMINES, or diphenhydramine, marketed as Benadryl, Unisom, and others, are very common over-the-counter sleep aids that can put you to sleep and reduce allergy symptoms. There is controversy in the scientific community about the role of antihistamines in dementia risk; however, some studies have shown there is an increase in risk potentially because they reduce the important neurotransmitter acetylcholine.

Morning Routine

Although I started with the evening routine, your morning routine is equally vital to your brain health and quality of life. A great thing about establishing a more robust morning routine is that it can very quickly positively change the cadence and feel of your days. After all, what you do in the morning sets the stage for the rest of your day—what you can accomplish, how inevitable stressors affect you, and how fulfilled you feel at the end of the day. It gives you more energy and bandwidth for everything else that happens. It also helps you tick a lot of Reversing Alzheimer's boxes before the day really gets going and you are more prone to be called away to various duties, obligations, and distractions. Plus, the rest of the day you—and your care partner—will be more relaxed, which means it will be easier to collaborate and extend grace to each other. And that means it will be easier to eat the foods, get the exercise, and do the activities that you aspire to do in order to take good care of your brain health.

At Marama, our morning routine is to get everyone out of bed and dressed, take empty-stomach medications and supplements, then sit down at the breakfast table by eight a.m. After breakfast there is a walk, followed by meditation.

My personal routine consists of brushing my teeth and then making and enjoying a matcha tea—outside, if the weather is nice, or looking out a window, if it's cold, so I get that connection to nature. Next, I meditate every single day, and I don't do anything else until it's done. I don't even get dressed until I've meditated. On those days when it's just not possible to meditate, like if I'm catching an early-morning flight, I feel a little off all day. I don't feel as present or as steady in the face of stressors. I'm grateful for those days, because they only add to my commitment to meditate every other day that I possibly can.

Just as with the evening practice there are a lot of boxes to check, yet one morning activity can fulfill multiple categories. I understand that if you're working, the morning routine can feel more condensed than the evening routine. Just remember that even fifteen minutes of doing something to support your brain health carries enormous benefit that can last all day.

Activity	Health support	Brain- engagement	Physical activity	Relaxation	Meaning	Nature
Self-care (brushing teeth, taking supplements, oil pulling)	X					
Meditation		X		X		
Spiritual practice (prayer)				X	X	
Going outside or looking out the window			X (if you go outside)	X	X	X
Exercise	X		X	X (if something like yoga)		X (if done outside)
Breakfast	X					

Upgrade Your Morning Beverage

One way to make your morning routine more supportive that doesn't require any additional time is to stop adding sugar to your coffee or tea and add some healthy fat to it, such as coconut oil, butter, ghee, coconut milk, unsweetened almond milk, or hemp milk. These will all provide you with some calories and a feeling of fullness without kicking you out of ketosis. If you are concerned about losing too much weight as you cut out carbs, consider adding half and half or heavy cream to your morning beverage. There are also great keto powders and immune-boosting powders you can add to make it even more nourishing (see the Resources section for my specific recommendations). Beyond what's in your cup, how you drink it can make a positive impact on your morning routine, too. Make it a point to sit down and resist the urge to scroll through your phone or to get dressed while drinking, and make that morning cup a mini exercise in mindfulness. Just allow yourself to pay attention and enjoy every sip. Another way to pump up the benefits is to make that morning beverage an opportunity to connect with a loved one and enjoy your cups together.

As I mentioned, you already have a morning routine—you probably get up, use the bathroom, brush your teeth, and get dressed every day already.

I'm suggesting that you simply add in either another link to this already established chain (for example, adding in meditation), or swapping out one link for another (such as making your morning coffee more nutrient-dense and a chance to practice a few minutes of mindfulness). Once you get used to that new link, you can continue to extend your chain by adding in one more link. For example, one of my patients goes on a short walk through her neighborhood every morning. At our appointment, she mentioned she'd been feeling her mood dipping, so we discussed what activities really give her a boost. She mentioned that she feels energized and much more positive when she swims in cold water. Since she lives near the ocean, she decided to commit to jumping in the water every day for one hundred days as part of her morning routine. I know this particular link is not appropriate for everyone, but it's a good example of how to think through the things that boost your mood and help you get the most out of your day, and then tying that thing to something you're already doing to help make it a habit.

Step Up Your Oral Care

As we've covered, your oral health is closely linked to your brain health, and the morning is the perfect time to take your oral care to the next level with the traditional Indian practice known as oil pulling, especially if you experience any bleeding or tenderness when you brush and floss, or if you've started to develop sensitivity because your gums have receded and exposed the more sensitive roots of your teeth. I've had patients who have reversed their gum recession after adopting an oil pulling routine; others have reported that it has helped with their teeth grinding and jaw pain.

Although one other possibility why your gums bleed when you floss or brush is as a result of taking fish oil supplements, which can have a blood-thinning effect. Still, if you have bleeding or inflamed gums for more than a day or two, go see a dentist; gingivitis is a recipe for brain inflammation.

To practice oil pulling, take a tablespoon of organic coconut oil into your mouth, swish it around your teeth and gums for five to twenty minutes (work up to more time), then spit it out. Coconut oil is mildly antimicrobial, and moving it around your teeth, tongue, and gums can extract any bacteria that may be lurking and reduce your oral infectious burden. I had a patient who was scheduled for surgery to correct her severe gum recession. She had tried everything the dentist had suggested, including using a WaterPik, switching her toothpaste and toothbrush, cutting out sugar, and brushing and flossing more frequently, but none of it had worked. She started oil pulling twice a day, and after about a month she no longer needed surgery.

(For the record, I do believe that a WaterPik is a great way to gently flush out the areas between your teeth and gums—I recommend oil pulling in the mornings and using a WaterPik at night. This is, of course, in addition to flossing and brushing.)

Organizing Your Days

Once you have your mornings and evenings in a nice, cognition-supportive routine, you can start playing with restructuring the middle of your day. Of course, if you're working full-time, your job and potential commute will likely make up the bulk of these hours, but keep an open mind and see if there is a day or two a week when you can weave in some movement, creativity, community, relaxation, or outside time—whether on your lunch break, an early evening, or perhaps even some time off that you negotiate.

Believe me, I understand that often the twenty-four hours we get each day doesn't feel like enough time to get everything done *and* get decent sleep. I find it helpful to remind myself that there are 168 hours in a week—even with eight hours a night for sleep and eight hours a day for work, that leaves fifty-six hours a week for everything else. That's well more than your standard full-time workweek. In 2023, the average American was spending seven hours a day staring at a screen—two and a quarter of those hours are spent on social media—every day. The time is there if you look for it.

As you're thinking through how to structure your days and weeks, here's a list of the things you want to find time for if you can. Remember that one activity can fit a lot of categories. Find one, two, or three things you can begin doing that will meet multiple needs. Each thing that you incorporate has the potential to help you feel better, more energized, and more clear-headed, so that adding the next new thing will be easier.

Daily Events

Things to consider weaving into your daily schedule include:

- Interaction with nature
- Cognitive engagement
- Creativity
- Physical activity
- Self-care, such as using a red light, prayer, meditation, or sauna
- Connection with others
- Relaxation

When you can weave these categories into your daily routines, your whole life—including your brain—gets more deeply nourished. You'll learn more about each of these in the chapters to come.

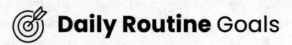 **Daily Routine** Goals

 Interaction with nature

 Cognitive engagement

 Creativity

 Physical activity

 Self-care

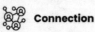 **Connection**

 Relaxation

WEEKLY EVENTS. Some things don't have to happen every day, but you still want them to be a regular part of your life—things like spending time on a project that adds meaning to your life or sharing a meal with extended family, as well as more mundane things like laundry, food prep for the week ahead, and appointments with various providers, from hair stylists to doctors. Having a regular slot in your weeks for these types of activities both helps you make sure you tend to them and gives you a space for them in your weekly schedule so that they're less disruptive to your daily routines.

For example, I counsel my patients to devote an hour or two to meal planning and prep on Sundays to make eating a ketogenic diet easier to maintain during the week. At Marama, we block out Wednesday and Friday afternoons for appointments.

ONE DAY OFF FROM CAREGIVING. I'll talk more about this in Chapter 10, but every caregiver needs one full day off from taking care of anyone else every week. This is a day to take care of you—to exercise, eat good food, have conversations with people who don't have cognitive decline, and enjoy your hobbies and activities. It is how you prevent overwhelm, lessen caregiver burden, mitigate your own risk of developing dementia down the road, and be equipped to provide the best care for your loved one.

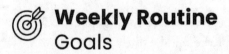

Weekly Routine
Goals

 Prepping and scheduling

 Meaning and purpose

 Appointments

 At least one day off

Connection over Correction

As big of a believer as I am in the power of creating a daily routine and scheduling the important pieces of your day to make implementing your Reversing Alzheimer's much more doable, I also know this: your days are often not going to go the way you planned.

Especially if you are a caregiver of someone with dementia, it can feel a little like herding cats to move from one activity within your routine to the next. That might be because you meet resistance, or your care partner is forgetful of what they should be doing to prepare, or perhaps you are all ready to go but then you get a surprise visit from incontinence. Especially when you are seeking to establish routines for the first time, or to modify an existing routine, acceptance is a hugely important tool to keep at the ready. You are going to have a vision of how the day will go, and it will not go that way, and it's okay. Being gentle and compassionate—with both yourself and your care partner—helps to cut through frustration. In fact, practicing self-compassion has been found to reduce the stress and burden of caregiving, as well as reduce the incidence of using dysfunctional strategies (things like losing your patience and yelling, which then makes the whole situation worse).

Bottom line: Remember that you are doing your best and so are they. If your morning routine or plan for the middle of the day goes awry, there's always the evening routine when you can try again.

To put compassion into practice, it helps to think about the phrases you'll say when things don't go according to plan—again, you can say these things to your care partner as well as to yourself. Here are some examples:

- I know you're doing the best you can.
- We can just try again later.
- It can be hard to try something new.
- I'm here to help.
- I'm sorry I _____ (pushed you too hard, treated you like a child, got frustrated, etc.).

Let's look at a particular piece of the daily routine—getting dressed. This simple task that you do most days without thinking about it can be very challenging for someone with dementia. Here are a few pointers to make this go more smoothly:

- Lay their clothes out in the order in which they need to put them on.
- Put their clothes on a surface where they are easy to see. For example, a pair of khaki pants lying on an off-white bedspread may not be clearly obvious, but dark blue pants will be.
- Put their socks and shoes in a place where there's somewhere comfortable to sit down.

My point in sharing this specific example is to demonstrate that when you're trying to encourage your care partner to do the next thing in the daily routine, a little forethought can make a big difference in how smoothly those transitions go.

Redirection is another helpful tactic—use your care partner's short-term memory loss to your advantage by bringing up the next thing in the schedule and presenting it as fun and exciting. End your sentence with the word you want them to remember. You may even notice they repeat that word in response. For example:

Let's go to the **car.**

It's time for **breakfast.**

Would you like to go to the living room or **outside?** (Providing options allows your loved one to feel more in control and free to choose. Listing your preferred outcome last will increase the likelihood, although not guarantee, they will choose what you prefer.)

Finally, you always want to remember what motivates your care partner and what their distinctive traits are—or what Teepa Snow describes in her wonderful book *Dementia Caregiver Guide* as "gems." Are they social, intellectual, strong, helpful? Show off their particular gem by appealing to what motivates them. I have one patient who was once an academic researcher and is now struggling with memory loss—she gets excited to try a new tool once she understands it intellectually. Another patient is a true helper. She can struggle to implement new ideas in her own life, but if someone else needs help with accountability, she will happily do it. So she posted in my private Facebook group asking if anyone there was looking for a coach. She said, "I know what to do, but I won't do it unless I'm helping someone else do it." So now someone whose gem is being social gets the opportunity to get their motivation stimulated while this patient gets to capitalize on her helping gem.

Another strategy for a helpful person is to explain that you need their help with whatever is next on your schedule. We had one gentleman living at Marama who would start to drift away from an activity, and we'd say, "Can you help us?" And he'd turn right around.

It's not about tricking or manipulating them in any way—it's about enrolling them in doing the things that will help their brain by tapping into their intrinsic motivations, as well as about reducing your stress.

To watch a summary video of this chapter and download the Reversing Alzheimer's workbook go to ReversingAlzheimersBook.com.

Reflection questions:
- What can you add to your morning routine that will benefit your brain and help the rest of your day go more smoothly?
- What can you add to your evening routine that will help you get the restful sleep your brain and body needs?
- What are the barriers to being able to take fifteen minutes in the morning for yourself?
- What are some ideas for working around those barriers?
- What are some compassionate statements you can use when things don't go according to plan?
- Is there a sleep-supportive supplement you want to try, either for yourself or your care partner?

CHAPTER 6

Move the Body to Strengthen the Mind

Betty had a MoCA score of 20 when she first came to see me. Her husband, Richard, wanted to help Betty get better, obviously—he had, after all, come to the appointment with her. But he was also a little dubious. He questioned whether she really needed to take all the supplements I recommended, and he didn't want to adopt a ketogenic diet himself, making it harder for Betty to do so on her own.

Betty wasn't making much progress until her daughter, son-in-law, and grandkids moved in with her and Richard for a few months. Betty's granddaughter was a nursing student with a big interest in health, and she would take Betty on brisk walks while quizzing her on family history and discussing the things the granddaughter was learning in school—a practice known as dual-task training, which you'll learn more about in this chapter. During the three months that Betty's granddaughter lived with them, her MoCA score got up to a 24—this was just with dual-task training and a few supplements, as Betty never did get into ketosis. Then the family moved into their own home. Without the support, motivation, and companionship of her granddaughter, Betty's MoCA score fell to 16 at our next three-month visit.

I share Betty's story to demonstrate the truly amazing brain-boosting power of movement. Honestly, exercise is such a powerful health intervention that if we could bottle it, we could dramatically reduce the incidence of chronic disease. It has so much more to offer us than burning calories—which is about the only benefit that many of us think about.

I also share Betty's story to illustrate how important it is to have support of your loved ones, especially if you are seeking to reverse cognitive decline, when the stakes are considerably higher than they are for those aiming at prevention.

Part of me wants to share only happy stories, but it's human nature to take some convincing to start doing things differently. I understand that this approach to preventing and reversing cognitive decline and dementia is at the leading edge, and not everyone understands or appreciates how powerful it can be. I hope that reading stories such as Betty's will help people who are more skeptical, like Richard, to be more supportive and engaged.

As it relates to exercise, Betty's story is also a great example of how really devoting yourself to one intervention can jump-start your reversal. And if you're going to choose one intervention to go all-in on, exercise is a great one. No matter what your current level of fitness is, by doing what you can and consistently expanding your capabilities, you will be taking great care of your brain.

Walking Is a Great Start—But It's Not Enough

Betty demonstrates how potent walking can be for cognitive health. Science backs this up: A 2022 article published in *JAMA* found that walking ten thousand steps a day reduces your risk of dementia by 50 percent.

While this dramatic reduction in risk is great news, you may be reading this book because you want to do more than reduce risk; you want reversal. If that's the case, getting your steps is a great place to start, but it's not enough on its own. If you're already noticing changes in cognition and you want to regain lost ground, you need to do more than just walk. Honestly, the same is true even if prevention is your goal. There's just too much potential upside to continually growing stronger and fitter to stick with just walking.

The overarching reason exercise is so beneficial to whole-body health, and brain health in particular, is that it is a beneficial form of stress known as *hormesis*. While too much stress breaks the body down, just enough stress challenges the body to grow back stronger, increasing your baseline capacity and overall resilience. That means that if you stick with one activity without ever varying the intensity, your body—and your brain—will acclimate and will stop adapting and growing stronger. The key to using exercise as a means to strengthen your brain is to continually do it differently than you have been doing it.

If you or your care partner never walked, starting with just walking to and from the mailbox will be an improvement. But you'll need to consistently build from there. While you don't want to overdo it, as too much exercise and not enough rest and recovery is too stressful to the body, the truth is that our bodies—including our brains—benefit from moving much more than the typical person does, and moving in ways that continue to challenge us.

In this chapter I'll share the truly mindboggling benefits of exercise, walk you through the types of exercise that we know to have the biggest positive impact on brain span, help you troubleshoot the most common barriers to exercise, and learn ways to talk to your care partner about exercise so that you can get them moving, too. By the end of this chapter, you'll have an incredibly potent tool for increasing brain span that just so happens to come with a laundry list of additional benefits. Let's look at those now.

The Amazing Array of Exercise Benefits

Because I know you're here to learn about brain health, let's look at how exercise is medicine for the brain first. Most obviously, exercise increases blood flow throughout the body, including to the brain. That means getting your body moving will deliver more oxygen and nutrients to your brain while also flushing away more waste products. Exercise also strengthens the heart and cardiovascular system, which helps improve blood flow even when you're not working out; it also reduces the risk of arterial plaques that might disrupt blood flow to the brain and contribute to dementia. Regular aerobic exercise at midlife has also been shown to increase the volume of the hippocampus, the brain region that plays a big role in learning and memory and that is often damaged in people with mild cognitive impairment and dementia. It's also been found to improve spatial memory and cognitive scores compared to people who did not exercise.

Where exercise's role in brain health gets truly exciting is how exercise changes the signals that your body sends to your brain. Exercise triggers the manufacture and release of several different kinds of signaling molecules—including neurotransmitters, signaling molecules known as *exerkines*, and other neurochemicals known as *neurotrophic factors*—that cue the brain to increase its function and capacities.

On the neurotransmitter front, exercise increases levels of serotonin and norepinephrine, which can help increase the brain's information-processing abilities.

Exerkines contribute to the formation of new blood vessels (a process known as *angiogenesis*). Vitally, they also beneficially influence the way your genes are expressed, helping to keep good genes turned on and bad genes turned off.

Neurotrophic factors are a family of proteins and peptides that foster the growth and health of neurons. The big cheese of the neurotrophics is brain-derived neurotrophic factor, or BDNF, which can trigger the development of new neurons as well as the formation of new connections between neurons. As such, it plays an important role in memory, learning, and mood. In fact, when BDNF levels are higher, the hippocampus is found to be larger, and when BDNF production has declined—as happens naturally with age—it is associated with the memory problems that accompany neurological disorders.

Another neurotrophic factor released in response to exercise is insulin-like growth factor-1 (IGF-1), which helps neurons differentiate themselves from one another, promotes neuroplasticity, contributes to the formation of new neurons and new blood vessels in the brain, and promotes spatial learning. Any one of these categories of molecules would be considered brain wonder drugs if they were manufactured in a lab and sold in pill form. Amazingly, exercise releases them naturally.

More specifically to dementia, research demonstrates exercise's ability to help improve cognitive function in people with mild cognitive impairment as well as full-blown dementia. These effects are described as "small to medium," but consider that exercise is free, very low risk, and something you can do at home with no prescription. It has also been found to have a moderate positive effect on the ability to perform standard activities of daily living—getting dressed, going to the bathroom. In other words, it allows us to maintain independence and dignity. That agency is priceless.

Of course, the benefits of exercise extend far beyond the brain.

- A POSITIVE HORMONAL FEEDBACK LOOP. When you challenge your muscles, they will grow back bigger. Because muscles are a hormonal organ, bigger muscles produce more hormones, particularly testosterone. Having more testosterone on hand helps you build more muscle, which then helps you maintain muscle mass and strength as you age. That means you become less prone to falling and better able to maintain your autonomy because you can do the daily tasks of living on your own.
- STRONGER BONES. When you challenge your muscles, you also challenge your bones to grow back stronger, as muscles pull on bones and bones respond to the forces placed upon them. Stronger bones mean that even if you do fall, you're less likely to experience a fracture, which can be debilitating as you get older. In fact, dementia and falls are responsible for more deaths in a senior population than cancer. The good news is that exercise reduces the risk of both of these things in a radical way.
- DECREASED STRESS AND IMPROVED MOOD. Perhaps you've had the experience of feeling a lot better about things after a good workout. That's due in large part to one category of neurotransmitters that exercise produces—*endorphins*. These feel-good hormones give your brain and mood a boost. Many physical activities are also meditation in motion—your thoughts quiet down as you either need to concentrate on where your body is in space (such as when you're playing tennis, doing yoga or Pilates, or taking a dance class) or you get into a rhythm (such as when you're walking, running, or biking). This mindful aspect of exercise helps take your mind off your problems and promotes focus and clarity.
- REDUCED PAIN. Those same endorphins are nature's pain relievers. Moving your joints through their ranges of motion increases the flow of synovial fluid, which lubricates the joints and reduces inflammation. And building stronger muscles takes pressure off your joints. I know the tendency is to cut out movement when you're in pain, but movement is what helps lessen pain. Of course, you likely have to modify your workouts until you're feel-

ing 100 percent again—I talk about how to find safe, good-feeling ways to exercise if you're in pain later in this chapter.

- BETTER SLEEP AND INCREASED ENERGY. Because movement challenges your body, it also tires you out. This helps you sleep more soundly, which then helps you feel more rested and energized. More technically, one of the hormetic effects of exercise is that it stresses your cells, cueing them to produce more mitochondria in your muscle cells. Mitochondria are the organelles within your cells that produce the majority of energy your body needs to function. More mitochondria equal more energy.

- IMPROVED EPIGENETICS. The belief that our genes are our destiny isn't true—it's our daily habits that shape our future, and the way they do that is through epigenetics. "Epi-" means "above," and epigenetics refers to the material that sits on top of our genetic code and dictates which genes are turned on and which are turned off. As we age, our epigenetics tend to change so that our bad genes (such as pro-inflammatory genes) get turned on, while our good genes (such as those that suppress tumors) are turned off. The great news is that regular exercise has been shown to contribute to positive epigenetic changes that reverse these typical age-related trends. It also promotes healthy expression of the gene that codes for BDNF. Basically, exercise helps you have the epigenetics—and the brain—of a younger, healthier person.

  Think of epigenetics this way: DNA is the equivalent of a blueprint of a house (and your body is the house). Your epigenetics determine how that home is actually built. When you choose to move your body more (without overdoing it, as intense exercise can negatively influence genetic expression) you help ensure that your epigenetics are working to keep your home sound.

In addition, exercise can teach you new things, whether you're learning a discipline like tai chi or trying to keep up with the routine in Zumba class. It can also help you spend more time outdoors—and research has found that exercising outside helps with focus and clarity more than doing the same activity inside. It can also be a great way to socialize, whether you're walking with a friend or family member, or developing a community at your gym or regular yoga class. When you take an outdoor tai chi class with a friend, you're addressing all three components (movement, connection, and time in nature) at once! Exercise truly can be a wonderful, enriching part of your life.

The one catch to exercise, as Betty's story demonstrates so clearly, is that it needs to be something you do regularly, or else the beneficial changes it creates will disappear.

Yes, exercise takes effort, time, and a little planning. But it is a free tool that you can use at home or when traveling most days of the week that has massive benefits. Those benefits only increase when you switch up the types of exercise you do to keep yourself continually at the edge of your capabilities.

Categories of Exercise—Some Familiar, Some Cutting Edge

There are four types of exercise that you want to prioritize. Four may sound like a lot, but they are not mutually exclusive. You can combine at least two types of exercise in one session—you can turn strength training into cardio by performing your strength moves in high intensity intervals, or you can make your cardio dual task by doing something that requires your mental focus while you move. There are absolutely ways to meet multiple fitness aims with one workout. But before you go mixing and matching, let's look at each of the categories on their own.

Aerobic Exercise

Aerobic exercise is what we think of as "cardio"—it gets your heart and blood pumping and includes forms of exercise such as walking, jogging, biking, dancing, and swimming. Aerobic exercise strengthens your heart, and what's good for your heart is also good for your brain, because your heart sends the brain the blood, oxygen, and nutrients that your brain relies on to function.

Your first goal with adding more exercise to your life is to get 150 to 200 minutes of aerobic exercise each week so that you get your heart rate into the vigorous zone of 70 to 85 percent of maximum heart rate. (You can calculate your target zone by using this formula: [220 − age] x .70 and [220 − age] x .85.) If you are just getting started, you may want to start in the moderate range, which is 50 to 70 percent of your maximum heart rate. Listening to your body and adjusting your intensity level based on your perceived exertion is one of the best ways to know if you are pushing yourself hard enough.

The recommended 150 to 200 minutes comes from nearly every health organization that sets guidelines based on decades of research from the World Health Organization, the American Heart Association, and the UK's National Health Service to the Centers for Disease Control. They all conclude regular physical activity reduced risk of heart disease, improved cardiovascular fitness, lowered blood pressure, supported healthy weight, prevented diabetes, and provided measurable mental health benefits. Each new study confirms these findings that at least 150 minutes of moderate to vigorous aerobic exercise per week reduces the risk of many chronic diseases associated with aging. That's essentially four forty- to fifty-minute sessions per week of anything that gets your heart rate into the target zone, or a twenty- to thirty-minute session six or seven days a week.

This target zone typically requires what's considered a moderate to vigorous workout, although what's vigorous to you depends on your basic level of fitness. (A slow jog might be an easy workout for someone who exercises regularly, and a major exertion for someone who's just getting back into exercise.)

Once you've determined your target heart rate, I recommend using a heart rate monitor—a wireless sensor contained in a thin strap that you wear around your chest, and that sends your heart rate to a display device that you wear on your wrist—to help you determine when you have reached it. Although some fitness trackers, apps, and special handles on some cardio machines do also claim to measure heart rate, heart rate monitors are the most accurate devices. You could also borrow a heart rate monitor and use it for a week or two to learn what your personal target heart rate feels like in your body and then use that knowledge as a barometer of whether you are exercising vigorously enough to reach it.

In general, when you are exercising vigorously enough to reach your target heart rate, you will:

- Notice your breathing—it will be deep and rapid
- Not be able to say more than a few words at a time
- Break out into a sweat within a few minutes

That means that slowly walking your dog, who stops every few minutes to sniff, really doesn't cut it. You'll need to walk quickly—as if you were running late to an appointment—and include hills whenever possible. Unless, of course, you or your care partner have been primarily sedentary. Then even a slow walk may feel relatively vigorous. If you're just getting back into movement, take it slow and use your heart rate as a guide, but know that your goal is to continually increase your tolerance for more vigorous exercise.

Examples of vigorous-intensity cardio exercise:

Brisk walking (as if you were late to an appointment)

Jogging or running

Singles tennis

Biking (fast and/or on hills)

Hiking

Jumping rope

Shoveling

Elliptical, stair climbing, or rowing machines

Zumba or other dance classes, like step aerobics, kickboxing, or hip-hop, that involve continuous movement to music

Hot yoga

Swimming

Rowing

Aerobics classes

Basketball

Soccer

If you're already getting regular cardio exercise—including walking—that is fantastic. Keep going, and make sure that it is vigorous enough to get your heart rate into that target zone, and frequent enough to add up to 150 to 200 minutes per week. Unless you are a devoted runner, dancer, or brisk walker, you probably need to up either the intensity or duration of your cardio workouts, or perhaps both. If you or your care partner hasn't been doing much in the way of cardio activity, this is the category of exercise to focus on first. It's like an umbrella insurance policy for your whole-body health, including your brain health. Focus first on making it part of your daily—or almost-daily—routine and then gradually seek to increase the intensity and duration.

BENEFITS: Increased blood flow to the brain, improved cardiovascular health, better mood, reduced pain

FREQUENCY: Daily (or as close to daily as possible) twenty- to thirty-minute sessions, or three or four fifty-minute sessions per week.

For everyone, while cardio is a great place to start, it's not the finish line. To keep your brain sharp and your body on its toes, you've got to mix up the types of exercise activities that you do. The next category to add into your rotation is strength training.

REBOUNDING: LOW-INTENSITY CARDIO WITH BIG BENEFITS

A rebounder is a mini trampoline, with a handle you can hold for more stability. Bouncing on a rebounder—even while sitting if balance is a challenge—is a great low-impact cardio workout that also promotes detoxification because the g-force created by jumping stimulates the flow of lymph, the fluid that travels throughout your body, delivering nutrients and carrying away waste products and toxins. Because of its detoxifying abilities, bouncing on a rebounder counts toward your daily cardio even though it's not high intensity. If you're easily winded by cardio exercise, rebounding is a great place to start. One note of caution: If you're struggling with incontinence, it can be helpful to empty your bladder first and wear some form of leak protection.

Strength Training

Strength training—also known as resistance training—is just what it sounds like, using weights or other forms or resistance to build muscle tissue. Strength training doesn't get the attention it deserves, especially for people at midlife and beyond, because it delivers so many key benefits that make aging a much more enjoyable experience.

Building muscle—particularly in the big muscle groups of the legs, hips, and torso—is directly related to brain health, because these muscles generate brain-derived neurotrophic factor (BDNF) and then send it to the brain. Remember, BDNF is like fertilizer for the brain, cueing it to create new neuronal connections and promoting neuroplasticity.

From a practical standpoint, strong muscles prevent falls, improve balance, and make it easier to maintain independence. They also prevent frailty, which can happen naturally as we age because we tend to lose muscle mass as we get older. Strength training also prevents losing too much weight when following a ketogenic diet, while also helping to change body composition, moving away from excess adipose and toward more muscle. The more you can maintain muscle mass in your biggest muscle groups, the better your overall metabolism, insulin regulation, and brain signaling will be. And the more muscle you build, the more these benefits increase. I personally find lifting weights to be a great tonic to my nervous system and outlet for relieving stress. For many of my patients, building muscle is an antidote to the weight loss they experience with the keto diet. The goal is to replace adipose or fatty weight with muscle weight.

You want to aim for at least two strength-training sessions per week. No matter your current relationship to strength training—whether you've never done it, or you sporadically hop on the resistance machines at the gym, or if you've got a regular routine that builds strength (such as yoga or barre classes)—consider working with a trainer or a physical therapist. These fitness professionals can help you develop a routine that will continually challenge your muscles in new ways, and help make sure that you use proper form and reduce the risk of injury.

Strength training doesn't have to involve your standard barbells and bench pressing your body weight—although you may be surprised how gratifying it can be to see the amount of weight you can lift increase. You can use resistance bands, light dumbbells, or even the weight of your own body in exercises like squats, lunges, and planks. Even climbing stairs or hills counts as strength training and cardio in one activity because they get your heart rate up as they also keep the muscles of the legs and hips strong. Think about it: the Blue Zones—areas that have the highest percentage of people living to age one hundred or older, including Costa Rica and Sardinia—are typically hilly. The people who live there are going up and down stairs and hills all day long as part of their everyday life. You just have to balance the benefit of climbing hills and stairs with a potential increased risk of falling.

Hormone therapy offers additional support for building muscle, particularly testosterone for both men and women—although, as I covered earlier in this chapter, your muscles also produce testosterone, so the more you lift weights, the easier it gets to build and maintain muscle. Talk to your provider about taking DHEA, which is a testosterone precursor and doesn't require a prescription, as your body will convert it to testosterone. For any type of hormone therapy, you want to work with a healthcare provider to make sure that makes sense for you.

DO-ANYWHERE STRENGTH-TRAINING MOVE

If you do only one strength training exercise, do a wall sit. It's a quick, free way to keep your legs and core strong. To do it, stand with your back against a wall and a sturdy footstool nearby to place underneath you in case you need to plop down on to it. Step your feet about a foot away from the wall, bend your knees, and slide your back down the wall until your thighs are parallel to the floor and there is a 90-degree angle between your spine and your thighs and between your thighs and your shins. (It's farther down than your muscles probably want to go, at least at first). Press your back into the wall and your feet into the floor and breathe deeply for as long as you can—aim for thirty seconds at first, if strength training is new to you, and work your way up to a minute, or even two, from there. For more of a challenge, hold your arms straight out in front of you at shoulder height, or raise them up alongside your ears.

Examples of strength-training exercises:

Yoga

Pilates

Circuit training gyms (such as Orange Theory and Curves)

Resistance band workouts

TRX workouts

Bodyweight workouts (squats, push-ups, lunges)

BENEFITS: Promotes brain signaling, neuroplasticity, improves glucose and insulin levels, prevents falls and promotes independence, boosts metabolism, strengthens bones, helps change body composition to more muscle, less fat.

FREQUENCY: Two strength-training sessions a week; if you get your heart rate up to your target zone while you do it (such as in a high intensity interval training session or class), it counts toward your 150 to 200 minutes of cardio.

Dual-Task Training

This next-level form of exercise combines physical movement with a cognitive challenge. The simplest form of this is walking and talking. What is a cognitive challenge will vary from person to person, but if you're in prevention mode, listening to a foreign language lesson or a nonfiction book while you walk outside or ride the stationary bike, and then pausing the recording to recap what you've just learned every few minutes is a good option. For some people, going to a Pilates or yoga class or other class where you really have to pay attention to the teacher's cues constitutes dual-task training—but not if it's something you've been doing for long enough that you can zone out. And if you have already started experiencing measurable cognitive decline, dual-task training may look like going on a walk while pointing out the names of the plants that you pass along the way, or having someone quiz you on the names of family members, or recalling family stories or important dates. Wherever you are, you want to be working right on your edge—you can almost feel the wheels of your brain turning in order to stay focused.

Dual-task training is a relatively new idea, but there is really compelling data that it helps people who have had a stroke or a traumatic brain injury recover their faculties. It has also been shown to help healthy older adults improve their gait, balance, and walking speed and reduce the risk of falls. And for people with mild cognitive impairment or full-blown dementia, randomized controlled studies have found that dual-task training results in small to moderate improvements in cognitive function. The use of dual-tasking to improve cognition in older adults has been pioneered at the Pacific Neuroscience Institute's Brain Health Center by Dr. David Merrill, Ryan Glatt, Dr. Corwin Patis, and others on their team. We have the benefit of learning directly from them and incorporating their insights at Marama.

There is significantly more cognitive benefit to combining physical and cognitive exercises than doing either exercise or cognitive games on their own. While it does take more effort than simply going for a walk, true to its name, dual-task training covers two bases at once. In fact, when it comes to things that benefit your brain, dual-task training is the most efficient thing you can do—remember Betty's story, from the start of this chapter? Those walks during which her granddaughter would quiz her on nutrition and family history were dual-task training.

This is such a great workout for your brain and body that you may find you feel physically more tired and sleep more soundly that night.

When you are doing dual-task training, you can keep your physical exertion level more moderate—you should still be able to speak in full sentences. That said, you do want to feel challenged—not pushing it so hard that you want to give up, but also not taking it so easy that you don't have to try.

As your cognitive function improves and you get in better shape, you'll have to find ways to add challenges so that you stay at your edge. If you have a setback such as an illness, injury, or other stressful event, you can dial back the intensity. Variety and variability will help keep your brain on its toes.

Dual-task training examples:

PREVENTION: Listening to an engaging podcast, audiobook, or foreign language lesson on a brisk walk or jog and periodically pausing the audio to go over what you've just learned; standing on a Bosu or wobbleboard while doing simple math or reciting a poem you're trying to memorize; trying a new fitness class where you really have to pay attention to the cues (yoga, Pilates, Zumba)

MILD COGNITIVE DECLINE: Taking a walk with someone who can quiz you on the presidents or state capitals or plant names

SEVERE COGNITIVE DECLINE: Taking a walk with someone who can quiz you on family member names, or engage you in retelling favorite stories

BENEFITS: Improves walking speed, gait, and balance; reduces risk of falls in older adults; and can boost performance on cognitive tasks such as memory and attention—all of which improves quality of life

FREQUENCY: Two to five times per week. As long as you are getting your heart rate into the moderate range, this can count as cardio, too

Contrast Oxygen Therapy

This relatively unique form of training alternates the amount of oxygen in the air you breathe as you exercise—an approach that encourages the tiniest blood vessels (known as your microvasculature) throughout your body, including your brain, to open up, resulting in greatly enhanced blood flow. It's similar to going to altitude to train and build your aerobic capacity, and it is incredibly valuable for cognitive function.

This type of exercise does require specialized gear. At Marama, we use the LiveO2 system, an oxygen mask that pumps in oxygen at either 80 percent saturation or about 8 percent. Wearing the mask while performing an exercise such as riding a stationary bike or using a rowing machine stresses your microvasculature in a beneficial way. When you sprint at 8 percent saturation, you force your blood vessels to expand, and then when you recover from that exertion at 80 percent oxygen, your newly dilated blood vessels soak up that extra oxygen and deliver it to your tissues, including your brain, and you flush away old waste products in greater quantities. In addition to increasing blood flow, contrast oxygen therapy kicks off processes that encourage the recycling of senescent (pro-inflammatory) cells, an increase in mitochondrial output so that you produce more energy (in the form of adenosine triphosphate or ATP) long after your workout is through, and the creation of more red blood cells.

You can buy the device, or go find a clinic near you where you can try it out. It does require you to wear a mask that is hooked up to a machine while you exercise, and when the oxygen saturation is low, it can be intense because you have to work harder to bring in enough air. In other words, contrast oxygen therapy is not for everyone. Some Marama residents just don't want to do it, and some people choose to exercise just with concentrated oxygen. But if you are willing and able, it can be dramatically helpful.

Clinically, I have seen that even when a patient makes no other changes, contrast oxygen therapy can have a big positive impact on cognition all on its own. One of my patients at Solcere came to see me because she was in a desperate situation. Laura had a physical disability and relied on her husband, Michael, for help with day-to-day living, such as shopping for and preparing food. The problem was that Michael was starting to show signs of cognitive decline, and Laura was panicking. They didn't have family nearby, and they were going to be in a difficult—and expensive—situation quickly. They needed a quick solution that was relatively easy to implement. She told me, "We don't have a lot of money or a lot of time, but we have a lot of motivation." Laura asked if there was just one thing they could do to protect Michael's cognitive function, what would it be? I told her I couldn't choose just one, and suggested the keto diet and contrast oxygen therapy. Because food prep was already challenging for them, Laura and Michael opted to start just with contrast oxygen therapy. They bought a LiveO2 system and a stationary bike for their home, and Michael started using it five times a week. Three months later, Laura wrote to me. Using online cognitive assessment tools (through Brain HQ and Apollo's ReCode—see the Resources section for more information about these), Michael's intelligence improved from 75th to 84th percentile; his memory went from 78th to 85th percentile; his people skills went from 86th to 94th percentile; and his navigation skills went from 87th to 96th percentile. In three months. With no other change. Even I, who have witnessed these kinds of improvements numerous times, was blown away that they all came from this one intervention.

I recognize that it is relatively expensive to buy the machine. (At this writing, a basic LiveO2 model costs about $5,000.) You have to have space for it in your home—or have access to a facility near you that you visit regularly, which will have costs of its own. And then, you have to be able to tolerate wearing the mask. But contrast oxygen is an incredibly powerful, low-risk tool that is highly underutilized.

For many people unable to do contrast oxygen therapy, just using EWOT or Exercising with Oxygen Therapy is enough to get the benefit. In this application, you skip the low oxygen and exercise with concentrated oxygen. Especially for those getting back into exercise after a prolonged sedentary break, this is a wonderful way to increase exercise tolerance quickly and reduce the amount of soreness after a new workout. It can be very beneficial for building confidence, getting more regular exercise, and delivering more oxygen to the tissues of the brain and body.

Types of contrast oxygen-therapy exercises:

Riding a stationary bike

Walking or jogging on a treadmill

Bouncing on a rebounder or mini trampoline

BENEFITS: Increased blood flow and oxygen saturation, improved mitochondrial function and energy production, lower levels of inflammation, improved cognition

FREQUENCY: Ideally, you'd do contrast oxygen therapy five days a week for twenty minutes at a time

Getting Started

Now it's time to leverage the incredible benefits of exercise for yourself. Where you start depends on you and your unique situations. In general, I recommend asking yourself these three questions to help you determine the best first step toward making any kind of change:

What's easy?

What's enjoyable?

What would make the biggest difference?

In general, the same rule applies that I've referred to throughout the book so far: you either want to start with low-hanging fruit, or tackle the one thing that would create the largest amount of benefit. Choosing either of these routes increases your likelihood of sticking with whatever change you're undertaking, because you'll be motivated by your successes and already enjoying some increases in energy and confidence that will help you keep going.

I tell people who haven't been exercising much, or even at all, to start with walking (aerobic exercise), and to make it your first priority to get even a small walk in every day, or nearly every day. This is typically easy and fairly enjoyable for most people. The hardest part of any type of exercise is just getting started—by aiming to add a walk to your daily routine, you will build a habit that helps you overcome this most common obstacle. From there, you can start to increase the duration and the intensity of these walks, weaving in some dual-task training to two or three of those weekly walks. As that becomes a regular part of your daily routine, seek to add one to two strength-training and/or contrast oxygen training sessions a week.

On the other hand, if you can do only one type of exercise, you want and need to see results quickly, and you're motivated to do whatever it takes, you can follow Laura and Michael's example and go straight to contrast oxygen therapy, embracing it as part of your regular routine. The increased fitness that adding oxygen, whether in alternating or constant levels, provides will make it easier to pick up new types of exercise.

If you have already been exercising regularly, your goal is to mix up your activities and weave in the types of exercise I've outlined in this chapter that you're not currently doing. You also want to find ways to up your intensity in whatever exercises you have been doing. If you're a runner, for example, you need to add in some strength training. If you've been taking yoga classes for years, you need to find ways to get your heart pumping and work up a sweat. No matter what exercise you're doing, novelty is also important. Your body quickly acclimates to the same challenges, and your mind can tune out when your routine is predictable. Choose activities that require you to stay present instead of just going through the routine and checking a box. If your goal is to reverse cognitive decline, or avoid the same fate as your loved one who had cognitive decline, you have to be willing to change.

If time feels like the biggest barrier to exercising more—or if you just don't love it—find ways to fill multiple needs in one pursuit. Exercise with a friend so that you get social time, and do it outside so that you are also getting natural light and fresh air. That way you'll get maximum benefit from the time you invest in movement.

A quick and efficient way to exercise is high-intensity interval training (HIIT), which has you work to your max capacity for a short time and then rest for a short time before repeating another burst of intensity. If you've heard of the seven-minute workout, that is an HIIT workout where you perform body weight exercises such as push-ups and lunges interspersed with brief periods of rest. A good HIIT workout will raise your heart rate and work the major muscle groups of the body in just a few minutes. It also increases stamina, burns fat, and decreases stress. My only concern with HIIT is that it can be intense, and you don't want to hurt yourself—and you don't want your care partner to get hurt. But if you're pressed for time, HIIT is a great way to get the benefit of exercise in just a few minutes. The best approach is to work with a personal trainer who can teach you the moves in a typical HIIT workout and give you a template to follow that is appropriate for your current level of fitness. Even if you don't do an official HIIT workout, you can maximize the impact of your aerobic exercise by pushing yourself to walk, run, or bike faster for short intervals followed by periods of walking, running, or biking slowly.

Wearing a fitness tracker can help raise your awareness of how much you're moving in a typical day, and seeing that number can motivate you to get some extra movement so that your step count climbs higher. My favorite tracker is the Oura ring—a low-profile band you wear around your finger that tracks multiple things, including steps, active minutes, heart rate, respiratory rate, sleep, and even your fertility if you are a female. It will also send you notifications that it's time to get up and move around if you've been sitting too long.

There are also apps—such as Challenge Hound and the Conqueror—that let you form a group of family and friends and then you all perform a virtual challenge together, such as walking from Florence, Italy, to Rome. Everyone records the number of steps they took each day (or you can set the app to automatically sync with certain trackers so that you don't manually have to enter your step count) and the map shows how far you traveled, as well as where the other members of your group are. It's a little friendly competition that is surprisingly motivating for finding ways to get more steps during the day.

Finally, the best way I have found to be consistent with my exercise is to schedule it and put it on my calendar. Make it just a regular part of your week (but don't forget to weave variety into that regular time slot!).

If You're in Pain

Sometimes exercise feels impossible. Perhaps you've recently had surgery, or an injury or illness, or you live with chronic pain. If you're recuperating from surgery or an illness, take full advantage of physical therapy—book as many appointments as your insurance will cover, and do your exercises every day at home in order to get as much value as you can out of it. Ask your physical therapist, "What's the most I can do? And how can I push this a little more?"

Across the board, movement—done mindfully, at an intensity that makes sense for where your body is at—promotes healing and reduces pain by increasing blood flow, lubricating joints, maintaining or building muscle (which then takes pressure off of your joints), stimulating the flow of lymph and thus improving immunity, and triggering the release of pain-reducing neurochemicals such as endorphins.

If you're experiencing joint pain, keep your cardio low impact until the pain subsides—swimming and biking are both ways to get your heart pumping with little pressure on your joints.

Pilates and the Egoscue technique are both exceptionally beneficial all the time, but especially when dealing with injury, recovery, or pain. Pilates was first developed by Joseph Pilates during World War I as a way to help rehabilitate bed-bound hospital patients—it is designed to accommodate and counteract physical limitations. Invest in a few one-on-one lessons with an experienced instructor who can help identify the exercises that will benefit you the most and show you how to make any modifications your current situation might require.

In my early twenties I had the privilege of working with people in their eighties or nineties who were scheduled for joint replacement or back surgery and were able to eliminate or reduce their pain by doing the exercises taught in the Egoscue method. It really opened up my eyes to see how doing very gentle exercises can take pressure off nerves and joints and relieve pain by placing the bones in optimal alignment. Egoscue is an easy and affordable place to start—you can begin with the book *Pain Free* and do the exercises included in the chapter that pertains to your unique challenge. There are also Egoscue clinics across the United States, and many do consultations via Zoom if there isn't one within easy driving distance of you—see the Resources section at the back of the book for more information.

Remember, what you don't use, you lose. If you want to stay mobile and able to live independently for as long as possible, you need to put your body through its paces.

Connection over Correction: How to Talk to Your Care Partner About Exercise

If you are caring for someone with cognitive impairment or full-blown Alzheimer's and you want to engage them in more physical activity, the best way to get them up and out of their chair is to make it fun. Take something that they already love to do—such as getting in the pool, playing some kind of a sport, attending a class, or walking a pet—and find ways to up the intensity while also maximizing the enjoyment factor.

If your care partner has been largely sedentary, really, you just want them to move more, and building that movement into a daily routine helps reduce any resistance they may have over time. In that case, you could have them write a letter to a loved one or a friend and then walk to the mailbox together to mail it—and then keep walking to the mailbox every other day to check for a reply. One patient of mine had a small stone sculpture of a duck in her yard—her husband would get her to take a walk by telling her it was time to go say hi to the duck. Perhaps there's a beautiful tree your loved one admires, or there's a playground nearby and your care partner may get excited to go watch the children playing.

For those who may already be wheelchair-bound, a favorite exercise is balloon volleyball. Just like it sounds, blow up a balloon and then challenge each other to hit it back and forth, keeping it in the air for as long as possible. Count the number of hits to add a little cognitive engagement and turn this into an easy dual-task exercise. Chair yoga is also accessible to those who feel most comfortable sitting and many chair yoga classes can be found online, eliminating the need for transportation.

If your loved one is social, make their daily movement a chance to connect—make a plan to meet up with friend for a walk, round of pickleball or golf, or exercise class where they can interact with other people.

You may find that your care partner is more willing to do more intense movements for a stranger rather than for you. A physical therapist, fitness instructor, or personal trainer can provide more than just expertise—they can provide motivation.

If your care partner is resistant to exercise, a powerful tactic you can use to avoid butting heads is to understand their biggest driving factor and then appealing to that. For example, if they're social, you can invite them to do it as a way to spend time together, or to see other people (in a class at the senior center, for example). If they're a helper (and a gardener), you can say, "I need your help identifying the plants along the sidewalk." If they're afraid of falling, you can say, "This is how you avoid future falls." And if they're devoted to living at home as long as possible, tell them, "Staying active and getting stronger helps you maintain your independence."

Of course, one of the most powerful ways we influence others is through our example. Whenever possible, do your exercises right along with them.

If you can't work out together, be sure to share with them about what types of exercise you've done since you last spoke to them and how it makes you feel. "Wow, Mom, I went to a Pilates class the other day and I felt an inch taller when I walked out of there!" Or, "I went on a walk the other day and saw a friend who was out watering her garden, and we had the nicest chat." Let them see you making exercise a regular and enriching part of your life—that way you can both reap the benefits of moving more.

To watch a summary video of this chapter and download the Reversing Alzheimer's workbook go to ReversingAlzheimersBook.com.

Reflection questions:
- How often are you and/or your loved one currently exercising?
- What's something you can start doing to increase the amount of time you spend exercising and the intensity of your exercise?
- What physical activities are easiest for you or your loved one to do?
- What physical activities are enjoyable?
- What type of physical activity would make the biggest difference?
- What physical activity will help you also spend time outside, learn something new, and/or socialize with others?

CHAPTER 7

Feed the Brain

It's hard to overstate just how important it is to change the way you eat if you want to protect your brain. One of my patients, Dean, is a perfect example of the power of diet to protect against cognitive decline. In his seventies, Dean has five grandkids. His dementia had been slowly progressing for about a decade when his daughter brought him to see me. He couldn't remember those grandkids' names, couldn't recall the names of the farm animals he regularly passed in the car at his home in Utah, and suffered from incontinence. His daughter was particularly heartbroken to witness his inability to call her children by their names.

After our initial meeting, Dean's daughter worked hard to get Dean into ketosis—or the metabolic state of burning ketones (a fatty acid) for fuel instead of glucose (a form of sugar). Dean's and his daughter's efforts paid off quickly. After about six weeks following a ketogenic diet, Dean's toileting issues went away. He could name the cows and horses they drove past. Best of all, he remembered each of his grandkids' names. It was a clinically significant and personally meaningful achievement.

While six weeks may seem like a short time for creating such miraculous improvements, in my clinical experience results like these are fairly common. For some of my patients, it's like their brain turns back on after only three or four days in ketosis. Seeing these changes so regularly firsthand has convinced me that while there are numerous tools in the new Alzheimer's toolkit, adopting a low-carb, high-fat diet can produce some of the most remarkable improvements. In fact, of all the strategies I outline in this book, I credit the ketogenic diet with a full 50 percent of the benefit of the Reversing Alzheimer's approach to promoting brain health.

The power of diet comes into even sharper view when those patients step away from this brain-supportive eating pattern. For Dean, whenever one set of his grandkids come to town, he eats pizza, ice cream, and cake along with them. And unfortunately, he also forgets their names again, and his incontinence returns.

I know that revamping your diet may sound complicated or challenging. In fact, in every presentation I do and webinar I lead, I get by far the most questions about the keto diet. But despite how complicated the ketogenic eating pattern might seem, it's actually fairly simple to follow, especially once you've figured out what to eat.

Keto Basics

The ketogenic diet is a high-fat, high-veggie, low-carb, and moderate-protein eating plan that has been used safely and successfully since the 1920s to reduce seizures in children with drug-resistant epilepsy. In the early 2010s, the ketogenic diet started enjoying a meteoric rise in popularity, thanks in large part to biohackers who were seeking ways to mimic some of the longevity-extending benefits of caloric restriction (eating a significantly smaller number of calories every day—an approach that has been found to extend life in fruit flies and mice) without restricting calories, which is really hard to do.

From there, the ketogenic diet earned a reputation as an effective weight-loss strategy, and a tool for lowering long-term blood sugar and insulin levels—and since one in every three Americans is either prediabetic or diabetic, the diet took off.

While it can be helpful with weight loss, keto actually isn't about weight at all. It's about restoring metabolic flexibility—the ability of your body to burn either sugar or fat—bring glucose and insulin levels back into a healthy range, reduce inflammation, and feed your brain with its preferred form of fuel.

In order to coax your body into burning fat in the form of ketones, the ketogenic diet guides you to eat far fewer carbs and sugars than is typical in the American diet. On a keto eating plan, you replace typical staples of the American diet such as bread, pasta, and desserts with plenty of healthy fats like avocados, nuts, seeds, olives, and olive oil, as well as colorful, non-starchy vegetables such as mushrooms, peppers, broccoli, cauliflower, and leafy greens, and high-quality animal proteins like pastured eggs, wild salmon, and free-range chicken.

Although this may feel like a big ask at first, it's not as hard as it might seem, because the foods on a ketogenic diet are nutrient-dense, filling, and delicious. Honestly, while I was testing the recipes that I included in this book, everyone I shared them with couldn't stop raving about how tasty and satisfying they were. I can tell you, unlike most diets, the keto eating plan is not about restriction. You are encouraged to eat ample amounts of the foods on the plan until you are full. As you continue to eat keto and wean yourself off the blood sugar spike–crash roller coaster, with its accompanying hunger pangs and cravings, I think you'll find that you feel fuller, longer, and that hunger becomes a less urgent sensation. That's because fat is such a long-lasting fuel, as each of us tends to have plenty of it already stored away so that our body never has to send the "must eat now!" signal that is so common when you're existing on carb-heavy foods.

Also, you or your loved one doesn't need to stay on a ketogenic diet continually. (How long to stay on it depends on your goals, whether it's prevention, reversal, or somewhere in between—more on this in a moment.)

Your Brain on Keto

As we've covered, while the brain is just 2 percent of your total body weight, it accounts for 20 percent of your body's energy use. In order to fill these huge energy needs, your brain has the ability to burn either glucose or ketones. That's right—in one of the many wonders of human design, your body evolved to be, essentially, a hybrid engine, able to burn whichever type of fuel is available. Yet because our modern diet is so carb-heavy—with breads, pastas, crackers, cookies, pizza, and bagels making up so much of our daily calories—your body has mostly stuck to burning sugar.

The problem with being a lifelong sugar-burner is that ketones are actually the brain's preferred fuel source: research shows when both ketones and glucose are available, ketone uptake in the brain increases when glucose consumption decreases. Ketones are more beneficial for the brain because glucose is a quick-burning fuel, like starting a fire with tissue paper. While being able to burn quickly can be helpful in high-needs situations when you require the energy to think and move quickly, using glucose as your primary fuel over a long period of time has a lot of downsides:

- Glucose continually needs to be replenished, so it requires a lot of energy to maintain the right amount in the bloodstream. This leads to a lot of insulin being released in an effort to manage glucose levels.
- It rises and crashes quickly, dragging your energy levels, mental clarity, and mood along with it.
- Glucose is also a dirty fuel, meaning it creates a lot of potentially harmful waste products during the energy metabolism process that occurs within your cells. These waste products can then cue oxidative stress and inflammation.
- As you age, your brain becomes less efficient at utilizing glucose and insulin, the signal that regulates levels of glucose in the blood, leading to what's known as insulin resistance—when your insulin receptors are so flooded with insulin that they stop responding to its signals.
- When you become insulin resistant, you have excess glucose and insulin on hand, which then accumulates in your capillary beds and essentially caramelizes your cells—including your brain cells—in a process known as glycation. Glycation can't be undone—once a cell is glycated, it stays that way.
- As glycated cells build up, it leads to the proliferation of harmful compounds called AGEs (advanced glycation end products), which can lead to cognitive decline. This process explains why Alzheimer's is known colloquially as

type 3 diabetes—it's a natural result of eating too many sugars and carbs, and the high glucose and insulin levels that occur as a result.

Ketones, on the other hand, are great brain food for a lot of reasons:

- The brain prefers ketones to glucose—it will burn them first in the rare instances when they are both present.
- They burn more slowly, more like a full-sized log in the fire. That means your energy levels are more stable and you don't have as many ups and downs as you do with glucose, which tends to spike and crash, dragging your energy levels along with it.
- Ketones not only burn longer, they burn cleaner, meaning the whole energy-creating process is more efficient, so your cells, including your brain cells, have more energy to pay attention, balance your mood, and make memories.
- Because ketones are longer lasting, burning them helps you exit that spike-and-crash glucose roller coaster. As a result, your moods can stabilize (no more getting hangry), your energy evens out, and your brain can function more consistently, with clearer and more focused thinking.
- Your brain's ability to metabolize ketones is unaffected by age.
- Being in ketosis increases apoptosis (programmed cell death)—a process that recycles those caramelized cells. (Exercise further helps the process by flushing away AGEs via enhanced circulation—an example of how each tool in our new Alzheimer's toolkit supports the others.)

If there's a downside to ketones, it's this: It can be a little challenging to get your body to switch over to making and burning ketones at first—getting into ketosis the first time may require some extra diligence, but once you've recovered your metabolic flexibility (the ability to switch back and forth between using glucose and ketones for fuel), it typically gets a lot easier to get into and stay in ketosis. But by sticking closely to the Phase 1 food list that I've included at the back of the book until you are firmly in ketosis (and I'll cover how to determine that later in this chapter), you'll grease the wheels on your keto train. Once the train is rolling, it just gets easier and easier to keep it going.

Studies on the Cognitive Benefits of Ketosis

Numerous studies confirm what I've observed at Marama and Solcere about the remarkable benefits of the ketogenic diet on cognitive improvement.

In one study, researchers with the National Institutes of Health conducted a six-week feasibility trial to determine if older adults with mild cognitive impairment could adhere to such a program for the duration of the trial. All volunteers participated in pre- and postcognitive testing.

While the test involved a small group of participants, all of them completed the trial—and all but one achieved a measurable level of ketones. Even more noteworthy, participants showed a statistical and clinically significant improvement on the cognitive assessment at the end of the trial. With such promising results, researchers are ready to move forward with the next phase of this study, which will involve a larger group of participants for a longer period.

In another study, published in *Alzheimer's & Dementia: The Journal of the Alzheimer's Association*, researchers gave one group of participants a ketogenic medium-chain triglyceride supplement twice a day, and a placebo to the control group. After six months, those who took the keto supplement showed increased ketone uptake, meaningful cognitive gains, and significantly improved brain energy supply as compared to the placebo group. (I'll cover later in this chapter whether using a similar supplement might be helpful for you or your care partner to take—for now, my emphasis is on showing the link between being in ketosis and enjoying improved cognitive function.)

Even more promising, a study published in *Alzheimer's Research & Therapy* tested the ketogenic diet on participants diagnosed with Alzheimer's disease. After two periods of following a modified ketogenic diet for twelve weeks, with a ten-week break in between, results showed patients improved in daily function and quality of life, as compared to the other group of AD patients who followed a low-fat diet.

Dr. Bredesen's team and my team at Solcere did two very similar clinical trials showing similar results, where the majority of participants with cognitive decline improved their cognition after a nine-month intervention (in Dr. Bredesen's study) and after a six-month intervention (in the study my team and I conducted). In both studies, participants were supported by health coaches to adopt a high-veggie, ketogenic diet.

At Marama, we test our patients' ketone levels regularly to determine what foods are or are not helping them get and stay in ketosis. As a result of our frequent testing regimen, I've observed that the more my patients' ketone levels rise, the more dramatically their cognition comes back online. Their MoCA scores support this observation—I've seen many patients whose ketone levels have stayed above 2 or 3 mmol consistently for several weeks increase their MoCA score by 10 points or more. That can mean the difference between being able to use the bathroom independently and requiring someone to accompany them, or between being able to engage in conversation and activities and spending most of the time sitting and staring into space.

If you could put these kinds of results into a pill with very few side effects and risks and bring it to market, you could make billions of dollars. Perhaps someday there will be such a medicine—in the meantime, you don't have to wait. You can begin choosing a new way to eat as soon as your next meal. In this chapter, I'll guide you through how to do it.

Bonus Benefits of the Keto Diet

Supplying your brain with ample amounts of the energy it prefers and flushing toxic compounds from your brain are pretty strong reasons to follow a ketogenic diet. There are so many additional health benefits. At the top of the list is a noticeable uptick in energy.

In addition to feeling like I'm witnessing their brains turning back on, I see renewed vitality in my clients at Marama every day as a result of cutting out excess sugar-laden processed foods and burning fat for energy. For example, when Rose came to Marama she was glazed over. She showed no emotion and sat in a chair all day with her head down. Once we got her detoxified from sugar and into ketosis, we witnessed a drastic change. She perked up and engaged with those around her, and even participated in exercise class. Additionally, her mood improved, as did her sleep.

Other health benefits of following a keto diet include:

- REDUCED RISK OF HEART DISEASE: According to the CDC, heart disease is the leading killer of men and women in the United States. Some of the top risk factors for heart disease include obesity, high blood pressure, and elevated triglycerides. The keto diet, as mentioned above, can help you lose weight if that's a goal of yours, as well as manage your blood pressure, increase HDL (good) cholesterol levels, and lower triglycerides. And what's good for your heart is also good for your brain.
- LOWER INFLAMMATION: The standard American diet is chock-full of foods rich in omega-6s—an essential fatty acid that is found in vegetable seed oils such as canola, soy, safflower, and sunflower, which is healthy in moderation but becomes inflammatory when you consume too much of it. On the keto diet, you reduce or eliminate the foods that contain omega-6 oils and focus on keto-friendly fare that's rich in healthier fats, including omega-3 fatty acids, which reduce inflammation. Reducing your sugar and carbohydrate intake and boosting veggie consumption reduce inflammation as well.
- DETOXIFICATION: Most of the toxins we absorb from environmental pollutants, pesticides, household chemicals, and personal care products are fat-soluble. Meaning, the body will store them in fat cells in an effort to protect your organs and other tissues from their damage. When you switch to burning fat, you can liberate those toxins that have been tucked away so that they can then be carried out of the body. This is why it's crucial to also eat plenty of high-fiber vegetables, so that your digestion stays strong and you can eliminate those toxins in a daily bowel movement. Don't forget to also drink plenty of water and exercise so that toxins can be excreted through your urine and sweat.
- LOWER BLOOD SUGAR AND INSULIN LEVELS: When you cut back on carbs, you lower your blood sugar levels and reduce the incidence of glycation. And with less blood sugar in circulation, you also release less insulin. Having less glucose and insulin circulating in your blood helps heal insulin resistance, which is often the first step in a cascade of metabolic imbalances that lead to chronic disease, such as diabetes and heart disease.
- HORMESIS: Just like exercise, ketosis is a form of hormesis, a beneficial stressor that cues your body to get stronger and more efficient. Specifically,

ketosis triggers the recycling of senescent cells—dysfunctional cells that are just hanging out, excreting inflammatory chemicals—and sends the signal to create new cells, neurons, and neuronal connections, increasing the adaptability and resilience of your system as a whole.

- ABILITY TO LIVE AS YOU WERE DESIGNED TO LIVE: Lastly, following the keto diet allows your body to be used the way it's designed. After all, your ancestors were forced to adapt to an inconsistent food supply—filling up on berries and grains in the warmer months and going long periods of time without eating during the winter, until they could successfully hunt an animal and fill up on its fatty meats. Periodically following a ketogenic diet mimics this state and helps you maintain that metabolic flexibility that helped our species survive and evolve.

Being in ketosis is actually quite freeing, because once you get off the roller coaster of eating carbs, burning carbs, and then craving more carbs, you won't feel hunger pangs and cravings. Instead, you'll feel full and satisfied for long stretches, and—once you adapt to eating in a different way and know which foods to reach for when you do feel hungry—you won't think about food as often. You won't even miss the refined carbs. Especially once you taste the scrumptious recipes I've included at the back of the book. (And if you do, there are now great keto-friendly bread options in the freezer section of your grocery store, such as those made by Carbonaut.)

Think Before You Eat: Mental Aspects of the Ketogenic Diet

The most important thing you need in order to be successful on the keto diet is a willingness to rethink what healthy means. We were told throughout the 1980s and '90s that a diet high in carbohydrates was good for us and that fats were bad—guidance that led us straight into the obesity, diabetes, and Alzheimer's epidemics that we find ourselves in today. The keto diet flips that faulty guideline on its head. It *prioritizes* healthy fats and doesn't restrict your intake of them in any way. It also demonstrates that the refined grains we've been told are foundational to a daily diet—with the USDA MyPlate recommendations still suggesting up to five ounces of grains per day, which is equal to two and a half cups of rice, five slices of bread, or five cups of cereal, which contain roughly 75 to 100 grams of carbs. The result is just too much glucose, too much insulin and insulin resistance, too much glycation, too many sugar crashes, too much inflammation and neuroinflammation, and not enough ketones.

Additionally, you'll need to think beyond your usual go-to packaged goods. Processed packaged goods may be convenient, but unless they are clearly labeled "keto-friendly," they will likely sabotage your efforts to get into ketosis. Even if bars are designed to fit within the parameters of a ketogenic eating plan, that keto snack mix should still play only a minor role in your daily and weekly food intake, because it's still highly processed and can keep your taste buds attuned to snack foods instead of whole foods. Much of the benefit of a ketogenic diet comes from drastically reducing your intake of highly processed foods. The more cooking and preparation you do, the better you'll do on the eating plan.

You may also have to change the way you cook, using ghee (also known as clarified butter), coconut oil, or avocado oil instead of canola or olive oil (you can drizzle extra virgin olive oil on salads and already-cooked vegetables, and can cook with it up to 350 degrees Fahrenheit, but above that temperature it oxidizes, so avoid it for high-heat cooking.)

If you're seeking to reverse cognitive decline, you want to stay in ketosis for three to six months to start, and then return to it regularly—I recommend aiming to be in ketosis more than you are not. If your goal is prevention, aim to be in ketosis for only about a quarter of the year, whether that's two days a week, one week a month, or three months out of the year. Sure, you may eat something that throws you out of ketosis once in a while. But when that happens, you know what you must do? Simply start again at the next meal.

Know that you will experience some ups and downs on this diet and also sugar cravings here and there. But understanding the improved cognition and increased energy that awaits you can help you stay committed.

What's on the Keto Diet?

There is a wide array of delicious foods on the keto diet.

- High-quality animal protein: grass-fed beef and bison, pastured chicken and eggs, wild fatty fish such as salmon, and shellfish
- Nonstarchy vegetables: lettuces, leafy greens, peppers, broccoli, cauliflower, asparagus, and mushrooms
- Nuts and seeds: hemp hearts, walnuts, macadamia nuts, pecans, almonds, nut butters, sunflower seeds, and pumpkin seeds
- Healthy fats: olives, avocados, coconut milk, olive oil, and butter and ghee
- Herbs and spices: salt, pepper, cilantro, basil, mint, rosemary, mustard

All these foods can be used to make delicious meals and snacks. I'm including plenty of recipes at the end of this book, including my favorites and our Marama residents' favorites to get you started.

I'm also including a full list of foods on the diet starting on page 308—you can start by eating any of the Phase 1 foods, and then when you've been in ketosis for two weeks, start adding in Phase 2 foods. (There are also Phase 3 foods, but those are for the times when you're cycling off the ketogenic diet.)

Some typical breakfasts include smoked salmon rolled up with a schmear of cream cheese; eggs served with sautéed greens and a healthy drizzle of pesto; avocado "toast" served on flaxseed crackers instead of bread; plain Greek yogurt with a handful of nuts and seeds stirred in; and coffee or tea with heavy cream. For lunch, enjoy a mixed vegetable salad topped with your choice of protein, olives, and a drizzle of olive oil. Hard-boiled eggs, cheese sticks, half a can of sardines, or a handful of nuts make great snacks. Cauliflower and broccoli doused with olive oil or ghee and sprinkled with sea salt then cooked in an air fryer as a side to dark meat chicken, wild salmon, or grilled beef makes for a delicious and satisfying dinner.

If you're craving carbs, there are carb-like foods you can eat such as cauliflower rice or zucchini noodles (also called zoodles). Additionally, check out the recipes for Keto Oatmeal, Brownie Fat Bombs, and Cauliflower Crust Pizza that can help satisfy your cravings.

Fats

Because we have been taught to fear and avoid fat, one of the most common mistakes people make when they first start the keto diet is not adding enough fats to their diet. That's a recipe for feeling hungry and possibly losing too much weight.

But not all fats are equal. Fried foods, processed foods, sugar-laced condiments, peanut butter, and grain-fed animal protein (grass-fed is healthier), as well as cakes and chips, are all examples of unhealthy foods with a prominent place on the standard American diet (SAD). Many of them are foods rich in omega-6 fatty acids, which, in abundance, can contribute to inflammation. That's because the fats that come in your food become incorporated into the membranes of your cells. Cell membranes continually break down and get recycled. So, if the fats that you eat are inflammatory, when those cell membranes are broken down, they can contribute to inflammation and a variety of inflammatory diseases, including dementia, heart disease, and metabolic disease.

On the other hand, foods with omega-3 fatty acids, such as wild-caught salmon, anchovies, grass-fed beef, and pastured eggs, do the reverse—they reduce inflammation. These foods are good fats.

Other good fats are extra virgin olive oil, avocado oil, and coconut oil. Coconut oil is a saturated fat known as a medium-chain triglyceride (MCT), a different type of fat that many people metabolize without gaining weight and one of the fats most easily burned as fuel. In fact, I like to start the day or a meal with two teaspoons of coconut oil—I eat them right off the spoon, but you can stir a bit of coconut oil into your coffee or tea. It fills you up and helps fuel your cells without impacting your blood sugar. Any way you can incorporate some coconut oil into your diet, do it—I'm including a Brownie Fat Bomb recipe that makes this delicious and easy to do.

(A note about coconut oil for those with the APOE4 gene: this gene affects your fat metabolism, making it difficult for you to metabolize saturated fats. I will discuss this exception and other contraindications later in this chapter.)

Here's a tip for storing your healthy fats—get them in glass bottles if you can. That's because, as fats, they're going to absorb fat-soluble toxins that are often present in plastic.

I also include full-fat dairy here as a source of healthy fat, although it's a good source of protein, too. Unless you are lactose intolerant or vegan, I advise keeping dairy in your diet when you're seeking to get and stay in ketosis. If you've restricted dairy in the past because of concerns of inflammation or other health issues, I suggest you try adding back sheep and goat dairy temporarily while in ketosis. Dairy is a quick and easy way to get high-fat, high-protein, high-caloric intake, and to feel satisfied. Eating it while following a ketogenic diet can help prevent the loss of too much weight and I want you to have as much variety in your diet as possible, and as much ease as possible to getting into ketosis.

Number of daily servings: three to four.

Protein

When you're starting a ketogenic diet, you need to eat more protein than normal, especially in the first week or so. This is because when your body doesn't have carbohydrates for fuel, but is not yet efficient at burning fat, it will use protein for fuel in the meantime. If you don't have enough dietary protein, your body will break down muscle as a protein source instead—and we don't want that.

A good baseline is to start with twice as much protein as you would normally eat or at least half of your body weight in pounds in grams of protein. For example, if you weigh 150 pounds, have 75 grams of protein minimum per day. I advise my clients to start with about 15 grams of protein in the morning, and then 7 to 10 grams every three to four hours after that. Two eggs have about 14 grams. Seven to 10 grams looks like this: a handful of almonds, a quarter cup of tofu, two ounces of beef or salmon jerky, one and a half ounces of pistachios, two to three slices of Brie, a single serving of plain Greek yogurt or cottage cheese.

If you're going with animal-derived proteins—things like eggs, dairy, meats, and fish—try to buy the grass-fed, pastured, wild-caught, and/or organic versions. Grass-fed red meat, such as beef, bison, and lamb, delivers higher levels of healthy omega-3s than their conventional, grain-fed counter-parts. Since one of the goals of a keto diet is to mobilize and detoxify toxins from your system, you don't want to add more back into your system—that's why buying organic whenever possible is a key part of the diet. (Be careful about processed meats such as sausage and bacon because many of them contain a lot of added sugar—which could kick you out of ketosis—nitrites, and food dyes; regular consumption of them has been linked to increased rates of cancer, diabetes, and heart disease. If eating them helps you get in and stay in ketosis, eat them in moderation, but avoid them as much as possible when you're not eating a high-fat diet.)

The same goes with fish, in terms of sticking to wild-caught, toxin-free varieties. To keep it simple, stick to wild-caught SMASH fish (salmon, mackerel, anchovies, sardines, herring) because other fish have potentially high levels of mercury. Farmed salmon, which you should avoid, for example, is typically grain-fed, given antibiotics, and raised in high-density fish farms at high risk of disease. Many of them contain dyes. That's why wild salmon is the only way to go if you have the choice. At Marama, we will do frozen wild salmon when fresh Alaskan salmon isn't in season. Of course, you can only do your best. If your budget needs a more affordable option, stick with sardines and anchovies.

Number of daily servings: Follow the formula I shared on page 142 to calculate how many grams of protein you should be eating each day. In general, you want to be sure you're including protein at every meal.

Veggies

I advise eating *a lot* of high-fiber, nonstarchy vegetables (think five to eight cups a day) when you're eating keto. This gives you the fiber you need to encourage a daily bowel movement (which will also help you detoxify) and the nutrients you need to help your body—and particularly your brain—work effectively. Say yes to greens, peppers, broccoli, cauliflower, mushrooms, and asparagus but skip the starchy, high-glycemic vegetables such as squash, sweet potatoes, carrots, and beets until you're ready to cycle out of ketosis and add in Phase 3 foods. Again, see the list of Phase 1 foods on page 308 for a complete list of veggies you can enjoy at the start of the diet.

Some vegetables can provide some of the comfort we associate with more carb-heavy foods—mashed cauliflower in lieu of mashed potatoes, cauliflower rice instead of rice, zucchini noodles (zoodles) instead of pasta, and kale chips instead of potato chips. Don't knock them until you've tried them! I think you'll be surprised how adding plenty of healthy fats, like cream, olive oil, or coconut milk, to your veggies will up the comfort factor.

Number of daily servings: five to eight cups a day, or two to three cups per meal.

Carbohydrates

In order to get into ketosis, you want to eat very few carbohydrates, especially in the beginning of the program, except for those that exist in small amounts in the nonstarchy vegetables, nuts, and seeds on the Phase 1 list. Think of ketosis as a light switch. The process of burning fat is either on, or it is off. Even small amounts of carbohydrates will quickly turn the switch off. Stick to the foods on the Phase 1 food list until your practitioner or health coach lets you know you can try adding in some of the Phase 3 foods.

If you're craving sweets, there are great sweeteners that don't raise blood sugar, including stevia, allulose, and monk fruit. They can be substituted for sugar in fat bombs, chocolate, and even low-carb baked goods so you never feel restricted. Also check out the recipes for Keto Celebration Cake, Berry-Cream Parfait, and Cardamom Almond Butter Fat Bombs, which can satisfy a sweet tooth.

Carbohydrates are not just breads and pastas. Fruits, root vegetables, and beans are also carbohydrate-rich food sources. So again, you will need to shift your thinking from grabbing an apple or banana, or having some carrots and hummus, as a snack because they can flip your ketosis switch to off.

Number of daily servings: Definitely fewer than 50 grams of carbs per day, spread out evenly throughout the day. You may find that you have to keep your carb count lower, to about 30 grams of carbs, to achieve ketosis.

Beverages

It's important to stay hydrated on this diet to address potential constipation and to replenish fluids in your body. Also, when you start keto, you'll be urinating more than usual as your body switches up its metabolism. Try to drink spring water because it has minerals and, as with animal products, you don't want to be adding toxins into your body as you're flushing them out. (I talk more about your best water options in Chapter 9.)

Other beverages that are keto-approved include coffee, club soda, green or black tea, and unsweetened herbal tea.

As for wine and other alcohol, I recommend eliminating them completely because they're hard on the liver, not good for the brain, and also interfere with getting a good night's sleep. Also, wine and beer will most likely kick you out of ketosis. If you absolutely aren't ready to give up alcohol yet there are keto cocktail recipes online. Decent options include vodka or tequila with club soda and lime juice to taste.

How to Get into Ketosis

When you're ready to start eating keto, refer to the list of Phase 1 foods on page 308 and stock up on all your favorites. Review the recipes at the back of this book—I've taken care to select Marama residents' all-time favorites as well as recipes that are easy, filling, and delicious. You can also refer to the Month of Meals on page 312 to get an idea of what it looks like to eat this way for a full four weeks.

When you begin, aim for about 50 grams of carbohydrates or less per day. Some lucky people can tolerate up to 70 grams and still maintain ketosis, while others have to keep their carb consumption to 30 grams or fewer. There will be some trial and error, especially to start, and that is okay. By regularly checking your ketone levels—I recommend once in the morning before your first meal of the day, and once again one to two hours after a meal to start—you will develop an innate sense of what your body needs to stay in ketosis.

Some people like to track their carbohydrate grams by Googling the grams of everything they eat and adding them up—and if you find data to be a helpful, motivating tool, by all means, go for it! But you don't have to do a lot of research. You can and should certainly check the carb information on the nutrition label of any packaged food you eat, but, on this diet, you're encouraged to eat whole foods and unprocessed foods that don't come in packages.

Just remember to also focus on adding in healthy fats so that you stay full and that your body has plenty of dietary fat on hand to help it start the process of manufacturing ketones.

As long as you stick with the foods on the Phase 1 list, and test your ketone and glucose levels, you'll know if you're in the range or if certain foods are kicking you out of ketosis or preventing you from getting into it.

If you're having trouble staying in ketosis or want to see if you can eat a certain food or beverage, then it may help to Google and count your carbs. Additionally, while the number of carbs is important to note, it's also important to spread your carb consumption throughout the day.

For example, I love kombucha (a fizzy beverage of fermented tea) for its taste and for its probiotics. But if I drink a big glass of it all at once, it will kick me out of ketosis. I've learned that if I sip it throughout the day, I stay on track. So I don't have to give up my kombucha, I just have to savor it and not gulp it down—likely there is a potentially nonketogenic food you love that you can continue to consume in a similar manner without derailing your ketone levels, too.

Another helpful trick when getting into ketosis is to use capsules or powdered ketones as a snack between meals or at any hint of carb cravings. Exogenous ketones come in supplement form and can significantly help raise ketone levels if you are struggling to get fully into ketosis.

HELPFUL SUPPLIES

It can be useful to work with a health coach to help you find foods, develop a plan, and troubleshoot any issues. Furthermore, an experienced health coach can give you even more tips and tricks than I can pack into this book.

In addition to a health coach, there are tools and supplements that can help and support you through this process.

» **KETONE AND GLUCOSE MONITOR.** You could buy two separate devices—one that measures ketones and one that measures glucose levels—or you can buy one device that measures both. I recommend the Keto-Mojo, as it does both. Also, the Keto-Mojo website is a rich source of tips, recipes, and information about the keto diet.

» **KETONE AND GLUCOSE TESTING STRIPS:** While ketone and glucose monitors come with starter supplies of testing strips, you're going to need a lot more to continue monitoring the impact of your food choices on your glucose and ketone levels over time.

» **LANCETS:** These tiny needles make gathering the drop of blood to test your ketones and glucose easy and painless. You'll need a plentiful supply.

» **KITCHEN TOOLS:** See Chapter 9 for a list of helpful kitchen tools.

» **PROGRESS TRACKING SHEETS:** Our easy-to-use Progress Tracker can help make this diet feel less overwhelming. See page 318 in the appendix.

» **SUPPLEMENTS:** Exogenous ketones can help nudge your body into ketosis at the beginning of the diet, magnesium citrate supplements can help replenish flushed minerals and minimize muscle cramping and other symptoms of the keto flu, and an organic greens powder can help you get beneficial and vital phytonutrients—particularly if it's hard to eat several servings of green vegetables per day. See page 301 for specific recommendations.

Common Keto Diet Misconceptions

Since you've read this far, you're probably interested or at least intrigued by the studies and information on how a keto diet can help prevent or slow and even reverse cognitive decline. But, maybe you've heard some things about this high-fat, low-carb diet that are giving you pause or concerns. I've probably heard the same things, and more, many times. This is what I tell my clients who have reservations about the keto plan.

Isn't eating all that fat bad for you?

The simple answer is: no. After all, your brain is made out of fat. Its neurons are sheathed in it. It makes sense then that your brain requires fat to function optimally. But I can understand why so many people have this concern.

We're still influenced by the food pyramid guidelines from the 1980s and '90s that called for eight to ten servings of grains a day, and little fat. Now we know that not only are those guidelines wrong, but also that they probably led to the obesity, diabetes, and Alzheimer's epidemics that we now find ourselves in. (Obesity rates have more than doubled since the 1980s.) We've since learned that we should've been eating the opposite of a high-carb, low-fat diet.

But it's important to note that eating "all that fat" is good for you only if you don't also eat all that sugar. It's when you eat a lot of both that you run the risk of overfeeding yourself, which results in having too much glucose and insulin on hand, leading to inflammation and glycation and gradual loss of cognitive health. Just stick to the Phase 1 foods, and you won't be at risk of consuming too many fats and carbs at once.

Ketosis is dangerous.

This misconception most likely comes from the fact that *ketosis*—the state of burning fat for fuel—sounds a lot like *ketoacidosis*—a serious medical complication of diabetes. In ketoacidosis, a lack of insulin prevents the shuttling of glucose into the cells where it can be burned for fuel, so the body starts burning fat, and then both glucose and ketones build up in the blood stream. Ketoacidosis can lead to serious complications and requires immediate medical attention. I explain the difference between the two in this way: Ketosis is a healthy sprinkle of rain, and ketoacidosis is a torrential downpour and destructive flood.

The ketogenic diet cuts out so many foods, I'll be hungry.

The keto diet is not about restricting calories—it's about switching your metabolic state. Because the keto diet encourages plenty of healthy fats, protein, and high-fiber vegetables, and because ketones are such a long-lasting fuel, being in ketosis gets you off the roller coaster of blood sugar spikes followed by crashes, and the cravings that cycle can bring.

I could lose too much weight.

While weight loss is a benefit of the keto diet for those who want to or need to lose weight, it's a concern for older people, especially older women, who don't want to become frail. Because there are so many rich and full-fat foods, it is possible to stay at your current weight by indulging in the higher calorie options on the keto diet. Personally, weight loss is not my goal, and when I go into ketosis, my weight stays stable. In fact, I typically develop some cellulite on my thighs if I have any cream in my daily coffee. Done correctly, the diet is calorie-rich.

Most often, people lose weight on the keto diet because they don't add in enough fats to make up for the calories those carbs were providing. You really can load up on avocados, olives, olive oils, whole (unsweetened) dairy, nuts, and seeds.

When I hear that a caregiver or a client is concerned about weight loss, I tell them to add organic heavy cream to their coffee, which is not only delicious but also a good way to add calories and fat to your diet. In fact, heavy cream not only helps keep your weight up, it also pushes your ketone number up. I also tell them that strength-building exercise and hormone replacement therapy, which I discuss in Chapters 6 and 11, respectively, can help prevent too much weight loss and also make it easier to add muscle, which supports bone health and reduces fall risk in addition to helping your cognition.

I'll have to be on a ketogenic diet forever.

No one should be on a ketogenic diet forever. Being in ketosis isn't a long-term goal. Rather, metabolic flexibility, where you can easily cycle back and forth between burning fat and glucose, is the long-term goal.

If you are experiencing cognitive impairment, or you feel like your memory is failing or not as good as it used to be, I recommend aiming to adhere closely to the diet for three to six months, and then cycling in and out of it. This gives you plenty of flexibility to loosen the reins and enjoy a more typical American eating pattern, to indulge on birthdays, holidays, and vacations, and then to get back to an eating style that's more beneficial for brain health. Spending just three to six months on a ketogenic diet will jump-start the brain's healing.

If you're not actively experiencing cognitive issues, I recommend following the diet about a quarter of the year as a preventative measure, which is what I do. I follow the keto diet for four to six weeks about two to three times a year. If you have a genetic risk, you should spend about a third of the year in ketosis. For example, you could follow the diet one month a quarter or ten days a month.

When you're not on the diet, however, resist the urge to resume indulging in processed carbohydrates and sweets on a regular basis, as studies show that highly processed foods increase your risk of developing dementia. You should continue to eat a healthy balanced diet, adding back into your diet some healthy carbs, such as beans, squashes, fruit, and whole grains. However, once you start incorporating these foods back into your diet, you'll probably want to back off the full-fat dairy. This is a great time to switch to a plant-based or vegetarian diet.

I'll get to eat all the bacon I want!

Bacon is technically a ketogenic food. That being said, bacon—as well as sausage, salami, and hot dogs—is a processed meat that can contain a lot of additives, often including nitrates and sugar, that are not healthy for you. As I mentioned earlier, processed meats are strongly linked to increased risk of cancer, diabetes, and heart disease. So, it's not really something you should eat regularly, no matter what diet you're following. But if eating bacon makes it easier for you or your loved one to enjoy this new style of eating, then it's okay to have it occasionally. Stick to eating bacon only while your goal is to maintain ketosis.

My cholesterol levels will rise.

Many people are concerned that eating more fats and animal products may raise their cholesterol. And certainly, if your cholesterol is high, you should consult your doctor or health coach before starting the eating plan. But my clinical experience shows that, while cholesterol levels may go up temporarily—particularly in the first three months of being on the diet, before your body has become adept at burning fat—cholesterol levels improve after that. Additionally, it's important to stick to the diet guidelines for the sake of your cholesterol because if you're eating animal products *and* carbohydrates and sugar, your cholesterol is likely to go up. Keep track of these numbers with the help of labs ordered by your provider at regular intervals—I recommend every twelve weeks for your first year using the new Alzheimer's toolkit.

How to Tell When You're in Ketosis

Technically, you're in ketosis when your ketone levels are at least 1 mmol, although ideally, you're maintaining levels between 2 and 3 mmol. Since you likely won't be burning fat right away, your readings will start lower and then slowly creep up. For example, you may see readings of .01 mmol or .02 at first, as your body burns off its glucose stores and starts manufacturing ketones. Mild ketosis is 0.5 to 0.9, and many people notice benefits at this ketone level. (See the box on page 147 for information on the measuring devices for ketones and glucose levels.)

Ketone testing strips can cost over $1 per strip, so you don't need to go overboard and test after every meal. I recommend testing ketones only twice a day: one test before your first meal of the day, and an hour before your second meal. And testing your glucose levels after meals to see if particular foods or beverages drive up your blood sugar. Fortunately, glucose test strips are less expensive than ketone test strips. You only need to register ketone levels over 1.0 once daily to have achieved ketosis.

Try to test your levels the same time every day. This way, you can understand if a particular food item was responsible for raising your glucose level, or lowering your ketone level and kicking you out of ketosis.

Some days you'll fall out of ketosis. That's okay. Don't stress over it. Just get back to following the diet and measuring your ketone and glucose levels to learn which foods will keep you on track, and which ones will kick you out of ketosis.

Nudging Your Body into Ketosis

If you're following the diet closely and still not getting your ketone level up above 1 mmol, there are some tricks to nudging your body into ketosis.

- DO AN OBJECTIVE ASSESSMENT. This would be a good time to actually count up the carbs you're consuming: review your tracking sheet that I've included at the back of this book (and in downloadable form at ReversingAlzheimersBook.com), and then an online nutrition database such as nutritionvalue.org to add up your total carbs to make sure you're not eating more than you think you're eating.
- MAKE SURE YOU'RE EATING ENOUGH FAT. Again, one of the most common mistakes people make with the keto diet is cutting down on carbs but not adding in enough fat. As I've mentioned before but it bears repeating: loading up on avocados, olive oil, coconut oil, olives, and full-fat dairy will help push you into ketosis. You can also try eating coconut oil straight off the spoon or swirled into your coffee, or eating fat bombs to get that healthy fat intake up.
- TRY SUPPLEMENTING WITH KETONES. Not all ketones need to be made by your body—you can take them in supplement form. They are called exogenous ketones, and they can come in drink, pill, or powder form. They can help you get over the hump at the beginning of the diet. I'll include my favorite exogenous ketone supplements in the Resources section. I generally recommend using exogenous ketones between meals or as needed when you have a craving for sugar or carbohydrates.

- IMPLEMENT A FASTING PERIOD. Intermittent fasting, where you limit your eating window to a twelve-hour period, i.e., from six a.m. to six p.m. or from seven a.m. to seven p.m., can also help you boost your ketone production by giving your body some time off from digesting and forcing it to create some ketones out of your stored fat to last until the next meal. As long as weight loss isn't an issue, consider fasting for longer. Some people find a sixteen-hour fasting period and eight-hour eating window helps them with sleep, energy, metabolism, and cognition. Be sure to leave three hours between your last meal and bedtime so your body gets more efficient sleep.

Troubleshooting

As you shift your primary source of calories from carbs to fats, your body will likely experience some side effects, especially in the first few days of the diet as your body goes through the transition from burning glucose to burning ketones for fuel.

While the symptoms are real, they typically don't last more than a couple of days—especially when you know these tips and tools that can help you get over the hump so you can enjoy the mental clarity, improved energy, and brain benefits that await you on the other side. Here are some common issues that arise and how you can manage them:

Fatigue and Brain Fog (aka the "Keto Flu")

The first few days, as your metabolism is shifting, your system undergoes a detoxification period from sugar. Many of us are literally physiologically addicted to sugar, and we go through a withdrawal period just like any addict does. Additionally, as the toxins that were once stored in your fat cells start moving through your system, you may feel like you're fighting something off before they make their final exit. This "am I getting sick?" feeling is commonly referred to as the "keto flu" because it can include symptoms of the actual flu, such as body aches and fatigue. Some people also experience muscle cramping and brain fog.

Another reason you can feel run down in the first couple of days is that, as you're flushing those toxins from your system, you'll likely end up urinating more frequently. As a result, you'll be depleting your system of sodium and other minerals more quickly than your body is used to. Those minerals fuel chemical reactions throughout your body, and, without them, it may feel like someone took their foot off the gas pedal of your body. Adding a scoop of calcium-magnesium powder to water can replenish those minerals, help with daily bowel movements, and reduce muscle cramps. (See the Resources section for my suggestions.)

In addition, your liver may be working overtime to process those toxins. Therefore, liver support supplements, such as those I list at the end of Chapter 11, will help move those toxins out of your system.

Throughout this short-lived transition, staying hydrated and getting enough rest and exercise can help you feel better as well as accelerate the process of getting into ketosis. Stay the course—these symptoms are signs that your efforts are working. Soon you should get to the other side, and your energy and clarity will return.

Constipation

Because of the change in your diet, you may experience constipation as your digestive tract adjusts. Not only can this be uncomfortable, but it can hinder the detoxification process that's happening now.

To combat constipation, drink plenty of natural spring water, eat a lot of colorful, nonstarchy vegetables, and exercise regularly (moving your body helps move your bowels). Remember, the target for vegetables is five to eight servings a day. The calcium-magnesium powder that can help ease the keto flu (and that I list in the Resources section) also helps make bowel movements more regular. If constipation continues to be a problem, see your provider for help.

Sugar Withdrawal and Cravings

When I recently went into ketosis with a coaching group, I spent an entire day dreaming about doughnuts. I don't think I've had a doughnut in more than fifteen years. My mind could barely concentrate on anything else. When this happens, it is helpful to stay committed by having keto-friendly snacks and meals prepared and at the ready.

The blood sugar spikes and crashes that follow after you eat sugar trigger a cascade of hormones that then makes you crave more sugar so that you have a steady supply of glucose on hand. It's natural, then, that when you step away from eating foods high in refined carbs and sugars you may experience some cravings. A fat bomb (such as the Brownie Fat Bomb or Cardamom Almond Butter Fat Bomb recipes that appear in the recipe section of this book) can really help nip those cravings in the bud, as can having a teaspoon or two of coconut oil or a protein-rich snack, such as a handful of nuts or seeds, some beef jerky, or a hard-boiled egg. Once your body has switched over to burning fat, your body no longer has a reason to trigger those cravings because your blood sugar will remain a lot more stable, and because keto-friendly foods provide a lasting sense of fullness.

Testing Strip Troubles

Pricking your finger in order to test your ketone and glucose levels can be challenging. To start, I recommend having lancets, Band-Aids, and alcohol prep pads handy. Wipe the spot you'll use with the alcohol pad—I recommend using the side of the finger, not the pad, because it's less sensitive—then quickly and confidently use the lancet to prick the finger.

I also recommend running your hands under warm water first to get the blood going so you can reduce the risk of having to prick your finger a second time.

Contraindications and Risks

There are certain health conditions or situations that should be closely monitored while following a ketogenic eating plan. And in some cases, such as pregnancy, the diet should be avoided altogether.

- ELEVATED CHOLESTEROL: In my clinical experience I see cholesterol levels go down after about three to five months on this diet. However, your levels may go up at first while your liver adjusts to manufacturing ketones.

    If you're concerned about cholesterol, it's important to adhere to the diet closely. Cholesterol levels are likely to be negatively affected if you increase your fat intake without also significantly reducing carbs and sugars.

    If you have familial hypercholesterolemia (the scientific term for genetic high cholesterol that runs in your family), bergamot, berberine, amla, alpha-lipoic acid, and niacin supplements can help you manage your cholesterol levels. Additionally, exercising regularly, taking care of your teeth, and getting enough quality sleep can also go a long way in improving your cardiovascular health and managing cholesterol.

- BEING UNDERWEIGHT: Being frail and too thin can be a health issue, especially as we age, and the keto eating plan can facilitate weight loss—especially if you're not eating enough healthy fats. Working with a health coach can ensure that you get the nutrients and calories you need to maintain weight while also switching your fuel source from glucose to fat.

- APOE4 STATUS: People with APOE4, a gene variant that affects how you metabolize fat and increases your risk of Alzheimer's disease, may need to avoid saturated fats such as coconut oil because it can increase your LDL (bad) cholesterol levels. Work with your provider to watch your lipid levels by testing them every twelve weeks. Watch for changes. If there is a concerning increase, work with your provider or health coach to make dietary adjustments.

- GALLBLADDER ISSUES: If you don't have a gallbladder or you have gallstones and you eat too much fat, you can trigger a gallbladder attack or experience nausea and vomiting. Fortunately, there are a lot of ways to mitigate the risks. In fact, I've had many patients who've had gallstones or their gallbladder removed who do very well in ketosis. But you will want to work with a health coach who can moderate your fat intake so you're getting the right amount at the right time.

- EATING DISORDERS: If you currently have, or have had, an eating disorder, an eating plan such as the keto diet where you are counting and limiting carbs could retrigger eating issues. Depending on where you are in your healing, it may be best to avoid a ketogenic diet altogether and focus on the other tools in the new Alzheimer's toolkit. Or, working with a well-trained health coach may help guide you in reestablishing a healthy relationship to food in general and starting a ketogenic diet, if that is a healthy choice for you.

- TYPE 1 DIABETES: If you are insulin dependent, keep in mind that following the keto diet can change your blood glucose levels and subsequently how much insulin you need. While type 1 diabetes is not a contraindication for the keto diet, it is definitely a condition that should be monitored by a healthcare provider who can help you adjust your insulin supply as needed.
- KIDNEY DISEASE: When you switch to burning fat for fuel, you may experience changes in your mineral balance. This can be an issue for someone with kidney disease because your kidneys are responsible for filtering toxins and balancing electrolytes and minerals. Additionally, eating too much protein can put a strain on your kidneys. On the flip side, reducing your sugar intake has the potential to improve kidney function. If you've been told you have stage three kidney disease or above, work closely with a healthcare provider to determine if the ketogenic diet makes sense for you, and what modifications you might need to make to support your kidneys.
- PREGNANCY OR BREASTFEEDING: I recommend avoiding the ketogenic diet while pregnant or breastfeeding. Building a baby and producing breastmilk requires carbohydrates. Additionally, the mobilization of toxins that could be passed to a baby at such a vulnerable time is too big a risk.

Ketogenic Diet FAQs

Why am I not getting into ketosis?

It can take anywhere from about three days to three weeks to get into ketosis when you're first getting started. The more carb-loaded your diet was before starting keto, the more sugar stores you'll need to burn through before switching to burning ketones. Also, your body might be rusty at running on fat, and it can take a little time for it to restore its metabolic flexibility.

A helpful starting point is to look over your Progress Tracker sheets to see if you may be consuming more added sugars or carbs than you realize. For example, some vegetables, such as broccoli and asparagus, are higher in carbs than greens and zucchini. You may need to limit these starchier vegetables if you're having trouble getting into ketosis.

Other factors that may increase blood sugar and interfere with ketone production are not getting enough sleep or exercise, and experiencing too much stress. And lastly, are you eating enough fat? A common mistake people make when they first go on a keto diet is cutting down on carbs without replacing those calories with adequate fats. Starting your day with a spoonful of coconut oil (unless you have the APOE4 gene variant, see page 156) can help nudge you into ketosis. Adding exogenous ketones can help push your ketone levels up as well in the beginning.

Do I really need to stop eating all fruit?

It depends. Some people can pop a few berries and not derail their metabolic state—I've found that I can have about six raspberries and still stay in ketosis, for example, but any more than that knocks me out of it. Other people find that even a few berries contain too many grams of carbohydrates for their bodies to maintain ketosis.

I advise avoiding all fruit until you've been in ketosis consistently for two weeks. Then you can start trying foods on the Phase 2 list, which include many fruits such as apples, blackberries, kiwi, and watermelon. Again, if you're able to snack on those fruits and stay in ketosis, then you're good. However, if your ketone reading shows that you're below 1 mmol, you'll probably need to cut back on the fruit.

One thing you can try is to spread out your fruit consumption throughout the day. Add a few blueberries in yogurt in the morning and have a couple of apple slices later in the day. Sometimes, if you don't have a bowlful all at once, you can stay in ketosis because you won't induce a blood sugar spike.

Are you saying fruit isn't healthy?

No. Fruit is a wonderful, healthy, unprocessed way to get carbohydrates and beneficial nutrients when you are not in ketosis. However, including multiple servings of fruit in your daily diet will likely prevent you from achieving ketosis.

How does the diet affect the medications I'm taking?

I've seen patients' health improve so dramatically that they no longer need many of the medications they've been taking for years. With lowered blood pressure and cholesterol levels, and improved insulin production, you run the risk of being overmedicated if you continue to take drugs for these conditions at the same dosages.

Check in with your doctor if you are taking medication for any health condition to see if you need an adjusted dosage or can stop taking it altogether.

Even people who are on antidepressants may find that their depression subsides or their mood stabilizes. Part of the brain benefits of the ketogenic diet is that it supports neurotransmitter synthesis. You may find that the medication that was once helpful in terms of your mood is now making you tired or manic.

Also, if you're on a stimulant antidepressant like Wellbutrin, you may need to switch to a nonstimulant if you find that you're losing too much weight. Bottom line: Check in with your health provider to discuss medication management while on the diet.

When can I start adding Phase 2 foods?

You can start adding Phase 2 foods when you've been consistently in the zone of 1 to 3 mmol of ketones for two weeks. Adding these foods will make the diet feel a little less restrictive, helping you stay on it longer. However, you should introduce foods such as apples, berries, nuts, and lentils slowly, making sure to test your blood sugar and ketone levels to see if these foods drop your ketone levels below 1 mmol. If they do, you can try eating smaller portions or spreading them out throughout the day. For example, try eating a few apple slices instead of an entire apple.

What if I'm a vegetarian or a vegan?

If you're a vegetarian, I highly recommend the book *The Ketotarian* by Dr. Will Cole. He does a great job of making keto accessible for vegetarians. One thing you should do is add nuts from the Phase 2 food list (see page 310) to your diet right from the start to ensure you're getting adequate protein.

If you're vegan, keto is still doable. However, I don't recommend staying in keto too long. Ketosis can become unhealthy for those following a strict vegan diet over time. It is very easy to become nutrient deficient when your diet is limited because you're restricting carbs and all animal products. I suggest following a keto diet for about a week at a time. You'll still experience cognitive benefits. And if you're a vegan or vegetarian, make sure you're taking supplemental B vitamins, especially B12. B12 is found only in animal products and is essential to the function of the central nervous system, the brain, and DNA synthesis.

What to Eat When You're Cycling Out of Ketosis

Whether you're seeking to reverse or prevent cognitive decline, your goal is not to stay in ketosis permanently. Your ultimate goal is to reestablish metabolic flexibility, where you are able to switch your fuel source from glucose to ketones, and back again, fairly quickly. That means you do want to have regular periods of time when you are burning glucose—and that means upping your carb intake during these times.

That being said, you don't want to go on big carb binges or revert to a carb-laden lifestyle, because then you'll undo more of the benefits of the time you do spend in ketosis. It will also make it more difficult to get back into ketosis when you're ready. When you're not in keto, it's time to loosen the reins but not go wild. If you do want to have some of your favorite foods, like pizza or ice cream, it's okay—just make them the exception, not the rule.

The list of Phase 3 foods on page 311 is the perfect place to look for foods to add to your regular rotation during periods when you are not seeking to be in ketosis so that you stay in a healthy eating pattern. They include a variety of fruits, beans, grains, and starchy vegetables. For a broader framework, Paleo, the Mediterranean diet, or Whole30 are good eating plans to follow when you're not on keto. All three diets are anti-inflammatory, and they include lots of healthy proteins, fats, and vegetables while limiting processed foods and sugars.

Connection over Correction

Here are some suggestions on how to communicate compassionately to your loved one so that your transition to a new eating pattern goes smoothly.

Introducing the Idea

As I've mentioned, if your loved one has dementia or mild cognitive impairment, they should aim to be in ketosis for three to six months in order to give their brain some time to heal. However, don't lead with that! Some things you can say:

- "It's an experiment. Let's see how things go."
- "Let's start with three days or a week."
- "We don't have to follow this diet forever."

Then, once you've sold them on trying it, focus on all the delicious, nourishing foods they can eat—don't dwell on the restrictions. Emphasize how filling and satisfying the meals will be, and how much fun it will be to try new foods together.

Sticking to the Diet

It's one thing to agree to try the keto diet, and another thing to stick with it. Make it as easy as possible to eat keto throughout the day by removing any sugary treats or carb-heavy foods from the house. If it's not there, it's a lot harder to eat it. Even better is if everyone in the household is following the diet—it will not only make it easier to prepare and eat meals together, but also, the ketogenic diet is good for everyone else's brain, too! Go on the journey and reap the benefits together.

In fact, one of the best activities you can do while on this diet is cook together. When cooking, get them involved in safe activities such as peeling vegetables or drizzling olive oil on salads. Make it fun and engaging, with music and good conversation. The more they're invested in the meal, the more likely they'll eat it.

As for what to say to encourage your loved one to try new-to-them foods, try things like:

- "I found this recipe that sounds truly delicious—I can't wait for us to try it."
- "Will you help me get dinner ready? I could use another set of hands."
- "I've heard that this is so-and-so's favorite thing to eat for breakfast." (Mention someone your loved one thinks highly of.)

Celebrations

Food and celebrations go together—typically our celebratory foods are sweet and starchy. One way to stay keto even on a special occasion is to flip the script on having a big family meal and suggesting that you celebrate with an experience—going on a hike, visiting a spa, or maybe singing some karaoke. Of course, you can still eat at these alternative festivities. But instead of cakes, cookies, and chips, come together over nourishing, delicious, and brain-healing foods—such as fresh fruit salad, keto avocado chocolate mousse, or coconut keto ice cream.

Here are some ways to talk about your alternative plans:

- "I've found a scrumptious dessert recipe that fits our new eating plan—I can't wait for us to try it at the party!"
- "Let's celebrate by doing something special that we don't typically get to do. I want us to make some memories in honor of this day."
- "Let's celebrate by feeding our brain something that makes it very happy."

Of course, sometimes cake happens. It's okay. Just forgive yourself and everyone else and get back to eating keto at the next meal.

Differences Between the Keto and MIND Diet

Many people have heard that the best diet for protecting cognition is the MIND diet. I stand by the keto diet as the best choice for your brain, but let's take a look at these two eating plans side by side in order to clear up any confusion.

The MIND diet is an eating plan that was designed to reduce risk of developing dementia and slow the progression of cognitive decline. It combines the Mediterranean and the DASH diets—both recognized as heart-healthy diets—into one. I can see how eating heart-healthy foods such as green leafy vegetables and olive oil, and reducing inflammatory foods, such as sugar and processed foods, instead of indulging in the standard American diet can be beneficial for your heart and health. However, the diet still allows significantly higher levels of carbohydrates in the form of whole and processed grains and fruit than the keto diet, and it allows for up to five servings of pastries and sweets a week. That's still quite a bit of added sugar to your diet on a weekly basis. You will also never get the metabolic benefits of ketosis on the MIND diet.

Sure, switching to the MIND or Mediterranean diet from a diet chock-full of unhealthy processed foods and sugar can help support your health. Yet even the level of processed carbohydrates and sugar allowed on the MIND, and even the Mediterranean and DASH diets, for that matter, can be detrimental to your cognitive health.

Also, the MIND diet recommends limiting salt in an effort to reduce blood pressure. Good sea salt can be an important source of trace minerals—especially for older women who need the support for their bones. Unless you have salt-sensitive hypertension, your body needs the minerals in sea salt, which include potassium, strontium, boron, and silicon, for balance and modulating blood pressure. (If you or your care partner has salt-sensitive hypertension, follow your doctor's guidance.)

Beyond all that, the MIND diet just doesn't appear to be effective at protecting and promoting cognition: A controlled trial that followed more than six hundred participants over three years found no difference in effectiveness than a slightly calorie-restricted diet.

And lastly, the keto diet can do more than reduce your risk of dementia. Giving your brain its preferred fuel source, ketones, can heal your brain and reverse decline. It's exciting to see people on the keto diet get their cognition back.

Similarities
Both include plenty of:

- Green, leafy, cruciferous, and other low-carb vegetables
- Poultry and fish
- Olive oil
- Red meat (although the MIND diet recommends limiting consumption to fewer than four servings a week)
- Nuts and seeds

Both recommend limiting or abstaining from alcohol.
Both help control blood glucose levels and can help with weight loss.

Differences
The MIND diet recommends limiting butter and whole-fat dairy, while the keto diet includes eating butter and whole-fat dairy.

The MIND diet encourages eating whole grains such as brown rice and wild rice, fruits, and starchy vegetables, while the keto diet restricts carbohydrates to 30 to 50 grams a day.

The MIND diet sets limits on certain foods—the approved foods on the keto diet are unlimited.

On the MIND diet, your brain is still using glucose as its primary fuel; on the keto diet, your brain uses ketones as fuel, which is your brain's preferred energy source.

Why Keto Is Superior When It Comes to Preventing Cognitive Decline
While both diets are healthier than the standard American diet and can help reduce your risk of heart disease, the MIND diet has carbohydrates

(at least three servings a day) and occasional sweets, and the ketogenic diet does not. Research shows that diets high in refined carbohydrates can negatively impact cognitive function in a variety of ways. And even eating healthy carbohydrates inhibits your ability to produce those brain-boosting fatty ketones that your body needs to get into ketosis. That said, the MIND diet does provide a healthy framework for eating during those times when you're not seeking to be in ketosis.

To watch a summary video of this chapter and download the Reversing Alzheimer's workbook go to ReversingAlzheimersBook.com.

Reflection questions:
- What resources and supplies do you need to embark on a keto eating plan?
- When can you devote some time to looking at recipes, shopping, and preparing food?
- What are your goals for eating keto? How long are you committing to eating a keto diet?

CHAPTER 8

Foster Cognition
with Activities

You've heard me say that brain health is use it or lose it—if you don't fire the neurons, they don't create connections. While the tools in the new Alzheimer's toolkit that we've covered this far have absolutely been supportive of brain health, they haven't targeted cognitive function in particular. In this chapter, we're covering the tools that are essentially bicep curls for your brain. These are activities that require you to use your noggin.

There are so many possibilities for how you'll incorporate the activities aspect of the Reversing Alzheimer's protocol into your life. I'm going to share as many of these possibilities as I can in this chapter—my point in doing so is not to imply that you should be doing them all! It's to provide plenty of options so that you can find the ones that appeal to you. Think of this as a brainstorming chapter. In fact, figuring out what combination of activities you'll commit to doing on a regular basis going forward is an exercise in creativity and brain engagement in and of itself. You'll be starting to flex your muscles in this category before you even pick up your first activity.

Here's the key takeaway for this chapter: Fun is key for brain function. Too many of us don't allow ourselves to do the types of activities I'm presenting in this chapter. It's all too common to feel like you have to complete all your obligations before you do things that are seemingly "just for fun." But as you'll learn, carving out time for these activities can do far more than nourish your brain—it can enrich your life. This chapter isn't about adding to your to-do list—it's about pursuing activities that you enjoy *and* that stimulate your mind. Take, for example, my client David, whose entire life opened up, thanks to one new activity he decided to pursue.

David came to see me when he was in his early sixties and at a low point. His mother's Alzheimer's had progressed to the point that she needed live-in care. David, who had had an illustrious career in teaching at the collegiate level, was out of a job. He had recently split up with his wife and felt that he had lost a lot of friends in the divorce. Now he was moving to San Diego, where his mother had retired and he knew no one. In addition, he was moving back in with his mom—not exactly an ego boost at this stage of his life. On top of everything, he was worried about developing dementia himself later in life, and he knew that the stress of caregiving made him an even more likely candidate for experiencing the same fate as his mother.

When we first started working together, David had high blood pressure, an underactive thyroid, and depression. We addressed his diet, got him on a regimen of supplements, and got him exercising more: David loved walking while listening to podcasts; he also got into strength-training and attending a weekly yoga class. Much to David's credit, he read one of the handouts I provided him that listed "Try something new" as a brain-health-promoting strategy. He decided to start learning Spanish using the language-learning app Duolingo.

When David came in six months later for a follow-up, he told me that he'd started meeting up with people to practice his Spanish in person. At the visit after that, he shared that he'd met a Spanish-speaking woman and they were dating. His ticking the box of "learning something new," and just doing a language program on his phone, had helped usher him into a whole new life. He and his girlfriend went out dancing, they traveled, and they had a community of friends. Best of all, he is so much happier. Now I struggle to get him into the office because his life is so full! (In other news, his mom is still with us, and still living at home, as was her wish to age in place.)

I can't guarantee that reading this chapter and doing one or more of the things I suggest here will result in a similar whole-life transformation for you, but I do know that committing to doing at least some of the ideas in this chapter can do a lot more than help you stay sharp (or recover lost function). It can help you have fun, express yourself, and perhaps even meet people. And, just maybe, change your life.

The Importance of Fun

In the research, the things I'm covering in this chapter are called *cognitive leisure activities*. That's just a fancy way of saying things that both stimulate your brain and are just for fun. Cognitive leisure activities have been found to be protective against cognitive decline: A 2016 meta-analysis of nineteen studies found a significant connection between regular participation in cognitively stimulating leisure activities and a reduced risk of cognitive decline later in life. It also found a positive correlation between the types of activities I cover in this chapter and memory, processing speed, executive function, as well as a slower rate of cognitive decline. An Icelandic study followed nearly three thousand older people for five years and assessed how different types of activities impacted their risk of developing dementia. It found that all categories of leisure activities were associated with a lower risk of developing cognitive decline, and that association became significant when the activity was cognitively engaging (whether performed alone or with a group) or creative. This study also found that the more frequently participants met up with family and friends, the lower their risk of cognitive impairment. What I take from these findings is that it's not enough just to challenge your brain—you need to make space for fun and companionship, too.

As I intimated earlier, fun is a key part of the equation, because it is what helps you stay out of defend mode, even as you're doing things that protect and challenge your brain. When you are having fun, you increase cognitive flexibility, improve attention, and are able to access more resources for processing and retaining information. In other words, fun can help you cope. This is wonderful news on any day, but when you're engaged in caregiving and feeling like you don't have any extra time and attention left over for anything that's not urgent, it's even more helpful.

The goal of this chapter is to nudge you into making time and space in your own life for enjoyable activities that can also strengthen cognition—whether you're caring for someone with dementia or you're seeking to prevent it for yourself. If you are a caregiver, you'll want to find an activity or two that your care partner will enjoy. Perhaps there are some you can do together. But you still need your own leisure, as prevention is vitally important for you, too.

From here on out, I'm breaking up the activities into categories: creativity, mindfulness, community, cognitive challenges, purpose and meaning, and health. I'll cover options in each of the categories, and at the end of this chapter, I'll also illuminate how you can choose activities that cover multiple categories and aims at once.

I've also broken out the possibilities according to cognitive state—whether your goal is prevention, you have mild cognitive impairment, or your loved one has severe dementia. Because you really want to stay in the sweet spot of being on your cognitive edge—you don't want activities that are either too easy or too challenging.

Creativity

Creativity has positive impacts on mood, stress, and anxiety for everyone. It encourages alternative ways of thinking, which makes you more adaptable and resourceful. Doing things with your hands can also be meditative and help to foster the state of concentration and absorption known as flow. And that's all before you factor in the joy, self-expression, and fulfillment creativity can bring.

Some creative pursuits are very quick, such as sitting down to play a song at the piano, or to write a letter, or to do a little coloring or drawing after dinner. Others require either some prep, or some cleanup, or both. You may need to order some supplies online and then devote some space in your home to making them easily accessible and providing an area to get your creativity on. I hope that you will find something that appeals to you and run with it. Because novelty is an important part of brain health, keep finding new ways to vary what you do so that you stay on that edge of doing new things.

If you want to get even more out of your creative endeavors, make something for someone you love. That way, you get the benefit of using your mind creatively and the physical and emotional rewards of doing something for someone else, which include lower blood pressure, and higher serotonin, dopamine, and oxytocin—basically, you're lighting up the brain's reward circuitry.

Even though I've made these suggestions of different activities for differing levels of cognitive function, I've absolutely seen patients with very low MoCA scores gain new skills over time—that's the power of doing creative activities regularly!

Art

FOR PREVENTION: Take a class in a new style of art—such as a ceramics class using the wheel; make a bird feeder out of wood; try dot painting; take photographs using a different style camera than you are used to; make stop-motion animation videos; try Zentangles (a good way for people who don't feel artistic to make—and experience the benefits of making—art); join your local arts association and gain access to classes, community, and maybe even an opportunity to show your work.

FOR REVERSAL OF MILD COGNITIVE IMPAIRMENT: Try DIY craft projects or wood models (do a search on Etsy or Amazon—we find many, many activities for Marama residents this way); do a tape art project; revisit a form of art making that you used to enjoy, whether that's watercolors, knitting, or crochet.

FOR REVERSAL OF DEMENTIA: Arrange flowers; paint; color; make pinecone birdfeeders; play with Play-Dough; paint with Do-a-Dot painters; wind balls of yarn; try needlepoint kits for beginners with big, nonsharp needles and thick thread.

Cooking

FOR PREVENTION: Research a new-to-you ingredient or cuisine and find recipes you want to try; take a cooking class; go to an ethnic market and select some new ingredients that inspire you; try a new cooking method (such as using a Moroccan tagine, air fryer, or pressure cooker);

start a supper club where you rotate hosting and cooking for a small group, which has the added benefit of creating community.

FOR REVERSAL OF MILD COGNITIVE IMPAIRMENT: Cook recipes you haven't made in a long time; learn new recipes in a cuisine you're already familiar with (such as enchiladas instead of tacos); try a new recipe for your favorite cooking appliance (something new for the grill or the slow cooker).

FOR REVERSAL OF DEMENTIA: Help select recipes that sound good to eat; taste the food as it's being cooked; measure; peel; stir.

Gardening

FOR PREVENTION: Plan a new garden bed, cutting garden, or veggie garden; try out new growing techniques (such as trellises, cold frames, or a simple irrigation system); plant a new vegetable and experiment with different ways to serve it.

FOR REVERSAL OF MILD COGNITIVE IMPAIRMENT: Select seeds and plants out of a catalog or a plant store; plant plants; weed; water.

FOR REVERSAL OF DEMENTIA: Care for a houseplant; start seeds indoors and keep them watered; harvest fruits and veggies.

Stories

FOR PREVENTION: Embark on writing your life story (or the great American novel); experiment with new forms of poetry; take a writing class; share something you've written at an open-mic night; make a scrapbook for your loved one with dementia; memorize a new poem each month.

FOR REVERSAL OF MILD COGNITIVE IMPAIRMENT: Write a letter to someone you love; start a pen-pal relationship with a far-flung relative or friend via electronic or snail mail; read or listen to the audio versions of memoirs of people you admire; relearn a poem you once knew by heart; create a digital photography book (use a service like Shutterfly, or visit your local CVS pharmacy, which offers simple make-it-yourself photobooks).

FOR REVERSAL OF DEMENTIA: Prompt your loved one by asking them questions about their life—even the stories you already know—and then write down their stories; use a magnetic poetry set to write poems; reminisce while looking through scrapbooks and reading old letters.

Music

FOR PREVENTION: Learn a new instrument; sign up for a music class; join a band; write a song; improvise on an instrument you already know how to play.

FOR REVERSAL OF MILD COGNITIVE IMPAIRMENT: Pick up an instrument you used to play; practice songs you used to know; learn new songs on a familiar instrument; write a song or collaborate on writing a song.

FOR REVERSAL OF DEMENTIA: Sing along to old favorites; play a simple instrument—such as the tambourine or maracas—along with a recording or with someone else who is playing the song.

Brain Engagement

This is the category that most people think of when they think of cognition-protective strategies—particularly things like crosswords, Sudoku, word finds, and digital brain-testing apps. While these activities can be useful tools, they're not that exciting or fun, and they are solitary activities. Plus, especially with crosswords, Sudoku, and word finds, if you've been doing them for a long time, you're not getting better at them and you're not creating new neuronal pathways as a result. The brain apps can be helpful, particularly because they are designed to identify your weaknesses and progressively challenge you to get better at them. But I'd rather you focus on activities that get you interacting with others, outside, engaging your senses, and learning new things, rather than being parked in front of a screen. (If you're going to do something on a screen, I suggest making it a language-learning app, so that you can put those skills to use interacting with other people out in the world, as David did.)

There are many other ways to enhance your cognition, as you'll see in my list of suggestions just below.

FOR PREVENTION: Learn a new language, whether using an app such as Duolingo or a class; learn how to code; learn new software programs or learn to use AI; force yourself to balance your checkbook or calculate the tip at dinner without using a calculator; when you encounter some kind of a problem around the house, such as a broken dishwasher, challenge yourself to do an internet search to guide you to fix it yourself; go to an escape room or murder mystery theater, or host an at-home mystery party with a mystery in a box (from companies such as Hunt a Killer or My Mystery Party); do challenging jigsaw puzzles; take an improv class; learn a new card game and start playing (like bridge, bunko, or poker); use a cognition-enhancing app (such as Brain HQ or Lumosity); host board game nights with friends and/or family.

FOR REVERSAL OF MILD COGNITIVE DECLINE: Keep doing whatever puzzles and games you've always done, and try out new types, too (if you've loved crosswords, try Wordle or Words with Friends, for example); use a cognition-enhancing app (such as Brain HQ or Lumosity); if you know a second language, find opportunities to speak it more frequently; aim to deepen any skills you already have—learn a new stitch in knitting, or master some new knots if you're a sailor; watch murder mystery movies and try to read the clues and guess the killer; play games you already know well with friends and/or family.

FOR SEVERE COGNITIVE DECLINE: Get out a typewriter and some envelopes and have your care partner "pay bills" (even though you've already paid them online); get out safe tools for handywork around the house, such as taking apart simple electronics; start conversations on topics your loved one knows well and encourage their contribution; use brain-enhancement apps (such as Brain HQ or Lumosity); play familiar, simple board games such as Chutes and Ladders or card games such as Uno or Crazy Eights; do jigsaw puzzles.

Community Building

I knew intellectually how important having a sense of community and connection was to health. Social isolation is, after all, one of the modifiable risk factors for dementia, according to *The Lancet*. But when we experienced our first resident to test positive with Covid in 2022, I witnessed irrefutable evidence of how crucial social connection is for well-being. As it happened, we decided to isolate residents from one another for ten days in order to limit the spread. (Residents still saw caregivers one-on-one, but none of their peers.) Thankfully, the isolation worked to curtail the spread of Covid—no other resident tested positive. But that isolation took other tolls. Three residents fell. Four developed new or worsening incontinence. Many started wandering at night, and every single resident experienced measurable declines in cognition. It took ten weeks to get back to baseline. The only thing that changed was that the residents were no longer interacting with one another or receiving visits from their families. That's how much we need to be with other humans.

It can be challenging to get your loved one the social interaction they need to be their best if their dementia is significant. Especially if they are older, as many of their peers and even family members may have died.

This is where committing to an activity with a communal component can really fill a void. Having a book group, a regular card game, or a volunteer commitment; going out on walks and chatting with neighbors along the way; or attending a class or adult day care at a senior center are all perfect opportunities to get that social connection.

Loneliness and social isolation have been determined to be as harmful to your health as smoking fifteen cigarettes a day. It is significantly associated with premature death, cardiovascular disease, elevated cortisol, an upregulation of inflammatory genes, depression, and, yes, dementia. Conversely, the less isolated you are, the better your health outcomes—such as blood pressure, inflammation, and cognitive function—tend to be. Truly, for overall health and brain health, it's absolutely vital to spend time in the company of others.

Insurance companies are recognizing how many of the chronic—and expensive—diseases of aging are associated with social isolation, and they are starting to devote effort—and money—toward keeping people engaged in social activities. One company, Grouper, reimburses clubs for every activity that their members participate in, helping to bring down the cost of membership. (See the Resources section for guidance on how to find clubs near you that have been subsidized by Medicare insurance through Grouper—some are even online, such as bridge leagues, so if you or your care partner are homebound, you can still experience the benefits of connecting with others.)

Community is a positive X factor—any activity in this chapter that you can do in the company of others will deliver considerably more benefit compared to doing them on your own. If you don't have a lot of time for activities, get the most bang for your buck by choosing something you can do with others.

FOR PREVENTION: Find a new hobby, such as sailing (taking a class can help connect you to other beginners who will be open to opportunities to practice); form or join a club, such as a regular mah-jongg, bunko, or poker game; join guided tours when you travel (such as Road Scholar, or your university's alumni association); start attending a regular class; participate in trivia nights and get to know the regulars there; make time to connect with friends and family members regularly—it's just as important, if not more important, than accomplishing some task; chat with people in line with you at the pharmacy or with the clerk at the grocery store.

FOR MILD COGNITIVE IMPAIRMENT: Check out your local community or senior center or library and find the community within the community—the tai chi class where people visit with each other afterward, or the mystery book club; consider adopting a dog and taking it to the dog park at a regular time of day to make friends with the other dog parents there.

FOR DEMENTIA: Check into adult day care options at your local community and senior centers; help them write letters to anyone they like (then you'll have extra incentive to get them to walk at least as far as the mailbox every day, to check for a response).

Mindfulness and Meditation

Mitch and Maggie are a husband and wife whom I met when they enrolled in one of my online coaching programs. Maggie had midrange dementia, with a MoCA score in the midteens, and Mitch was her caregiver. Mitch was struggling to get Maggie to change her diet, exercise, and do her Brain HQ. But she was open to doing the Kirtan Kriya meditation I always suggest to new patients, so Mitch made it his number one priority to make sure they did it every day.

After a couple of weeks, Mitch came on our coaching call and said, "I can feel my brain changing." He noticed that he was feeling a lot less scattered and a lot more focused. Maggie seemed sharper, too—she was responding quicker when asked a question. Most importantly, she was less resistant to the other things Mitch suggested. As a result, they were both feeling more connected, and Mitch felt he had more capacity to be creative and understanding when Maggie did dig her heels in about something. Their relationship was better than ever. They were both less stressed during the day, which meant fewer arguments. Everything just felt a little easier. Mitch described the Kirtan Kriya as opening up some kind of lock that he hadn't been able to pick before.

I love Mitch and Maggie's story especially because it so beautifully shows how you get extra benefit when you and your care partner meditate together—you each get more relaxed, which then helps the rest of the day go more smoothly, and your connection can grow stronger.

I'm also not surprised by their story, as I credit meditation with being one of the most powerful tools I've used over the last twenty years to guide me and steady me at various turning points. At one point I really sat down to evaluate all the things I've done to take care of my mind—such as seeing therapists, journaling, and attending retreats. That's when I realized that meditation is the thing that has provided the maximum return on my investment of time and money. So I committed to meditating every day—not just as a way to cope during times of high stress, but as a way to optimize every day. After about twelve months of daily practice, I've noticed a massive amount of change in how I respond to things. My days are so much smoother. I take things less personally and can more easily be creative and productive. And when I don't complete something I set out to do, I feel much less angst about it. I feel it makes me a better parent because I'm less reactive. For caregivers in particular, the ability to calm the mind, create space, and think creatively is valuable and powerful.

Meditation in general has been shown to have truly mind-boggling impacts on overall health and brain health in particular. On the health front, it can lower or decrease blood pressure, inflammation, the perception of pain, symptoms of irritable bowel syndrome, post-traumatic stress disorder, and fibromyalgia. It can also help individuals overcome addictions. More specifically to the brain, meditation has been shown to increase overall brain volume, and the thickness of the lining of the hippocampus. It has also been shown to decrease thickness in areas of the brain associated with emotional reactivity and rumination. It also enhances brain function by increasing focus, attention, and memory.

Kirtan Kriya is what our residents at Marama do, too. Where in other sections of this chapter I've suggested different activities for different levels of cognitive function, for mindfulness, I recommend that everyone do Kirtan Kriya. It's just so simple, and it has an active component that makes it easier to do even on days when you feel your mind is moving in a million different directions. It also has an impressive trail of research that demonstrates its effectiveness in people with cognitive decline and their caregivers. In these populations, regular practice of the Kirtan Kriya has been shown to increase memory, improve sleep, and decrease depression and anxiety. Fascinatingly, it has also been shown to beneficially alter the way our genes are expressed—down-regulating inflammatory genes while upregulating genes that influence the immune system and that regulate levels of glucose and insulin.

A common thing I hear from people after I've suggested they try Kirtan Kriya is a concern that it's against their religion. But meditation isn't a religious practice or a prayer, it's a tool that helps quiet the mind and makes you calmer, clearer, and more aware. It changes your physiology away from attack and defend and toward rest and repair. That being said, it's also not for everyone. If you just can't get behind the idea of doing the Kirtan Kriya, there are plenty of other ways to get into a more mindful state, many of which I've listed in the examples below.

EXAMPLES: Bible or other holy text study, breath work, gratitude meditation, guided meditations (from apps such as Headspace, Calm, or Insight Timer), Kirtan Kriya, journaling, mindfulness meditation, prayer, yoga nidra.

As I covered in Chapter 5 on the value of creating a daily routine, meditation is a great addition to your morning routine, for a few reasons. First, it ties meditating to something you already do without a lot of thought—such as brushing your teeth or having your first hot beverage—which makes remembering to do it more seamless. Second, meditating in the morning, before the day really gets going (and may get away from you), makes it more likely that you will actually meditate on a regular basis. And third, meditating in the morning positively influences the rest of your day, as Mitch and Maggie's story illustrates so well.

If the morning doesn't work for you, meditating as part of your wind-down routine at night is also beneficial—it helps you shed the stresses of your day so that you can be in a more receptive state for sleep.

Another resistance I often hear—particularly from my own mom—is "it's too hard to sit still, I can't quiet my mind." It's normal to feel this way. And feeling like your thoughts are racing is a sign that you stand to gain a tremendous amount from meditation. Even if you try and feel like nothing is happening, something *is* happening. You are retraining your brain.

KIRTAN KRIYA INSTRUCTIONS

The Kirtan Kriya is a structured form of meditation that combines vocalization with hand gestures. During the meditation, you'll repeat the syllables "saa," "taa," "naa," and "maa" over and over again while touching a different finger to your thumb. This little bit of movement helps you stay present. And the syllables are drawn from the Sanskrit mantra "sat nam," which means "true identity."

While I'm including the instructions for performing Kirtan Kriya here, I find the easiest way to do it is to follow along with a YouTube video—I've included a link to my favorite in the Resources section.

» Sit in a comfortable position with your spine tall and your hands resting in your lap.

» Close your eyes.

» As you sing "saa," bring the index finger of each hand to touch your thumbs.

» As you sing "taa," touch your middle fingers to your thumbs.

» As you sing "naa," touch your ring fingers to your thumbs.

» As you sing "maa," bring your pinkies to your thumbs. All the while, imagine the sound flowing in through the very top of your head and moving out through the middle of your forehead (this gives you an added level of concentration).

» Continue this way, chanting each syllable out loud in full voice for two minutes.

» Next, whisper the syllables as you continue the hand motions for two minutes.

» Then repeat the sounds silently as you continue the hand motions for four minutes.

» Return to whispering the syllables (while continuing to do the hand motions) for two minutes.

» Finally, resume singing the syllables out loud for the final two minutes.

» At the end of the twelve-minute cycle, finish up by raising your arms over your head as you take a deep breath in, and then exhale as you let your arms sweep out and down to return to your lap.

Health Promoting

Some of the activities that help the brain be its best are more passive, but they are still valuable tools. The activities I list in this section work on promoting relaxation, detoxification, and cellular renewal. They do require purchasing a device. If cost is an issue, consider going in with another family so that you can share the cost, or choosing just one to start with for now and adding others as your budget allows.

- RED LIGHT THERAPY: We use two different types of red light therapy (which I cover in depth in Chapter 12) at Marama—a larger, full-body light to reduce inflammation and aches and pains and to promote blood flow all over the body, and a smaller one that is designed to target the brain that is worn on the head. (I include information on the specific products we use in the Resources section.) Our residents use both types of light five to six days per week, for about twenty minutes at a time. The brain-specific red light device can be used while you are engaged in other things, such as meditating, cooking, or doing a creative activity. The more general red light requires you to be stationary—you can use it while you read, meditate, or simply relax.

  Our staff—many of whom are in their mid-twenties—use the brain-specific red light, too, and they report that their perception of anxiety and stress goes down significantly after using it. You certainly don't need to be experiencing memory loss to get a benefit out of it.

  Because the red light mimics the light emitted at sunrise and sunset, it's ideal to use these devices in the morning or the evening.
- SAUNA BLANKET OR SAUNA CHAIR: These devices are a great way to work up a sweat and get rid of toxins. Compared to a traditional sauna, they take up very little space, use very little electricity, and are simple to clean and store. (See the Resources section for the brands I recommend as they are low in electromagnetic fields [EMFs] and volatile organic compounds [VOCs].) Using a sauna just before you exercise—even for ten minutes—will help you get your heart rate up faster and sweat more. When you first start using a sauna, it may take twenty or even thirty minutes before you break a sweat. As you begin using the sauna regularly, that amount of time needed to start sweating will come down.

Adding Meaning

Having a sense of purpose in life not only makes it easier to get out of bed in the mornings and to keep going during tough times—it also can protect against dementia. One study of more than nine hundred older people found that those who scored the highest on a purpose assessment were about 2.4 times less likely to get Alzheimer's than those who scored the lowest. Having a strong sense of purpose was also associated with a lower risk of developing mild cognitive impairment, and a slower rate of cognitive decline. Other studies have shown that engaging in purposeful activities—such as mentoring young children—is associated with larger hippocampal volume.

Even if your loved one already has advanced dementia, finding ways to infuse their activities with more meaning can amplify the benefits of those efforts.

There are two main ingredients to infusing your activities with more purpose—(1) taking on a bigger, longer-term commitment, and (2) helping others. Here's an example of what I mean: I have had the honor of working with a group of former professional football players—a population that is vulnerable to chronic traumatic encephalopathy (CTE), a disease of the brain that develops as a result of multiple head injuries and concussions; CTE is often accompanied by dementia. While we haven't studied CTE specifically, because we are doing so much to support the brain at the cellular level, it makes sense that Dr. Bredesen's approach that we use at Marama would be beneficial for professional athletes with a history of traumatic brain injuries. As part of their treatment plan, we discussed how they could amplify the benefits of their activities by committing to a longer-term project that incorporates an element of giving back. That's how we decided to reach out to local high school football teams to begin the process of establishing a mentorship program that would enable these NFL veterans to counsel their younger counterparts—and get some exercise along the way, too.

It needn't be this formal: A friend's mom who has some mild cognitive impairment enjoys checking in on neighbors in her senior living community. When someone returns from a trip to the hospital or a skilled nursing facility, she will coordinate a meal train for them and visit them to make sure they have everything they need, as well as enjoy some companionship. In so doing, she's creating an outlet for her nurturing energy. She's also keeping her brain sharp by exercising her planning and organizational skills and staying connected to her neighbors.

These two stories show how giving back and committing to a longer-term project can and should be customized to your interests and personalities. Of course, the scope of this project will vary according to cognitive health.

PREVENTION: Join a mentorship program or alumni organization; volunteer on a project with a specific goal (such as raising funds for a new library, or lobbying to pass a law on an issue you care about); if you're an animal lover, adopt a pet or agree to foster animals in need of a new home.

MILD COGNITIVE IMPAIRMENT: Make something for a grandchild, such as a scrapbook, recipe book, or knitted blanket; become a pen pal; care for a pet; tend a garden.

DEMENTIA: Care for a plant, fish, or pet; make cards for people who are sick, collect flowers and give them away.

Keep in mind that purpose isn't something you pay attention to only when your plate is clear and you have extra bandwidth—it's something that can help you cope with and grow from challenging circumstances. If your time, energy, and resources are truly limited, look for meaning in the things you do every day. Caring for a loved one may not feel purposeful in every moment, but when people look back on their caregiving experiences, they tend to view them as some of the most important and fulfilling times in their lives. Aim to remind yourself of the purpose that caregiving can provide.

Checking Many Boxes at Once

If you have read this far in the chapter and are wondering how on earth you're going to find time to do all these many different types of activities, know that you can meet multiple goals in one pursuit.

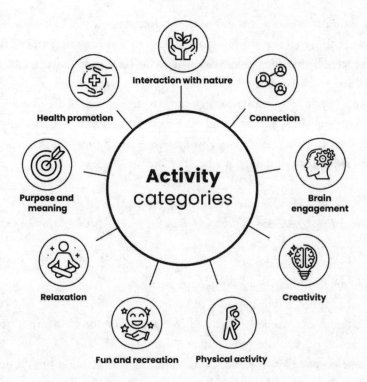

Whenever you feel strapped for time, prioritize activities that check multiple boxes. For example, if you've been doing cognition-enhancing apps or jigsaw puzzles, swap that out for something that stacks multiple interventions into one activity. Ballroom dancing includes community, touch, cognition-enhancement (learning steps as well as rhythm), and exercise. If you decide to train for a competition, you add purpose to the mix—even just wanting to show up so that you don't let your partner down can add a layer of purpose. Other fitness classes, such as Zumba, Pilates, yoga, tennis, and pickleball also add in those cognitive and social components. If you exercise outside with other people, you also get to check the nature box.

No two people will have the same roster of activities because there are so many variables that go into determining what will work best for you, including your current state of cognitive health, your degree of athleticism, and how much time and money you have available to devote. Finding the right activities mix is a choose-your-own adventure. The only thing you really shouldn't choose is to do nothing. Remember, you can always start with one thing that meets a lot of needs. Once you get started on one thing, you'll kick off that virtuous cycle, when you have more energy and more motivation to keep adding in new things as you go along.

If you need more inspiration, go back to the wheel of life exercise that you completed in Chapter 4 and take a good look at the scores you gave yourself for fun and recreation; think of an activity that will help you take better care of this vital part of a healthy, balanced, enjoyable life.

To watch a summary video of this chapter and download the Reversing Alzheimer's workbook go to ReversingAlzheimersBook.com.

Reflection questions:
- How much fun are you having currently?
- What kinds of activities sound fun to you?
- What activities would be easy and convenient for you to incorporate?
- What activities would provide maximum benefit?
- Where do you have wisdom, skills, and insight that might benefit others?
- Are there people who would benefit from your mentorship?
- What will keep you cognitively engaged, socially engaged, and maybe even physically engaged?

CHAPTER 9

Create a Brain-Nourishing Environment

When I first walked into the residential care facility that I would eventually convert into Marama, there were three televisions blaring in the common area—one was tuned to a twenty-four-hour news channel, one was showing an infomercial, and the third was showing a sporting event with loud whistles being blown every few minutes. I could hardly hear myself think! Beyond that, the scent in the air had the detectable undertones of eau de cleaning products—a mix of synthetic fragrance and bleach.

As I envisioned what this space could be, the TVs and the toxic-chemical-laced air were the first things I imagined gone, because stress and toxicity are the top two aspects of a home environment that influence brain health. The flip side of this truth is that a nontoxic, serene environment goes an incredibly long way toward supporting cognitive ability. When that environment is set up in a way that encourages a health-supportive routine, the work of taking care of your brain becomes a lot less effortful. You aren't tempted to turn on the TV, because it's not the main focus of the room, and there is plenty of space for enriching activities. The clear surfaces, natural light, and chemical-free air all help you get into a rest-and-digest state and out of defense mode. Your home becomes a source of support and renewal.

One of my patient's experiences really demonstrates the power of the environment to support healing. Bob had mild cognitive impairment, and his wife, Diane, really wanted them to travel while they still could. She booked a trip to Europe, and off they went. But the travel was very disorienting to Bob. He started having a lot of trouble finding the right words. He was on edge. He wasn't sleeping well. Bob also caught Covid while they were away, and it hit him hard—likely because the stress of being away from home had lowered his resilience. While he was ill, Bob was unsure of where he was. His words came out as gibberish. Diane feared that Bob was losing ground that he wouldn't be able to regain.

Once he was well enough to travel home, Diane got Bob back on the Reversing Alzheimer's plan—eating keto, getting regular exercise, and living in an environment where he could relax and rest. That's where he made his full recovery from Covid—and where his mental faculties returned. In fact, at their next visit, Diane shed tears of relief and told me, "I have my husband back!" At that visit, Bob even told me he'd heard that Viagra can protect the brain, and could I prescribe him some of that? (He's right—Viagra helps with blood flow to more parts of the body than just the genitals; it helps get more blood to the brain, too. However, the science is mixed, as one study found there was cognitive improvement with regular use and one refuted that claim.) Clearly, being back home in a stable, healthy environment and in his routine had made a big difference.

Bob's story shows how both disease and recovery from disease is affected by multiple inputs. Being in an unfamiliar environment, getting away from the ketogenic diet, plus getting exposed to a virus all worked together to set Bob's cognition back significantly. Being in a familiar and restorative environment, eating well, and returning to a daily routine got him back on track. While this story doesn't mean you should never travel once you're exhibiting some level of cognitive decline, it does show how your environment can dramatically influence your health. (A general rule of thumb is that the more severe the cognitive decline, the more important having a predictable and familiar environment is.)

Reducing Exposure and Promoting Renewal

As I've mentioned, the two main priorities of upgrading your environment are to reduce toxic exposure and to create surroundings that make it easy to relax, rest, and do the things that promote overall health.

You may not be thinking of your home as a potential source of contamination, but many threats may be lurking there. I don't want to alarm you, but the list of potential toxins within a home is long, and it includes mold, pet dander, chemical gases and particulate matter from cleaning products and fireplaces, and contaminated tap water, for starters. The hopeful aspect of this news is that you have so much potential to make your environment healthier. In fact, reducing any toxic exposures goes 75 percent of the way toward restoring health. We know that toxins are an important part of the Alzheimer's story. No matter how well you eat, how often you exercise, or how deeply you meditate, if you are exposed to some toxic actors every day of your life, your chances of being able to reverse Alzheimer's drops dramatically. You simply can't get truly better if you have to defend against contaminants every day.

In this chapter, I'll walk you through the action steps you should take on a room-by-room basis, so you know exactly what to do, and the reasons why those action steps deserve a spot on your to-do list, so that you also understand the reasoning.

Keep in mind that these actions can be done gradually, and once you do them, you don't have to keep doing them. They are one and done. Well, "one and done" is not entirely accurate. Everything in this chapter applies to the home of the person you're caring for, as well as your own home (if you live separately; if you and your care partner live together, it truly is one and done!). After all, you want to be able to reap all these benefits for yourself if you are the caregiver. So if you live in a separate home from your care partner, think of it as two and done.

I know that it costs more money and takes more time to evaluate the products you bring into your home from a nontoxic perspective. My hope is that by creating a simple checklist for every room in the house, a list you can gradually work your way through, this important effort will become a lot easier.

FIRST STEP: TAKING STOCK

To help you identify what in your home or your care partner's home needs attention, do a little mental inventory of what it's like today.

Is it comfortable?
Is it safe?
Is it enjoyable?
How much natural light does it get?
Is there a safe and enjoyable outdoor space?
What parts of the home are most relaxing?
What parts are most cluttered?

   Whatever your answers are, just note them without judgment. Make a list of the parts of the home that need attention. This will give you a starting point, and it will help you track your progress as you go.

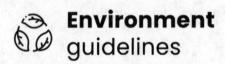

Environment guidelines

 Nontoxic

 Comfortable

 Incorporates nature

 Natural scents

 Natural light

 Few distractions

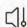 **Quiet, soothing sounds**

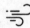 **Air quality**

 Uncluttered

Throughout the House

SAFETY FIRST: This is a process you'll likely have to revisit again and again. If you are caring for someone with significant cognitive decline, you want to make sure that you've removed trip hazards such as slippery rugs and exposed cords and made a plan to work around other things you can't remove, such as stairs, steps, and raised thresholds, shower edges, or sliding-door tracks. I've also included specific safety information for each room in the rest of the tips.

NATURAL ELEMENTS: Nature is incredibly soothing to the nervous system. For this reason, you want to give careful thought to how you can incorporate elements of nature throughout your home. That could mean changing the orientation of your seating or your desk so that you have a more direct view outside, bringing in more plants, hanging art that reflects the natural world, and using natural materials such as wood, wool, cotton, leather, and stoneware throughout your home. I also encourage you to make sure at least some windows open easily so that you can let in fresh air whenever the weather allows. Inviting in plenty of natural light is also extremely helpful, as natural light regulates the body's master clock, which then beneficially influences sleep, appetite, mood, and energy. You could perhaps get shades that open from the top down, so that you can allow light to come in at the top but still have privacy because the lower half of your windows are still covered. You can hang easy-to-open curtains so that you can whisk them shut at night and open in the morning.

AIR QUALITY: It's a sad truth that indoor air is typically significantly more contaminated than outdoor air. This is partly the reason why I suggest opening windows and doors whenever the weather allows—because not only does it invite nature into the house, it also flushes out stale, potentially contaminated air. Houseplants are also fantastic for cleaning indoor air—even very easy-to-grow versions, such as spider plants, snake plants, and aloe vera plants.

To cover the rest of your indoor-air-quality basics, I recommend investing in at least one air purifier that you can use in the room where you spend most of your time—typically the bedroom. Especially if you live in a colder climate, where you can't open the windows for long periods of time, if you have any inkling that you might have mold, if you live near a freeway or airport where there could be a lot of residue from petrochemicals in the air, if you have a pet that sheds, or if you simply notice that there is soot that accumulates on your windowsills or fan blades. (I share the air purifiers we use at Marama in the Resources section.) Whatever air purifier you buy, they are only as good as their filters are clean, so you'll need to replace those filters every few months. If you're thinking your HVAC system has a good-enough filter on it, make sure you're cleaning or changing that filter to keep it functioning the way it's designed.

If you have a fireplace, I recommend having it evaluated by a fireplace specialist to make sure it's properly sealed; otherwise, you run the likely risk of having particulate matter from the logs and the smoke getting in your indoor air and, thus, your lungs.

SCENTS: Avoid artificial scents—from things like plug-ins, candles, and air fresheners—as they are highly toxic and, thanks to the wiring of the olfactory system, can take a shortcut to the brain. The scents in your house should come from cooking, fresh flowers, air coming through open doors and windows whenever possible, and maybe essential oils (if you like those scents, they are by no means necessary).

DECLUTTER: We all have clutter—things pile up no matter how devoted you are to living minimally. The problem with clutter isn't that it doesn't look picture-perfect. It's that it tends to be overstimulating. It's like every item that's not put away represents a task that needs doing, and, even more taxing, a decision that needs to be made. It's very hard to relax when there is clutter around. Even if your home has been cluttered for years and you've gotten used to it, any items that are lying around are still cueing your nervous system that there are things that need tending to. Because it's happening every day, it's like constantly living with a low-grade stressor.

The great news is that decluttering reduces stress. To make decluttering easier, it's helpful to have at least three boxes or bags on hand as you start to declutter a room—one for things you'll donate, one for things you'll store, and one for trash and/or recycling.

Once you go through the items that are lying around, get rid of the things you don't need, and find a home for the things you do, you can relax more deeply whenever you're in that space.

For the items you keep that are used every day, give them a place to reside that's clearly visible—things like reading glasses or a wallet or purse. You can even label drawers and cabinets as reminders of what's being stored out of sight—this may help your loved one feel assured that the things they need are indeed there.

SOUND: Are there ways you can make the majority of sounds you can hear in your home soothing sounds? Set up a speaker to play calming music, perhaps get a water fountain in the yard to create the beautiful background sound of moving water, keep the television off except for rare occasions when you're watching a favorite show or movie (and don't leave the twenty-four-hour news station blaring all day).

The Kitchen: Source of Nourishment

The kitchen is where we feed ourselves and our loved ones; as such, the focus on optimizing this vital room is on removing sources of chemical contamination in items of cookware, food storage containers, and cleaning products, as well as organizing the fridge and pantry in such a way that eating a nutrient-dense, ketogenic diet is as easy as possible.

Your cookware is important because when pots and pans are heated, they can release toxic chemicals into your food. I know that nonstick pans are super convenient, but the chemicals used to make the nonstick coating are extremely toxic, and the coating is easily damaged by using metal spatulas or cooking spoons, so that pieces of it can flake off and get mixed in with your food. You also want to avoid cookware made with aluminum. While we don't know that aluminum contributes to Alzheimer's, it has been found within the tangles in the brains of people who have died with dementia. It makes sense to avoid it. The best choices for cookware are stainless steel and cast iron.

Plastic is the other material to eliminate as completely as possible from your kitchen. That includes cups, plates, food storage containers, utensils, and plastic wrap. Switch to glass storage containers (including Mason jars, which you can even use in the freezer), glass or ceramic cups and glasses (especially for those that will hold hot liquids), silicon storage bags, and beeswax-coated wraps instead of plastic bags and plastic wrap. Corelle is a highly durable and toxin-free form of glass—you can find plates, bowls, coffee cups, and some baking dishes made out of it. It also has the benefit of being lightweight and affordable.

From a safety perspective, fire and knives are the big risks in the kitchen. You may want to consider hiding the knobs on the stove, and any sharp knives, in a locked drawer to reduce the risk of injury or fire.

As for making it easy to stick to a healthy eating plan, get any highly processed, sugary foods at least out of sight, if not out of the house altogether. Put easy-to-grab snacks—such as a nuts, seeds, celery sticks, guacamole, flaxseed crackers, soups, and fat bombs—in clear containers either in a cupboard or in the fridge at eye level. "Eye level is buy level" is an apt phrase used by the food marketing industry because what we see, we tend to want. Food companies pay a premium for shelf placement that puts their products at eye level—use this tactic for good by making keto-friendly foods the first thing you see when you wander into the kitchen looking for a snack.

Helpful Cooking Appliances

These counter-sized appliances can make food prep a lot simpler and healthier:

- Air fryer (look for one made of stainless steel and avoid plastic)
- Instant Pot
- Spiralizer for making vegetable noodles
- Toaster oven (often included in the air fryer)

Kitchen Checklist

- Replace nonstick cookware with stainless steel, cast iron, or ceramic.
- Purge as much plastic as you can and use glass storage containers, silicon storage bags, beeswax-coated canvas food wrap, or Corelle dishes instead.
- Consider hiding knives and the knobs to the stove in a locked drawer.
- Make keto-friendly foods front and center and either give away or hide unhealthy foods.
- Replace conventional cleaning products with nontoxic versions each time you run out.

Water Quality

Water is a vital element for the body, which makes sense once you know that between 55 and 60 percent of your body is actually composed of water. In the brain, this percentage is significantly higher—it's 80 percent water. For that reason, you want your water to be as free of contaminants as possible. This means that drinking the water that comes out of your tap is probably not your best choice.

Of course, we don't want bacteria and other threats in our drinking water, but the typical chemical additives that most water suppliers put in the water—such as chlorine and fluoride-halogens—that are meant to protect our health can also add to our toxic burden. In addition, there are substances present in our public water supply that include toxic chemicals from fertilizers and pesticides, other chemicals from manufacturing and the burning of fossil fuels, and trace amounts of medications that end up in the wastewater. Sometimes, there is a massive breakdown in water infrastructure that results in undrinkable water, such as has happened in Flint, Michigan, and Jackson, Mississippi.

It's difficult to talk about water quality because it's not just a health issue, it's also an environmental issue and a social justice issue (lower-income communities tend to house more utilities that produce more pollutants). There's no easy answer to the conundrum of how to get easily accessible, affordable, and high-quality water. Water is such a vital component of health, however, that it's worth the time, energy, and money you may have to spend in order to find the best water option that's available to you. In general, the cleanest water is spring water. After that is filtered water. Although there are considerations for both types of water.

Spring water that's shipped in glass bottles (so that chemicals from plastic bottles don't leach into the water) is generally the purest, best-quality water you can get. Spring water is bottled at the source, which means it has fewer opportunities to become contaminated before it ends up in your glass. And yet, buying spring water in glass bottles isn't an elegant solution, I admit, because water is very expensive to ship for multiple reasons: it's heavy, as are the glass bottles, and the process burns a lot of fossil fuels that then go on to contaminate the environment even more. It also costs a lot of money to keep a steady supply at home. Perhaps there's a company that sells spring water in glass bottles from a spring near you that makes this option less taxing on the environment and your wallet. You can also check the website findaspring.org to see if there's a source of spring water near you where you can go and collect it in your own glass bottles.

Water filters can be a next-best option because they can take water from the tap and remove contaminants from it. This, too, is an inelegant solution because different filters remove different contaminants, and they all have their plusses and minuses. Carbon filters—like those that are in most refrigerators and countertop pitchers—are good at removing a handful of contaminants, including lead and disinfection by-products. They are also relatively inexpensive. But there are many contaminants that they don't reduce, including fluoride and many heavy metals. Also, if you don't change the filters frequently enough, all the contaminants they have caught in the past can start leaching back into your water. Reverse-osmosis filters remove the greatest range of contaminants, but they also remove all minerals—so you'll need to add trace minerals back into your water so that your body has the electrolytes it needs to actually retain the water. (You can do this by adding small amounts of sea salt into the water, or a liquid mineral supplement—see the Resources section for brands I recommend.) Reverse-osmosis filters also waste a lot of water—it takes two to four gallons of water to produce one gallon of drinkable water, although some newer models are more efficient. Where I live, in California, we simply don't have the water to waste. For this reason, I buy my water either from a local spring, or have it shipped from Mountain Valley—a company that delivers spring water from Arkansas throughout the United States. It is my biggest environmental impact. I justify the environmental cost because I have watched the levels of petrochemicals and chemical fertilizers—particularly glyphosate, the active ingredient in Roundup—in my own and my patients' lab work come down dramatically when we switch to spring water.

There is some hope on the horizon for higher-quality water with fewer environmental consequences. Paris, for example, uses ozone and UV light to treat its water instead of chemicals, and the result is some of the cleanest municipal water in the world. Some US cities have started using UV to treat their water, although it is typically still used in conjunction with chlorine, as is the case in New York City's water supply.

Water quality varies widely from well to well, town to town, and state to state. The first stop in assessing your tap water is to visit the Environmental Working Group's Tap Water database (at www.ewg.org/tapwater/) and look up your zip code to see the quality of your water. If you have good quality water, drink away. If you don't, the next step is to have your water tested through a lab, especially if you're on well water. From there, you can research which type of filter works best for you, or your best source for securing spring water in glass bottles.

No matter what kind of water you choose, avoid storing it in or drinking it out of plastic. Stick to stainless, ceramic, or glass only for your water containers. For example, if you find spring water sold in plastic bottles, I personally would keep looking, especially if you live in a hot climate where those bottles could have gotten warm, which causes them to leach more chemicals into the water. Keep in mind that a lot of standard bottled water is tap water. Some big box stores, such as Walmart, sell refillable bottles of reverse-osmosis, UV-treated, and remineralized water (such as those sold under the brand name Primo). This is likely an affordable and accessible source of high-quality water for most people, although they use plastic bottles. Although somewhat complicated, I recommend buying a large-capacity stainless steel, glass, or ceramic water jug that you can pour the water into once you transport it home.

You could also work with a healthcare provider to test your urine and determine what chemicals are present in it—seeing some numbers may inspire you to invest the energy and money in improving your daily water.

As you can see, there really is no one perfect solution. And yet we know that toxins play a big role in Alzheimer's, and water helps not only by flushing toxins out of the body but also by not introducing toxins in the first place. Also, because I'm asking you to move more and get plenty of exercise, the amount of water you need to stay adequately hydrated will only increase. Any opportunity you have to reduce your toxic burden is worth the hassle. Remember, you want to do everything you can to stay out of defend-and-fight mode and in repair-and-regenerate mode.

Water Checklist:
- Look up your local water at the Environmental Working Group Tap Water database (www.ewg.org/tapwater/), or visit the website of your local water supply and look up their most recent water quality report.
- If you are on a well, or if your local water doesn't get a good rating, have your water tested.
- Consider having your urine tested for contaminants to help determine how urgently you need to upgrade your water.
- Decide if you'll filter your own water or if you'll secure water from a spring, a company that sells spring water in glass bottles, or perhaps a refillable source of highly filtered and remineralized water (such as that sold at Walmart).
- Commit to drinking and storing water only in glass, stainless, or ceramic containers.

Bedroom: Place of Healing

The bedroom is where you restore yourself, and where you rinse your brain each night. Since you spend a third of your life in bed, your bedroom is a crucial room for your environment-setting efforts. Many of the things that are important throughout your home are extra important here, simply because you spend so much time here. The bedroom is the most important room in the house for plants and/or an air purifier so that the air is as contaminant-free as possible; it's also the room that benefits the most from a decluttering session, as this is where you go to retreat, not to worry about getting things done.

There are four main areas of focus in the bedroom—the bed itself, temperature, light, and noise.

Bedding

Many sheets, pillows, and mattresses use chemicals such as formaldehyde, flame retardants, and pesticides. Then you spend hours at night with these chemical residues right up against your skin, and breathing them in, at a time when your body is doing the crucial work of detoxing. New conventional mattresses are more likely to be off-gassing toxic chemicals, but even older mattresses carry risks—primarily mold, which can often develop between the mattress and the box spring. If your mattress is more than ten years old, it's likely time for a new one. I've listed my favorite mattress companies in the Resources section.

Whenever possible, make your bedding organic—your mattress, pillows, and sheets. In addition to reducing chemical exposures, you'll also likely be more comfortable, as synthetic sheets can trap body heat and make it difficult to sleep restfully. At Marama we use organic sheets from Target, and they are wonderful—they feel great, are long-lasting, and aren't expensive.

Temperature

Sleep experts advise that a nighttime temperature of somewhere between 65 and 69 degrees is the most conducive to restful sleep, although if you enjoy the sensation of sleeping under heavy blankets or comforters, you may want it even cooler than that. Higher temperatures make it harder to sleep—you get hot, you sweat, you wake up to throw off the covers, then you get cold, which wakes you up again. If you use a device to track your sleep, it can be very illuminating to see how well you sleep when your room is set at different temperatures—then you can find the ideal thermostat setting and warmth of bedding for you.

Light

The pineal gland is a tiny gland that's located deep within the brain that regulates your master clock, including your sleep-wake cycles. The pineal gland is highly influenced by your exposure to light. Blue light—emitted by alarm clocks, night-lights, streetlights outside the window, or electronic devices—is stimulating. If there is any amount of blue light coming into your bedroom all night long from outside, consider blackout curtains. Wearing a sleep mask can also increase your experience of darkness. If you do need a night-light, get one in the orange or red spectrum to help support reaching deeper sleep and getting right back to sleep after a trip to the loo.

Noise

Sounds can either prevent you from falling asleep or cause you to wake up. A white noise machine can mask a lot of noises, whether it's the trash truck that wakes you up early every Monday morning, loud neighbors, or a snoring partner. Earplugs can also help, and putting them in each night can become part of your bedtime routine that signals to your body that it's time for sleep.

Bedroom Checklist:

- Declutter the room.
- Bring in a couple of plants for relaxation and air purification.
- Consider an air purifier; get rid of air fresheners.
- Make sure anything that is illuminated at night emits a light that's dim, and preferably in the red portion of the light spectrum (e.g., an alarm clock with red numbers instead of blue or green).
- If you have reflux or sleep apnea, try elevating the head of your bed by placing the head of the bed on bricks.
- Upgrade to organic bedding.
- Block out light with blackout curtains or a sleep mask.
- Mask noises with a white noise machine, a fan, or earplugs.

The Bathroom: Important for Cleansing and Independence

The bathroom is one of those places where you maintain dignity or lose it. You want to support independence in the bathroom for as long as possible, because a lot of shame and embarrassment can arise when toileting issues start to crop up.

Depending on how severe the cognitive impairment, simple things like putting a "restroom" sign on the door—a picture of a toilet or a shower— can help. Either getting a bidet toilet or installing a bidet attachment (which are available on Amazon for less than $50) can help someone tend to their own toileting needs for longer. If your loved one is missing the toilet when they aim, consider painting the wall behind the toilet a bright color to enhance the contrast, thus making the toilet easier to see. You may also consider installing a softer toilet seat and handrails to help with getting onto and up from the toilet. You might start keeping incontinence supplies on hand—such as panty liners, pads, or even panties (I like the washable organic cotton panties designed to catch urine leaks made by Knix). I recommend acquiring these things before you think you need them. Finally, getting a chair for the shower is a helpful idea because showering takes energy, causing fatigue for those who don't spend much time on their feet, and being in hot water can cause a drop in blood pressure and dizziness.

The other big piece of setting up a brain-friendly bathroom is choosing nontoxic personal care products and cleaning products. The most important of these are any products that you use on your skin, from shampoos and conditioners, to lotions, and especially cosmetics, as any toxins in the product can be absorbed into your bloodstream, without the benefit of being filtered by your liver.

I've included a list of my favorite personal care and cleaning product brands in the Resources section. A great resource for evaluating the potential toxicity of any personal care product is the Environmental Working Group's Skin Deep database, available at www.ewg.org/skindeep/.

Bathroom Checklist:
- Add handrails, a shower chair, a bidet or bidet attachment, and incontinence supplies before you need them.
- Gradually replace all personal care and cleaning products with nontoxic versions.
- Remove any bathmats that tend to slip or bunch up—look for those that have a rubber backing with no tassels or fringe.
- Be sure to run the fan after warm showers to encourage any lingering water to dry completely, and have your bathroom evaluated for mold.

Living Room: A Place to Socialize and Have Fun

The living room is where you spend time with others and is often the room where a lot of waking hours are spent. As such, you want it to be comfortable, soothing, and conducive to doing the activities that we covered in Chapter 8. What you don't want it to be is an open invitation to plop down and watch TV for hours at a time. Yet this is what most living rooms are, as the TV has a place of prominence, and every piece of furniture is placed so that you have a prime view of the screen.

A top-level question to ask yourself about the living room is, how can I make it harder for the TV to take center stage, and how can I make it easier to do the activities that are so fun and so good for brain health? For example, can you put your TV inside a closed cabinet? An even more extreme example, which I use in my own home, is keeping the TV in a closet—we have to clear off a place for it, pull it out, carry it into the living room, and then plug it in in order to watch it. Sometimes we have to find an extension cord. There are a lot more steps than simply grabbing the remote and pressing a button. If you make things you don't want to do more effortful, you'll think twice before you do them. By the same token, keeping things out, like puzzles, books, or drawing supplies will make it easier to choose those brain-enriching activities. Or maybe you'll be inspired just to sit and have a conversation with your loved one. When you create a little friction to the well-worn path, you make it easier to do things differently.

From a practical standpoint, incontinence can become a factor when cognitive impairment is present. At Marama, we have leather couches and chairs because they are easy to wipe off. Microfiber is also easy to clean and has a softer feel than leather. You can also use waterproof mats on the seats, just taking care to avoid plastic and vinyl, because they can be uncomfortable, can off-gas toxins when new, and can stick to your legs.

Living Room Checklist:
- Declutter the room.
- Add potted plants for relaxation and air purification.
- Consider an air purifier; get rid of air fresheners.
- Make a plan to make the TV a less prominent presence in the living room.
- Set out the materials for a few activities that encourage brain enrichment instead of zoning out.
- Assess whether you need to think about preparing for incontinence at this time.
- Remove trip hazards like rugs and wires.

Outdoor Areas: A Chance to Connect to Nature

Spending time outside is such a healing thing to do—the fresh air, the natural light, and the view of plants, trees, birds, and maybe your neighbors are all uplifting both physically and mentally. Your body will produce vitamin D in response to being in the sun, and connecting to nature is a great reset for the nervous system. If there is an accessible outdoor space, it's so worth it to spend a little time on making it a comfortable, compelling, and safe place to be.

The biggest safety concern is that the area is secure. People with dementia are known to wander, so you want to be sure that there is a fence, with a gate that can lock. Of course, you also want to tend to anything that could be a fall risk—are there railings for any stairs? Rugs, pots, toys, or hoses that could trip them up? A lip on the sliding-glass door that you could perhaps cover with a ramp?

Another important aspect of outdoor safety is not using any chemical fertilizers, pesticides, or herbicides. If you worry about cockroaches, silverfish, fleas, ticks, lice, ants, or other bugs, try using diatomaceous earth—a nontoxic powder that you sprinkle around outside that will kill anything with an exoskeleton. Diatomaceous earth won't harm bigger animals, including cats, dogs, and humans, if they accidentally ingest it. You do need to reapply diatomaceous earth after it gets wet from dew or rain.

Beyond that, you want your outdoor space to be set up for comfort and engagement. Are there chairs in a shady spot? Is there a bathroom that's accessible? Is there something to engage your loved one when they're outside, such as a garden, hummingbird feeder, birdbath, or perhaps a fountain?

Other things to consider keeping handy outside:

- A basket with a blanket or two in case it gets chilly
- A cooler for drinks and snacks (so that you don't have to run inside and leave your care partner outside alone)
- An umbrella so that you can create some shade if it's too sunny and hot
- A big container or small raised garden bed where your care partner can get their hands in the dirt and care for plants.

Outdoor Space Checklist:
- Be sure the perimeter is secure, and install a lock on the gate or add a fence, if necessary.
- Stop using chemical fertilizers and pesticides.
- Address any potential trip hazards.
- Keep a few supplies outside to make your care partner more comfortable and engaged while outside—such as blankets, a bird feeder, an umbrella.
- Think about how you might be able to get your care partner gardening and taking care of plants.

The Laundry Room: A Room for Cleanliness

The laundry room is where we go to clean our clothes, yet it's often a room that we neglect on cleaning day. The biggest things to be aware of in the laundry room concern mold and synthetic fragrances. Let's start with the biggie—mold.

Most front-load washing machines develop mold around the rubber gasket that forms a seal with the door. That's bad enough, because you can inhale mold spores and mycotoxins any time you're doing laundry, but worse yet is that they can get on your clothes, towels, and sheets, and then you're breathing them all day long. I am a huge proponent of old-fashioned, simple, top-loading washing machines. Not only do they tend to last longer, there are no built-in mold traps. I understand that most people have a front-loading machine. If you have one, and you can't replace it with a top loader for whatever reason—space, cost, etc.—you can have the gasket replaced. Then, every time you finish up a round of laundry, wipe down the inside of the door, the outside and underneath of the gasket, and leave the door propped open until everything is fully dry before closing the door. If you think I'm being alarmist, go and look at your front-loading laundry machine right now. I was having this conversation with a friend of mine, who then went to visit her dad at his Florida condo. When she went to do a load of laundry there, she saw that the gasket of her dad's front-loading washing machine was black with mold. Living in a humid climate, like Florida, makes your chances of developing mold even higher, but this can happen with front-loading washing machines in any climate. She texted me immediately and said, "You're right!"

Beyond mold, the residue of your laundry detergents, fabric softeners, and dryer sheets can embed themselves in your clothes, which lie right against your skin. Synthetic fragrances tend to be very aggravating to the nervous system. Switch your detergent to something fragrance-free and nontoxic. (Again, see the Resources section for some of my favorite nontoxic brands.) Use dryer balls instead of dryer sheets. The ultimate purpose of your clothes is for protection—making these switches will help them truly keep you safe from exposure to the elements as well as safe from exposure to toxins.

Laundry Room Checklist:
- Clean the gasket of your front-loading washing machine to remove any existing mold, then dry it completely after each use to prevent the future formation of mold.
- Consider a top-loading washing machine.
- Switch to natural, nontoxic, fragrance-free detergents.
- Skip the dryer sheets and use wool dryer balls instead.

Mold: Hidden Danger to Health, Particularly Brain Health

One of the larger home-based threats to brain health is something that isn't always easy to see—mold.

It's not necessarily the mold itself that is a threat, it's the mycotoxins—which are known neurotoxic and immunosuppressive chemicals—that mold produces. In fact, there is a prescription drug made from mycotoxins—called CellCept (mycophenolate mofetil)—that is given to organ transplant patients to tamp down the immune response and reduce the odds that the body will reject the new organ.

Mycotoxins are a well-known threat in the animal husbandry industry; they are commonly found in moldy barns and can impact the mortality of animals raised for food. There's a lot of effort in that industry to make sure mycotoxins are reduced. Yet in humans they don't get as much attention. In part, that's because mold is often growing behind walls, under carpets or mattresses, or below floorboards, where we can't see it. You could un-knowingly be exposed thanks to some form of water damage, such as a burst pipe, a slow leak behind the refrigerator or under the sink, or maybe the gasket around the toilet, if it has lost its seal. Mold can start growing quickly, and within forty-eight hours it can have spread farther than a re-mediation company knows to remove.

Mold is a complicated financial issue. Even if you do discover that you have mold in your home, it's difficult to fix because there are a lot of in-terests and stressors at play—often a landlord, an insurance company, the people who live in the home—and no one wants to pay to fix it.

Another confounding factor is that symptoms of mycotoxin exposure in people are so systemic and vague that it can be hard to link them back to mold. They include digestive changes, pain, headaches, mental confusion and cognitive decline, joint pain, chronic cough or chest congestion, and fatigue. Some people are extremely sensitive to mycotoxins and can quickly develop multiple symptoms, while someone else will not have any symptoms— although it can definitely still be negatively impacting their health.

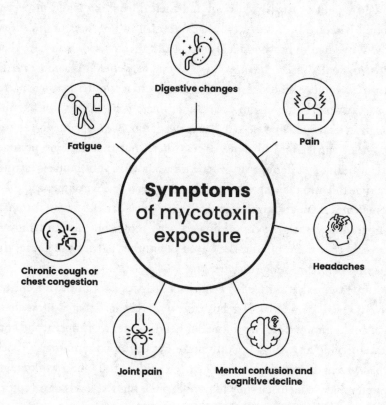

Over the years I've worked with thousands of patients who are highly sensitive to mold exposures. I've learned a ton from Dr. Bredesen, and he and I have also learned a lot from Dr. Neil Nathan. I have been studying with Dr. Nathan and seeing mold patients since 2015. Dr. Nathan published a book called *Toxic* in 2018, and it has proven to be a profoundly helpful resource for patients affected by mold. I highly recommend his book for patients and practitioners looking to understand the complexities of treating mold. It's an area that is too often ignored by conventional medicine, but as our climate grows more unpredictable and we experience more intense storms and subsequent flooding, I fear it's a subject more and more of us will have to learn how to mitigate.

I fully get it. Dealing with mold can feel scary and overwhelming. As I'm writing this we are dealing with mold at Marama. After several atmospheric rivers dumped huge amounts of rain on California, we had some water damage. We thought we had fixed it all and then during our mold inspection we found baseboards and drywall that were still full of moisture in several rooms. We've had to move residents out of the affected rooms to have them repaired, as well as delay the move-in of several residents. It is a chore no one wants to have to do. It's expensive to fix, and it often requires tearing apart at least part of your home. It can even contaminate your clothes, linens, rugs, and mattresses, which may need to be replaced, too. I've had patients feel very stuck—they can't afford to move or remediate, but they're being poisoned and their health is suffering. Yet getting rid of mold in your home is essential to brain health and making your home a safe, healing environment.

Sometimes there are workarounds. Remember Darlene from Chapter 1? Her bedroom was highly contaminated with mold, but her husband was able to seal that room off and they lived in another part of the house; that shift really helped her cognitive health.

It wasn't quite that simple for a more recent patient of mine. Phoebe had relatively severe dementia. Her husband was skeptical that a lifestyle approach could improve her cognition, but her daughter was hopeful and committed to trying anything. In addition to her cognitive symptoms, Phoebe also had severe diarrhea. The family agreed to do a full blood workup, and her mold report came back showing some of the highest levels of mycotoxin I'd ever seen. In fact, the family told me that they had experienced major flooding in the bathroom and the basement. But the husband wasn't experiencing any reactions to the mold, and he was attached to the house—they'd lived there for fifty years and had raised their family there. We were at a standstill in terms of addressing the mold until the family went on vacation. Phoebe's symptoms all got dramatically better after the first day or two away—and they kept getting better the longer they were gone.

When the family returned, her husband was ready to try moving Phoebe into a different area of the house. I get that it can take some convincing to pull the trigger on mold remediation. After all, it's a massive undertaking, a big expense, and a fraught decision-making process. Sometimes just getting away for a week or two can give you the insight you need to make these tough decisions. For patients who have financial constraints, I'll often recommend a camping trip. For those who need more support, visiting a loved one can be a way to at least test if a toxic environment is contributing to your cognitive decline.

Because mold can be difficult to see, asking yourself these questions can help you determine if either you or your home should be tested for mold exposure:

- Has your home ever had water damage? From a leak, burst pipe, or a storm, for example?
- Even if your current home hasn't experienced water damage, have you ever lived in a home that had? (Even if you were exposed ten or fifteen years ago, those mycotoxins can still be in your body, and they are worth getting rid of.)
- Do you have one or more vague symptoms—such as fatigue, brain fog, chronic cough, or the tendency to catch every virus that comes your way?

If the answer to any of these questions is yes, you should get tested and take steps to remediate them. (See the Resources section for services that help test and remediate your home.) Remember, the most important step is to minimize or eliminate any current exposure—that will make treating any previous exposures a lot more effective.

If you have been exposed to mold, these strategies can help mitigate that damage:

1. HAVING A BOWEL MOVEMENT EVERY DAY. That means drinking plenty of filtered or spring water, getting ample movement, and eating plenty of high-fiber foods, such as flaxseed crackers, almonds, celery, and avocado (as well as the Keto Oatmeal recipe on page 280).
2. TAKING A BINDER. A binder is a molecule that binds to a toxin and helps escort it out of the body. There are many different binders—including

chlorella, charcoal, clay, silica, and modified citrus pectin—that generally bind to a specific toxin. You may want to get a urinary mycotoxin test to identify the particular toxin you need to remediate. Although if you are sweating regularly, drinking plenty of filtered or spring water, and having a bowel movement every day, your body is already doing a lot of detoxing on its own.

3. SUPPORTING YOUR BODY'S NATURAL DETOXIFICATION PRO-
CESSES. Certain foods provide ample amounts of the nutrients your body needs to fuel the detox process. They include beets, cilantro, cru- ciferous vegetables (arugula, bok choy, broccoli, Brussels sprouts, and cabbage), garlic, ginger, greens of all kinds (collards, kale, mustard greens, spinach), green tea, lemon juice, and onion. Eat these at every meal or have green tea with breakfast if you're not ready to face the other foods on this list.

4. HYDRATING. Many toxins are excreted via the kidneys and urine, so drinking plenty of spring or filtered water is important because it facilitates this process.

5. TAKING LIVER-SUPPORTING SUPPLEMENTS. Your liver is responsi- ble for processing most toxins—filtering them out of the blood and then manufacturing bile that then sweeps the toxins into the digestive tract where they can be excreted through your stool. You can take one or more supplements of the compounds that support the liver, including gluta- thione (an antioxidant produced naturally by the liver that helps your cells excrete waste products—I recommend taking it as a spray or drops that you place under your tongue for better absorption), n-acetyl cysteine (NAC, an amino acid and antioxidant), milk thistle (an herb that sup- ports liver function), curcumin (the active component in turmeric that supports detox), and/or detox teas.

6. SWEATING. The skin is an organ of elimination—it excretes toxins through sweating. So make sure you sweat regularly—whether in a sauna or steam room (or sauna blanket or chair, as I covered in Chapter 8), sitting in the sun, or going on a brisk walk, perhaps while wearing extra layers if the temperatures are cool. Just remember to pay extra attention to your hydration, and even sprinkle a little sea salt in your water to replace any lost electrolytes.

7. DEEP BREATHING. Your lungs also dispel toxins, so doing five minutes of deep abdominal breathing helps with detox. Breathwork also calms the nervous system, which helps you enter the rest-and-digest state—and that's when your body can focus more on cleaning up any messes that may be present.

8. SPENDING TWO OR THREE DAYS AWAY FROM HOME, IF YOU SUSPECT YOU HAVE MOLD BUT AREN'T SURE. Ideally, you'd go camping, where you can spend as much time outside as possible, but even going to stay at someone else's house or a hotel is helpful. If you feel noticeably better away from home—if there are any symptoms that resolve, whether it's fatigue, brain fog, achy joints, scratchy throat, or itchy eyes—that's a good indication that you may have mold in your home.

Getting Started

Hopefully you have already done a scan for safety, as I outlined in Chapter 1, and you've started to switch out the items that are in view to include activities and foods that are part of the new Alzheimer's toolkit. If you haven't yet done these things, I suggest starting there.

From there, there are two places to turn to next:

- The room you spend the most time in—that could be the living room, the kitchen, or the bedroom. The results you create in that room will help motivate you to keep going.
- The spot with the most urgent issue—such as mold, leaks, a fall risk, or a door that your loved one has been using to leave the house and wander (a common occurrence in dementia patients).

Regardless of where you start, start small. You don't want to try to clear out your entire house in one day, or even in one weekend. Take one step, or work on one small project at a time, so that you have enough time to fully clean up once you're done and you're not living in chaos as you work your way through the house. You can likely clean out two or maybe three kitchen cabinets in one session and still have time and energy at the end to put the items you're giving away in a box that you carry out to your car, and then place everything you're keeping back in the cabinets.

When it comes to replacing your current cleaning and household items for less-toxic versions, you don't need to go out and buy everything new, nor do you have to throw away everything you already have. As you run out of things, simply replace them with something more natural and less toxic. For example, once you use up your standard laundry detergent, you can replace it with something less chemical-laden. The same goes for your dish soap, body lotion, floor cleaner, mattress, and sheets.

Like everything else in the new Alzheimer's toolkit, it's also extremely helpful to carve out space for refining your environment in your schedule. Whether you can do thirty minutes every night after dinner, or devote one full day or half day a week, or perhaps even a full weekend this month and next, when you put it in your calendar, you make it much less likely that something else will crowd out the time, and much more likely that you will actually do it.

Connection over Correction

Any home environment is a form of communication that speaks volumes, as creating a loving, thoughtful, supportive environment is an expression of love. When you talk to your loved one, or to the people you live with, about refining your home environment, focus on the ways that your efforts will help everyone feel better when they're at home, both because the space will feel more relaxing and be more conducive to spending time together, enjoying each other's company, and because decluttering will make it easier for everyone who lives there to feel their best day-to-day.

Typically the hardest part of this home makeover process is encouraging someone to get rid of things. Most importantly, you don't want to purge items that belong to your care partner without talking to them first. Explain that you are creating more space for enjoyment and relaxation and suggest donating these items or giving them to a specific person—that way your loved one can feel like they are helping someone else, and that positive emotion can help make the process easier.

If you or your care partner doesn't want to part with an item, take a picture of it, then pack it up and store it away, either in a box on a shelf or in a storage unit. You can put the pictures of all the items you're storing in a little album—both so you can show the photo to your care partner, who may be wondering where it is, and so you can remember exactly what you packed away.

To watch a summary video of this chapter and download the Reversing Alzheimer's workbook go to ReversingAlzheimersBook.com.

Reflection questions:
- What will you do first?
- What things do you need to do or buy? Start a list.
- What room do you or your care partner spend the most time in? What's a good first step for making this room more restorative?
- What need is most urgent? For instance, is there mold you need to address? Or something that is significantly increasing the risk of falling?
- When can you devote some time to this work? Block it out on your calendar.
- Who can help you with these tasks?

CHAPTER 10

Care for the Caregiver (Meaning You)

When I meet with a new dementia patient, I know that I am treating their caregiver in addition to treating them. Of course, not every caregiver is on board with the idea of prioritizing their own health at that moment—mostly, they want to do everything they can to help their loved one get better. But dementia is almost like a virus. It doesn't affect just one person. It can reach out and impair the cognitive health of the people who care for the patient, too. And you are also important, as a person in your own right, not just as a caregiver. The better care you take of yourself now, the better care your loved one will receive. To be blunt, if you are not caring for yourself, you are not going to be a good caregiver.

Taking care of someone with Alzheimer's is such a big and important job that it's easy to lose yourself to it. That tendency is precisely what I hope this chapter will help you rewire. Because if you don't also care for yourself, your effectiveness and your health will suffer, which will only make things worse for the person you're caring for.

In my clinical experience I have witnessed that caregivers get more motivated to take better care of themselves when they understand how their well-being affects the people they love. So if you don't want to put the time and effort into taking better care of yourself for you, do it for the people who love you and rely on you.

The truth is, you need to have balance in your life in order to show up fully for the person you are caring for—to have the wherewithal to handle the daily tasks, the long-term planning, and the big-picture decision-making, all while maintaining the equanimity and compassion to be patient and kind. I mentioned this in the beginning of the book, but if you are reading because you are caring for someone with dementia, everything I outline in this book applies to you, too. That means that part of your responsibility as a caregiver is to treat your own care as a main focus, not a side project.

If that sounds impossible, this chapter will give you plenty of ideas and insights on precisely how to do it. But first, for a little bit of motivation, let's take a look at the health risks that caregiving can bring.

The Risks of Caregiving

I'm guessing you already know that caring for someone with dementia is taxing. You may not realize just how detrimental to your own health it can be. I'm sharing this list so that you can see the potential costs of *not* tending to your own well-being during this time. There are two hopeful notes to keep in mind as you read it: (1) The risks of each item on this list can be mitigated by making sure you get plenty of sleep, nourishment, exercise, connection, relaxation, and time for adventure. And (2) caregiving also has its unique and powerful rewards, which I'll cover in the next section. But let's take an honest look at the potential downsides.

- CAREGIVER BURDEN: Whether you're living with your care partner, and providing day-to-day care, or living at a distance, and providing mostly financial and/or logistical support, having someone in your life who has dementia is often hard in multiple ways—emotionally, physically, and financially. Many people find that their sleep, diet, physical exercise, and fun suffers. It's a burden that works in two directions: it's common to give up the things that help you stay healthy, and to feel a big weight of responsibility, frustration, and guilt. While caring for an Alzheimer's patient is similar in many ways to caring for a child, it's also less predictable than raising kids. Children hit milestones and gradually become more independent. With Alzheimer's, patients lose their independence, and there are no benchmarks that align with a predictable timeline. That unpredictability can make the experience stressful and uniquely challenging. Collectively these outcomes are referred to as "caregiver burden." This multifaceted phenomenon plays a role in the increased rates of depression and stress experienced by dementia caregivers, and a decrease in a general sense of well-being and quality of life. Caregiver burden is precisely what this chapter aims to reduce.

- IMPAIRED COGNITIVE FUNCTION: Research has found that dementia caregivers have significantly lower scores on tests of cognitive function. This may be linked to the fact that many caregivers report poor sleep, which can impair your ability to process and respond to information, and thus can influence how safely you are able to perform complex caregiving tasks.

- POOR SLEEP: Between 50 and 70 percent of dementia caregivers report regular sleep disturbances. After all, stress and worry can make it difficult to sleep well. And if your care partner wakes up in the middle of the night, you may be required to wake up with them, too.

- DEPRESSION: Depression and dementia are closely linked—having depression can increase your risk of dementia, and having dementia can increase your risk of depression. On top of that, caregivers of people with dementia experience depression more frequently than the general population, and depression in a caregiver can in turn affect the status and prognosis of the dementia patient.

- ISOLATION: A common feeling among dementia caregivers is that people who aren't also caring for someone with dementia can't understand what it's like, which understandably can lead to feeling isolated from others. Also, your devotion to your loved one can make it hard to ask for help—I can't tell you how many family members of patients have expressed the idea that they should be able to do everything on their own. On top of that, your caregiving duties may be preventing you from getting together with friends or doing things that get you in the company of others, such as working out at the gym, attending church, or participating in some other social activity.

- LACK OF TIME: Few of us feel as if we have extra time in our schedules. So of course, adding appointments, daily care, and spending time with your loved one can easily create or intensify what's known as time poverty, which is the sense of never having enough time to do all the things you need to do. Time poverty has been found by Harvard researchers to have a bigger negative impact on well-being than unemployment, with a particular adverse effect on creativity, relationships, and mental health. Time poverty also makes it more likely that you skip the things that promote health, like exercise, cooking nutritious foods instead of grabbing highly processed convenience foods, and sleeping.
- STEEP LEARNING CURVE: Part of the caregiving burden is due to the fact that there is so much to learn. So many patients and families tell me, "I didn't know anything about Alzheimer's, and then all of a sudden I felt like I needed to know everything." Being on the learning curve can also make you feel vulnerable, like you might be being taken advantage of by a senior living facility, or you're not feeling confident to make a decision about treatment options, or you don't even know where and how to get help.
- DEMENTIA RISK: Devastatingly, all these negative effects combine to create an increased risk of developing dementia yourself—up to a sixfold increase compared to non-caregivers. Which is not to say that caring for someone with dementia definitely means you are getting dementia, too. It's really when the sense of caregiving burden is high, and you don't exercise as much, sleep as well, or make healthy food choices, that this risk is at its highest. The takeaway? Everything in this book, and especially in this chapter, is as important for you and your cognitive health as it is for your loved one and their cognitive health. Whether you realize it or not, you are in prevention mode.

The Positive Side of Caregiving

And now for the good news: There are good things that come from caregiving. In fact, a growing body of research has documented that caregiving actually bestows important gifts. Some of these benefits are more emotional, such as deepened relationships and an increased sense of purpose. Others relate to physical health, including living longer and experiencing greater overall well-being than non-caregivers.

When I interviewed gerontologist and author of *Positive Caregiving* Sarah Teten Kanter on my annual Reversing Alzheimer's online summit, she explained that caregiving provides a lot of opportunities to experience positive emotions, such as compassion, love, gratitude, and reminiscence, and that these emotions carry health benefits of their own. That likely explains why some research has found that many caregivers say that the positive aspects of caregiving help them deal with any negative effects they may experience.

Teten Kanter also pointed out that caregiving is something most people will experience at some point, and that it is an experience that many caregivers look back on as one of the most meaningful parts of their lives.

I know it can feel like your life is no longer your own because of your caregiving duties, but this time of your life will eventually end. Keeping in mind the temporary nature of every phase of life can help make it all feel more manageable, and perhaps even help inspire you to savor the meaningful pieces.

I've also seen the family members and friends who are caring for my patients enjoy a significant uptick in their own physical, mental, and cognitive health as a result of implementing the Reversing Alzheimer's protocol along with their care partner. If they hadn't needed to care for their loved one, maybe they never would have learned to take better care of their own health, too.

As much as we may complain about growing old, and despite the fact that we may lose a lot of our faculties—mental and otherwise—as we do, aging is a privilege denied to many, as is caregiving.

I'm in no way trying to minimize the difficulties that can accompany caregiving, nor am I telling you that if you just think positively, everything will be okay. What I am trying to say is that it's important to acknowledge all the aspects of caregiving—the good as well as the bad, and that paying attention to the good can help mitigate the negative effects of the bad.

Caregiver Nonnegotiable: At Least One Day Off

If there's one thing I know for absolute certain about Alzheimer's, it's this: Taking care of someone with dementia is not a one-person job. Trying to do it all yourself without ever taking a break is impossible. It will only increase your caregiver burden and put you on the path to burnout, which can then take a toll on your own risk of developing dementia and render you less able to care for your loved one.

It's for this reason that I tell every caregiver I encounter that there is only one nonnegotiable piece of any caregiving plan, and that is that you take at least one full day a week off from caregiving.

Why? In addition to staving off your own burnout as well as giving you some time to care for yourself, putting in place a "my day Friday" (or any other day[s] of the week) will force you to line up some help. Even if you think you don't need any assistance now, it is only a matter of time until that changes. Your care partner could fall or become ill, or you could. You could also need to go away for work, a family event, or just for fun. And if, when that time comes, you don't have another caregiver who's already gotten to know your loved one, you could find yourself in a real bind of needing to hire whoever's available, or perhaps not being able to find anyone who is available. Don't wait until you're desperate. I've seen far too many families with a caregiver who's been doing the bulk of the work who suddenly can no longer do it, for any number of reasons. Then the family ends up backed in a corner, paying too much for someone who doesn't do it right.

You need time to do whatever sounds good to you without feeling guilty or like you are shirking your responsibilities. Taking a day off from caregiving gives you the space to get exercise, meet up with a friend, engage in a hobby, get a massage, and enjoy yourself. It's so important that you have a regular opportunity to see people you love and do things you enjoy. Remember, caregiving is finite—you want to have a life, and a healthy self, to get back to when this phase of your life is over.

To make this one day off possible, refer back to the list of places to look for support in Chapter 4. Find someone who can be your regular backup so that your loved one can begin developing a relationship with them, your backup can start learning your routine, and you can get a day off to recharge and increase your resilience.

SIGNS YOU NEED MORE HELP

Of course, you may need more than one day a week off. The two things to look out for that suggest you need more help so that you can have more time off are:

» You're not able to tend to your own diet, exercise, stress management, and sleep; these are just as important for you as they are for your care partner.

» When envisioning your ideal week, all you can imagine is being on vacation. Yes, caring for someone with memory loss is hard, but if all you can think about is getting out, it's time for a break so you can come back feeling refreshed. Both you and your loved one deserve that.

Tools and Techniques

Whether you realize it or not, you already have ways of coping with the stress that caregiving can give rise to—it's just that they are likely not that helpful in the long run. That may be skipping out on sleep, drinking alcohol, blaming others, blaming yourself, or deciding that you just need to try harder. All these can ultimately only add to your caregiver burden, not lessen it.

Here I'm providing a laundry list of tools and techniques that can help make a positive difference in both your day-to-day reality and your long-term health. Each of them can provide relief in some way, whether it's something quick, like pausing to take a deep breath, or something longer lasting, like finding support in fellow caregivers. You certainly don't have to do them all. Use this list as a brainstorming tool, and use the reflection questions at the end of this chapter to help you determine which ideas you want to try.

Reframing

This is a shift in your thinking that helps you deal with the unexpected with more equanimity—such as when your loved one is not listening to you. It's very easy to be judgmental in these moments, and to feel victimized, as in "Why are they making my life harder?" Especially when you're caring for a family member, with whom you have a long history. Ultimately, making it about you and judging the other person leads to more disconnection, which can breed upset and an escalation of the challenge.

I have learned so much from Teepa Snow, author of *Understanding the Changing Brain* and *Dementia Caregiver Guide*. An occupational therapist with decades of experience, she is funny, insightful, creative, and highly skilled at understanding and communicating with those suffering with dementia. I highly recommend Snow's YouTube videos and books to anyone who cares for someone with dementia. Although I'll leave a deep dive into her work up to you, I do want to at least introduce you to her, because she is *the* expert, and these concepts, so that you will hopefully be inspired to learn more from her.

What I've learned from Snow is that whenever you're in that place of judgment, there is an invitation in that moment to notice that you've gotten upset, and then reframe your loved one's behavior as the communication of an unmet need.

Determining an unmet need requires some curiosity and some detective work. In any situation, take a step back and objectively ask, "What's going on here?" For example, if your care partner isn't listening to you, instead of concluding that they are choosing not to hear you, stay open enough to investigate if their hearing aid is turned up, or needs a new battery, or if there's too much background noise.

Also consider this person's history. Did they clean homes for a living, so now they constantly feel like they need to tidy up? Or were they a financial adviser, and so they want to take over the bill paying even though they no longer have the capacity to do so? Or did they have a partner, child, or other family member who meant a lot to them and now they are looking for them? Sometimes there are patterns that link back to when this person had their full cognitive capacity.

Once you can identify that unmet need, you have an opportunity to fill it, at least partially. Because when those needs are tended to, it will make everyone's experience easier and more enjoyable—including yours.

POSSIBLE UNMET NEEDS

Here are some things to consider that may be influencing your care partner's behavior.

Physical needs
Being hungry
Being thirsty
Being tired
Being wired (from caffeine, sugar, or overstimulation)
Having to urinate or defecate, or having had a toileting accident
Being too hot or too cold
Being in pain
Not being able to hear
Feeling unsafe or threatened

Emotional needs
Anger
Sadness
Frustration
Difficulty communicating
Loneliness
Boredom
Being reminded of something from the past

Releasing Expectations

This is probably one of the hardest things about loving and caring for someone with dementia—little by little they lose the ability to do things they once could, whether that's log into an online account, manage finances, remember your name, or brush their teeth. As painful as these losses can be to witness, what makes them more upsetting is when you expect your loved one always to be able to do what they once could. That's why, even though you hold out hope that they will be able to do some of these things again after following the protocol outlined in this book, it's helpful to everyone—especially you—if you can let go of the expectation that they continue to be the person they were. By releasing the expectation, you can relieve yourself of at least a bit of the disappointment that comes from being let down when your expectation isn't met. Maintaining a spirit of curiosity can help. Saying things to yourself such as, "I wonder how this will go," can help you meet your care partner where they are that day. Don't forget to enjoy and celebrate when your loved one does regain capacity.

Self-Compassion

I'm listing self-compassion before having compassion for your care partner because self-compassion tends to have a ripple effect that helps you become more compassionate toward others. Self-compassion has also been shown to reduce the perception of caregiver burden.

An important way you can implement self-compassion is to continually remind yourself that you're doing your best. That may not mean you're doing a perfect job, or even a great job—some days, you may need to phone it in because you didn't sleep well the night before, or you're not feeling well, or you have to focus on work that day, and that's okay. But it does mean that you are doing the best you can in that moment. Just the fact that you're reading this book means you are trying to take the best care possible of your loved one. Also, the fact that you are willing to be a pioneer and learn about the things that can prevent or reverse the downward slide of dementia and put in the work to help your loved one get better suggests to me that not only are you doing your best, you're doing a phenomenal job. It's not easy to be at the forefront of a movement.

Another important tool is to become aware of how you talk to yourself. We all have moments when we get frustrated, say the wrong thing, or do something we later wish we could take back. I think we can agree that no one is perfect. So when things do go wrong, begin to notice what you say to yourself about it. It helps you become an observer of your own thoughts, which then creates a window of opportunity to be more intentional about what you tell yourself. In these moments, try talking to yourself the same way you would talk to a friend—someone you care for, and whom you're trying to encourage. If they made a mistake, I'm guessing you wouldn't criticize them. You would just remind them that they're doing their best. Resist the urge to say harsh, judgmental, or downright mean things to yourself.

To break it down into steps:

1. Notice when your thoughts about yourself have become unkind.
2. Remind yourself that everyone in this situation is doing the best they can—including you.
3. Ask yourself, What would I say to a friend who was in this situation? Or, What would a friend say to me if they saw what just happened? And then speak to yourself that way.

Another way to show yourself compassion is to consider your own unmet needs. (Refer to the box on page 220—all those same unmet needs we listed for your loved one apply to you, too.) Are you hungry, tired, thirsty, frustrated? Some needs you may not be able to fulfill immediately—like a need for several days off from caregiving—but being really clear and honest about what you need will help you right the ship.

If you aren't sure what your unmet needs currently are, go back to the wheel of life exercise you did back in Chapter 4 and think about how you could create a little bit more balance in your scores. This may mean scheduling a weekly or monthly massage for yourself, or hiring someone to care for your loved one a couple of times a week, or getting your siblings more involved.

If you still aren't sure what you might do to feel more supported, go take a look at your morning and evening routines that you outlined in Chapter 5, and see if there's something you might add to these bookends of your day to help you feel more grounded. Maybe that's spending some time alone, meditating, journaling, or doing some form of mindful movement like yoga or tai chi. Finally, consider what practices you may have tried that helped, but that you got out of the habit of doing. What is worth revisiting?

For more on the power of self-compassion and how to apply it in your own life, I highly recommend the book *Self-Compassion: The Proven Power of Being Kind to Yourself* by Kristin Neff.

Compassion

Compassion can be difficult to access in the midst of caretaking—maybe you feel stressed because you have a lot to get done and your loved one isn't in a cooperative mood. It's easy to slip into judgment and aggravation in those trying moments, but there is another option: having compassion for the person you're caring for. In those moments when perhaps you're feeling triggered or upset, try imagining your loved one as a young child. There are, after all, a lot of similarities between caring for someone with dementia and caring for young children. They can both struggle with language and have strong opinions and desires that perhaps they can't fully express. Both are reliant on others for care. There are, of course, many differences between children and people suffering with Alzheimer's. Older adults have experienced autonomy, and they are larger—you can't simply pick up your loved one the way you could a small child. To have compassion for a person with dementia means to help them hold on to their dignity and autonomy as long as possible, so long as it's safe.

Forgiveness and Self-Forgiveness

Forgiveness is an incredibly powerful act that helps you let go of negative emotions like anger, disappointment, and resentment—all of which can make life in general, and caregiving specifically, more challenging, especially when you are having those feelings toward your care partner. The release that forgiveness fosters can usher in tremendous healing. Sometimes even the original offense is not as harmful as the resentment that you may be holding on to before you forgive. You may feel that you've been legitimately wronged, and that you can't possibly condone the other person's actions, but when you hang on to your upset, the hurt lasts longer, and you give that other person the power to continue negatively influencing your life. Forgiveness may seem difficult or even impossible to access, but you do have agency.

If you're open to the idea of forgiving someone else or yourself but it just doesn't seem possible, focus on having compassion for yourself and others for a while, and try again in a few days or weeks, as compassion can help open your heart enough to let some of that stored upset and resentment out.

A HAWAIIAN PRAYER FOR FORGIVENESS

"I'm sorry."

"I love you."

"Please forgive me [or, "I forgive you," depending on the situation]."

"Thank you."

If you have the opportunity, say it while looking into the eyes of the person you are forgiving and just keep repeating it.

For very personal and potentially profound healing, go into the bathroom, look at yourself in the mirror, and say these words to yourself with sincerity.

Gratitude

Taking the time to write down things that you appreciate or are grateful for has been shown in studies to reduce anxiety, boost optimism, and enhance a sense of connectedness and life satisfaction in as little as two weeks.

To put the power of gratitude to work in your life, in the evening, write down three things that happened today that you are grateful for—it could be a moment you had to yourself, a really good cup of coffee, or a sweet thing a loved one said to you. It could even be as simple as the fact that you woke up today. They don't have to be big things, although certainly, if something big and wonderful happened today, put it on your gratitude list! But bringing your attention to even the little things will help you start noticing more things you're grateful for in the days to come.

Consistent gratitude practices support neuroplasticity by changing how we experience life so that we focus on what we do have instead of what we don't have. In study after study, we find people with a gratitude practice experience more positive emotions, sleep better, are kinder and more compassionate, and have a stronger immune system. In particular, caregivers for their spouse who practice gratitude experience better psychological well-being compared to those who don't.

There are many quick, simple ways to get started with a gratitude practice:

- Journaling regularly about what you are grateful for, big and small.
- Thinking about someone you are grateful for.
- Writing and sending thank-you notes. Handwritten letters expressing thanks for wonderful qualities and how someone has affected your life positively engenders gratitude.
- Incorporating gratitude into your prayer or meditation practice.
- Creating a gratitude jar and filling it with little slips of paper with what you are grateful for. Go back to the jar when you need an emotional lift.
- Gratitude rock, marble, or another small token that fits in your pocket. When you touch it use it as a reminder to think of something you are grateful for.
- Going for a gratitude walk. Take a walk with the intention of taking it all in and observing everything around you and finding thanks for little things along the way.
- Giving thanks before each meal.

To really make an impact, make a point to slow down and really feel the gratitude. Consider adding this to your morning or evening routine so you create a ritual and you can more easily commit to the practice.

Don't keep your gratitude practice a secret. It always feels good to learn you've made a positive impact in someone's life. When you think of someone you are grateful for, tell them! As your gratitude practice takes hold you may even notice you are more aware of what you are grateful for in the present moment throughout the day. Embrace this. Your practice is working. As with many things in this book, the most important thing is to just get started.

Stress Relief

Remember that your nervous system can either be in a defensive state or a relaxed state, which is when repair can happen. Any practice you can do to nudge you out of the hyper-vigilant, stressed-out state, you can then redistribute those physiological resources away from fighting and defending and toward rebuilding and renewal. When you are chronically stressed out—for your brain that means few resources are going toward creating new infrastructure, such as neurons, connections between neurons, and memories—it's easier to feel overwhelmed in the face of any kind of new stressor. By committing to a relaxation practice, you help foster that cognitive infrastructure that makes everything feel more manageable.

In Chapter 8, I covered my favorite, evidence-based form of meditation, the Kirtan Kriya. I'm going to make yet another plug for it here because it is just as powerful for caregivers as it is for people who are experiencing memory loss. Give yourself these twelve minutes of doing the practice (see the Resources section for a link to my favorite YouTube video that guides you through the full practice). Just for these twelve minutes, don't worry about emptying the dishwasher, calling back whoever needs to be called back, or answering that email. You will more than make up those twelve minutes of lost productivity with increased clarity, focus, and overall sense of ease.

Another tool I haven't yet covered is the Gupta Program, an online neuroplasticity training program that aims to retrain hypersensitivity in two particular regions of the brain—the amygdala and the insula—so that you can get out of the defensive state and into the repair state. Ashok Gupta, who developed the program, has published studies that show that the Gupta Program provides significant relief in symptoms of fibromyalgia and long Covid. The program offers a free twenty-eight-day mini course and a six-month paid full program at guptaprogram.com, and it is something I highly recommend to any caregiver or any person struggling with dementia, although it is best suited for those patients in the earlier stages of cognitive impairment. (The Kirtan Kriya is great for anyone at any stage of cognitive decline.) I have seen it be profoundly helpful for people.

A basic practice from the Gupta Program: Whenever you notice yourself getting upset or stressed, say the words "Stop, stop, stop" out loud, and then smile, even if it's a completely fake smile, because the muscular actions required to smile stimulate the production of neurochemicals that can help to calm the nervous system. It also increases the time between the triggering event and your reaction to that event, which gives you more of a choice in how you're going to respond and can help you avoid knee-jerk reactions that perpetuate the release of stress hormones. Just doing those two things— saying "stop" and smiling—can be a very effective place to start.

Touch

Physical touch, when consent is given and you feel safe, can be profoundly relaxing. Humans, after all, are social creatures. We are wired to live in community with others, and touch helps regulate our autonomic nervous system and can put us in that relaxed state where healing and repair can happen. A 2020 pilot study found that dementia caregivers who were assigned regular massages saw a significant reduction in caregiver burden and an improvement in mood and well-being—and that those caregivers who did not receive massages or any relaxation training saw their depression scores rise significantly over the course of the trial.

Taking time to touch and be touched can be a highly effective and enjoyable part of your self-care strategy, whether you get a massage or pedicure, cuddle with a pet or loved one, or even give yourself a massage (using a foam roller, massage balls, or a massage gun).

Mini Breaks

This is different from taking off one day from caregiving every week. This is taking mini breaks on a daily basis to give yourself the experience of downtime and not being "on." Whenever you get someone else to relieve you of your caregiving duties, or whenever your care partner is sleeping and you are not, it is so tempting to use that opportunity to dive straight into your to-do list. And I implore you, whenever you get these chances, to make taking a break your priority—not getting things done. Go for a walk, read a book, or lie down on the couch and close your eyes, even if it's just for fifteen minutes. If you are continually in "doing" mode, you are perpetuating that hypervigilance that diverts resources away from rebuilding and repairing. If you have children, you likely remember the advice to nap when the baby naps. It's the same concept here. When your loved one is being cared for, care for yourself.

Caregiver Support System

Connecting with friends and family is a wonderful and important thing to do. It's a great outlet for fun and connection, but it's not a true support system, because most caregivers report having the feeling that no one they know truly understands what it's like to be caring for someone you love who is losing their cognitive function.

Having a network of fellow dementia caregivers gives you the opportunity to commiserate with people who get it (just don't get stuck doing only that), bounce ideas off people who are in a similar situation, and continually be reminded that you're not alone. It could be a local support group or a virtual one. Good places to look for possible caregiver support groups include your local senior centers, hospitals, churches, and meetup.com. For virtual support groups, check out the Alzheimer's Association (www.alz.org), Hope Health (hopehealthco.org), Smart Patients (smartpatients.com), and the Facebook groups Caregiver Nation and Memory People.

If you're following the guidance in this book and have hope that your loved one is going to improve, you will likely run into people who think your hope is misguided at best, and possibly even dangerous. It's so helpful and reaffirming to be in a group of people who are also caring for someone with dementia, and preferably people who are also following this protocol. You want people who are ahead of you on the path to cheer you on, and to cheer on the people who are coming behind you. It can be hard enough to implement this protocol all on its own; when the people you love are telling you it couldn't possibly work, it's even harder. I'm including in the Resources section guidance on how to access a few support groups for people who are implementing a Bredesen-based protocol like the one outlined in this book.

Guidance for Making Hard Choices

I believe that there is always hope for regaining cognitive function. But hope takes resources. It takes commitment, energy, time, support from family and friends, and money. Some of these resources are tangible, and some are intangible. They are all finite. So at some point, you may have to ask yourself, "How much am I willing to pay for that hope?"

We have a patient at Marama who did very well financially when she was working, and has no heirs, so it makes all the sense in the world for her friend, who has power of attorney, to devote money to her care. I hate that health status is so often closely linked to financial status, but it is our current reality. By spending the money that is available for this purpose, that friend is also reducing her own caregiver burden—which is a good thing, because we don't want the disease to take down two people.

If you, like the vast majority of people, don't have unlimited funds, you have to consider the cost of your own health, stress levels, and relationships when you are making decisions about the care of your loved one. For example, I wouldn't want to lose my relationship with my brother in order to be right about how to care for our parents. If you are feeling like the costs of following the Reversing Alzheimer's protocol may be too much, I get that it's a complex and heart-wrenching decision, but the cost/benefit (or cost/hope) analysis needs to be acknowledged.

To help you do that analysis, these are the things that give me more confidence that someone with memory loss can get better:

- A YOUNGER BIOLOGICAL AGE. I don't believe in hard-and-fast rules of chronological age. I've seen some patients in their late eighties and into their nineties who were more vital than some others in their sixties and seventies. In general, the healthier and more robust someone is physically, the more hope I have for their recovery.

- LESS DISEASE PROGRESSION. Again, there are no strict rules here, as I've seen many exceptions to each guideline I'm sharing, but once MoCA scores dip below 16, so does my hope.
- GREATER WILLINGNESS. You can be young with only mild cognitive impairment, but if you aren't willing to make new choices about what to eat and do on a daily basis, the likelihood of making lasting changes is lower than it is for someone who is open to change.

All these factors point to a deeper truth: the sooner you start, the better. If you're having a hard time convincing your mom or dad to be more proactive about their own cognitive decline, channel that concern and energy toward yourself and stop banging your head against the wall with someone who's clinging to resistance. Your example may inspire them to make changes—or it may not. But at least someone in your family will benefit.

It's vital to remember that dementia itself, as well as the Reversing Alzheimer's approach, is unique to every individual, as is the process of determining when the costs of hope are too high. In the next section, I'll share some approaches you can take when discussing whether and how much to adopt the changes I outline in this book with the people in your care partner's life who may not be as hopeful as you are.

Connection over Correction

One of the biggest challenges I see to implementing the Reversing Alzheimer's protocol is the dynamics within the family. While there are some families who work together beautifully, my experience suggests that having a united front is rare.

To give you an example of what a spirit of collaboration looks like, as well as the results it can foster, one of my recent patient's MoCA scores went from an 8 to a 13. Her husband and her daughters all show up for every single visit—even if someone needs to dial in on speakerphone—and they share the duties according to their availability. They say things like, "Kara, you take mom to dance class," and "Kelly, you talk to the sleep doctor."

Witnessing them work together is almost like watching a game of volley-ball. They make a beautiful team, and they also make it a point to laugh and find humor where they can. It's so heartwarming to see.

Maybe your family is a little less touchy-feely—you can still find ways to work together in a powerful way. For example, my partner's mother has dementia, and he and his siblings keep track of all her appointments, notes from those appointments, and meds in a shared Google sheet. It's still very collaborative and accommodating of the fact that they each have constraints on their time and finances.

It's an understatement to say that not every family is like these two examples.

Maybe you as the daughter or son want to take a proactive approach, while the spouse of the person who is declining doesn't want to acknowl-edge that there's a problem, or doesn't want things to change, or doesn't want to take on more of a caregiver role.

Sometimes the health decision-maker and the financial decision-maker are two different people who don't agree. Maybe one sibling is financially stable and another isn't, and they feel that investing in their parent's health is risking their inheritance. Maybe one family member wants to wait for a pharmaceutical treatment. These are all completely legitimate feelings and concerns. The dynamics can play out in an infinite number of ways and get more complex the more people are involved.

If you're an only child or are feeling like you don't have the support of a big family, consider yourself lucky because you also don't have a lot of opposing opinions. There's a simplicity in being the sole decision-maker—although I recognize that there are challenges in everything falling to you, too.

Whatever your family situation, resist the urge to get so excited and confident that you get attached to doing things "the right way." Keep in mind that if your loved one has moderate dementia, with a MoCA score under 16, and your sibling is highly resistant to devoting any resources toward reversing that decline, there may be hope, but it may not be worth it to jeopardize your relationship with someone who will be around for the next several decades. In every family there's a different cost-benefit analysis. Destroying relationships in your family—especially with people in your generation or younger—may not be worth it.

To watch a summary video of this chapter and download the
Reversing Alzheimer's workbook go to ReversingAlzheimersBook.com.

Reflection questions:
- Do you feel that your life is balanced?
- Are you able to come from a place of strength, or are you feeling more needy, or even desperate?
- Do you have the support you need?
- If you feel you need more support, have you identified the resources that could help?
- Are you developing compassion for yourself and others?
- How burdened do you feel by caregiving?
- How could you lessen the burden?
- When you consider the costs of having hope that your loved one will get better, what feelings arise?

CHAPTER 11

Partner with Your Provider

My ultimate goal in writing this book is to share the extensive number of cognitive health-boosting tools you have at your disposal that you can implement on your own. I want you to recognize just how much power you have over your—or your loved one's—brain span. And yet, partnering with a trained healthcare provider can take your efforts even further by helping you in a variety of ways, including collecting and interpreting data via labs, identifying any root causes (such as infections or deficiencies), formulating and monitoring a plan, ordering prescriptions (whether it's a sleep study to evaluate your sleep apnea risk, bioidentical hormones, or a medication to address an underlying condition), or referring you to other trusted care providers, should you need them. I would be remiss if I ended this book before helping you understand the many different types of providers you could work with, and the specific ways they could help.

One word of caution—many of the types of providers I recommend in this chapter are not likely to be covered by your insurance. Even if they are, your deductible and rates of coverage may be such that your out-of-pocket costs will still be high. I'll walk you through how to evaluate how ready you are to partner with a provider, because it will likely be an investment.

That said, if cost or access to providers and/or labs is an issue, stay focused on the tools in the new Alzheimer's toolkit that you *can* do, and only do the things in this chapter that are within reach for you at this point in time—such as scheduling an appointment with your primary care physician, asking for the labs that your insurance will cover, and identifying the supplements that you can commit to start taking regularly, for example. Once you've been working your plan for two to three months, come back to this chapter and see if it's time to start partnering with a provider to help take your results to the next level.

The Types of Healthcare Providers to Consider

There are four basic types of providers you could partner with. Let's look at them one by one so that you can get a broad overview of your options. I include information about how to find each of these kinds of providers in the Resources section.

- BREDESEN-TRAINED DOCTORS. My top choice is for you to work with a doctor—either a medical doctor (MD), doctor of osteopathy (DO), or naturopathic doctor (ND)—who has been trained in the ReCODE protocol that was designed by Dr. Dale Bredesen. These providers are well versed in assessing and rebalancing the upstream causes of cognitive decline. They may or may not accept private insurance, Medicare, or Medicaid.
- NON-BREDESEN-TRAINED PHYSICIANS, who are still well versed in using lifestyle medicine (exercise, nutrition, stress reduction, etc.) to address the root cause of disease, are my second choice. These physicians include:
  ◊ FUNCTIONAL MEDICINE DOCTOR, who ideally has been certified by the Institute of Functional Medicine. Functional medicine takes a systems-based approach to maintaining health, and its practitioners are trained in using diagnostic labs to create a personalized treatment plan that incorporates diet, exercise, stress reduction, supplements, and more.
  ◊ NATUROPATHIC DOCTOR, who has undergone a four-year degree program to learn how to address the root cause of disease by supporting the body's systems for self-healing. They are typically well educated in nutrition, exercise, detox, and supplements, and may also have a specialty (such as hormones).

◊ CHIROPRACTOR, who attended an accredited chiropractic college, will also have training in nutrition. Not all chiropractors extend their practices beyond physical manipulation, but some do.

◊ AN ACUPUNCTURIST OR DOCTOR OF CHINESE MEDICINE often incorporates nutrition and supplements into their patients' treatment plans and can help address common imbalances. The treatment itself is very effective at dialing down stress and triggering the relaxation response.

   Typically, these providers are not covered by insurance, meaning that you have to pay for them out of pocket, although more and more plans do offer some coverage for chiropractic care and/or acupuncture.

• A PRIMARY CARE PHYSICIAN (PCP) is conventionally trained in preventing and managing chronic diseases. They are covered by all forms of insurance and can give you access to a significant number of labs. If money or access is an obstacle to working with a Bredesen-trained provider or an out-of-pocket provider such as a functional medicine doctor or naturopath, you can still get a lot of insight and support from your PCP. They are also your point person to help you navigate urgent situations, such as acute illnesses or injuries. Ask your PCP if they are open to working in tandem with another provider, whether it's a Bredesen-trained physician, another healthcare provider, or a health coach.

If you go this route, you may also want to consult with some specialists, depending on which areas your physician hasn't been trained to address, such as:

• A DOCTOR CERTIFIED IN MENOPAUSE MEDICINE by the Menopause Society, or an endocrinologist, as they may be able to guide you on hormone therapy.

• A NEUROLOGIST, who can order brain imaging for you. Although, I do caution that the typical patient interaction with a neurologist isn't always helpful. Most neurologists want to help, but they're totally unfamiliar with this approach. Even if your neurologist is familiar with a more lifestyle medicine approach like the one outlined in this book, they'll still need to limit your visit to mere minutes, and they aren't trained to support you in a lifestyle intervention. As much as they want to help you, the system isn't set up to allow them to. Perhaps by being open with them about your goals and the tools you're using to meet those goals, you may open the neurologist's mind to what's possible in terms of preventing or treating dementia.

- HEALTH COACH. These professionals are well trained in behavioral change and can help you implement the treatment plan that you, or you and your doctor, have developed together. That plan in and of itself can be overwhelming, and that's before you run into some kind of challenge—like an illness, or a move, or a particularly stressful time—that makes it extra hard to stick to your program. A health coach helps you brainstorm workarounds to challenges, celebrates your successes with you, and helps you tailor your treatment plan to fit within your daily life.

  Some health coaches have even been trained in Dr. Bredesen's ReCODE protocol, and thus they also have the experience of having helped many families who are facing the same issues you are. That also means that they have a database of resources, strategies, and stories to share with you.

  At a minimum, consider working with a health coach for the first three months of your program—that's about how long it takes to establish some new habits and encounter some unforeseen hiccups.

- BREDESEN-TRAINED REGISTERED DIETITIAN OR NUTRITIONIST. A nutritionist or registered dietitian can also help you navigate a new way of eating, although most were not trained in the ketogenic diet. Some of these professionals do become certified in Dr. Bredesen's ReCODE protocol; however, I recommend sticking to this subset of registered dietitians and nutritionists to help you personalize the dietary guidance in this book to your unique goals and circumstances.

A Typical Timeline of Visits

In my practice, I have a general rhythm to how often I like to see patients—other Bredesen-trained providers will often have a similar schedule. If you are working with a non-Bredesen-trained provider or a PCP, you can suggest this timeline to them.

Day 0: Baseline Visit and Initial Labs

- An appointment with your provider; labs may actually occur a few days before or after meeting with your doctor

  At this visit, you and your provider are getting to know each other, capturing a snapshot of where you're beginning this journey, and talking about your goals. You'll want to bring a full list of medications and supplements that you're currently on, as well as copies of any recent labs, scans (such as MRI or mammogram), and assessments (such as your MoCA score or the results of other cognitive function tests, if you have them).

  At this visit your provider should request a number of labs—see the boxes on pages 244–245 and see how many on that list this provider can or is willing to request for you.

Months 1 to 1½ (4–6 Weeks After Initial Visit): Follow Up to Review Labs

- With your provider

  It can easily take four weeks to get the results of all your labs back, so it's a good idea to schedule your follow-up visit for six weeks after your initial visit to give that process plenty of time. It's worth calling your provider's office before you go in to this appointment to make sure that all lab results are in, because those results—as well as your goals and your current lifestyle habits—will help your provider create an individualized care plan at this visit.

  Once you have your plan, be sure to update the list of things you are currently doing—the supplements and meds you're taking, the dietary changes you're making, the exercise you're getting, and every change your provider suggests.

Months 4 to 5 (12 Weeks After Last Visit): Repeat Labs

- Lab or nurse visit only

  It'll take another twelve weeks or so to start to see measurable changes, so these labs should start to capture those improvements. Some things will change more quickly for example, your fasting glucose level or thyroid levels—while others take more time, such as cholesterol levels. But after three to four months of working the plan, making the changes that you're able to make and getting in a new rhythm, this second round of labs should deliver some good news. And for those measures that don't improve, or that change in a negative direction, now you and your provider have great information for how to further refine the plan.

Months 5 to 6 (2 to 4 Weeks After Last Visit): Follow Up to Review Labs

- With your provider

Again, it can take some time for all the lab results to come back; call your provider's office to make sure they've all returned before you go in for your appointment, and for lab results that come either directly to you or from another provider, make sure your doctor's office gets those results five to seven days before your appointment so that your provider has a chance to review them before you are sitting in front of them. You could also ask to repeat your MoCA at this time. I don't usually retest everything that we did at baseline, just the things that I'm expecting to see change because of some aspect of the treatment plan.

Months 8 to 9 (12 Weeks After Last Visit): Repeat Abnormal Labs

- Lab or nurse visit only

Again, we're typically testing only the labs that were abnormal before. We want to measure progress.

Months 9 to 10 (2 to 4 Weeks After Last Visit): Follow Up to Review Labs

- With your provider

At this point, your provider is hoping to see that your toxin levels are down, and your hormones, vitamins, and nutrient levels are stabilized.

Once you're there, we wait another six months to test labs, just to ensure they remain stable. After that, you can go to more of a maintenance phase, during which you're pulling labs and tweaking your plan only every year or so.

Thereafter, meet to update your plan and repeat any necessary labs every six months, eventually moving to once a year.

Your provider may have a different timeline in mind—particularly if you aren't working with a Bredesen-trained provider. If that's the case, you can certainly hand them a copy of this timeline and say, "This is what I want," and see if they will follow that for you. Regardless, at least when you first start working with a new provider—or really targeting your cognitive health with your existing primary care doctor—you want to have all your labs back so that your doctor can get a full picture of your baseline and identify that areas where you need to focus.

While this timeline is helpful, you may get knocked off of it. After all, life happens. You may get sick, or go through a stressful period, or your provider may leave the practice and you have to find someone new. There are any number of variables that could prevent you from following this timeline to a T. Just get back to it as soon as you are able.

Preparing for a Visit

Meeting with your doctor, whether they are Bredesen-trained or not, can be stressful, emotional, and feel like a blur, particularly when you feel your cognitive health is on the line and you may be paying out of pocket, as that sense of time ticking and wanting to get your money's worth can only increase the stress level.

It's important to head into one of these visits with an open mind and expectation that you will be able to work collaboratively. Remember that everyone in the room, including you and your doctor, are doing the best they can. You may not always feel you're on the same exact page, but you do form a team. Beyond that, here are some other tactics to consider:

- BRING SOMEONE WITH YOU. Whether you are there to check on your own cognitive health, or you're going with your loved one, you want to have another person there who can be a fresh pair of eyes and ears. There is often a lot of information to process, a lot of things you're being told to do, and a lot of questions you'd like answered. It can also be emotional, so consider bringing another family member, caregiver, friend, or even a health coach to help take notes, and make sure you ask all your questions and get answers. If you aren't sure who could do this for you, maybe there's someone from church or a senior center who is willing to support you. The people I see in my practice who often do the best are the ones who come with a team.

- BRING A COMPLETE LIST OF ALL MEDS AND SUPPLEMENTS. There can be some interactions between medications and supplements—for example, vitamin K, which I typically prescribe along with vitamin D supplements because it works in concert with vitamin D to direct calcium into the bones (and not into arterial walls), can interfere with blood-thinning medications. So if you're on a blood thinner for any reason, maybe because of atrial fibrillation or a history of blood clots or strokes, there is still an option to take a consistent amount of vitamin K every day, but you'd likely want to moderate the amount of blood-thinning medication you take based on that consistent level of vitamin K. As long as the doctors know about it, there are safe ways to do these things together. You just want to make sure that you're communicating.

  You also need to create an easily accessible and easily modifiable place to store this information, because it will change as you go. Consider keeping a Google doc or Excel spreadsheet or list in the Notes function of your phone with everything you are committing to doing and taking so that you can share the same information with every doctor you see. You'll want to update this list every time you see any doctor, such as a cardiologist, endocrinologist, neurologist, gastroenterologist, or other specialist so that you can share the list of everything you're doing—from meds, diet, exercise, other interventions—with every provider you see before each appointment in time for the support staff to get the information loaded into your electronic health record. Generally, five to seven days before your appointment gives them enough time to get it integrated into the system on the doctor's end, and then they will have that information in the right spot at the right time.

- BRING A SNAPSHOT OF YOUR LIFESTYLE. Prepare lists of a day or two of your typical diet, type and amount of exercise in a week, how much sleep you're getting, how much socializing you do, the activities you do regularly, and your daily routine so that you can share an accurate snapshot of the things you're doing to take care of your health. (The Progress Tracker I include at the back of this book and in downloadable form at ReversingAlzheimersBook.com is useful here.)

- NOTE YOUR CURRENT SYMPTOMS. Add to your list the symptoms you're currently experiencing—what's different? What's better? What's worse? How is your digestion, sleep, and stress?

- SEND ANY LABS AND QUESTIONS IN ADVANCE. At your first meeting, bring any lab results from the past one to three years so that your providers can have a better perspective on recent trends. Better yet, send them to your doctor's office five to seven days before your appointment so that the staff has a chance to upload them to your electronic health record. The same goes with the questions you have for your provider—the more advance notice they have, the better prepared they can be to answer them. That doesn't mean that if you think of a question you want to ask the day before or day of—or even during—your appointment that you shouldn't ask it; you just want to help your provider have everything they need to be able to serve you best in the moment.

You want to call ahead and ask if all the labs are back and if the doctor has seen them. This will save everyone time and frustration, as it's harder to create an individualized plan without them. Also, some labs are easier to interpret than others. I have patients who bring me labs I've never seen before. If I've received it five to seven days ahead of time, I can make time to look it up and understand it. If not, I'm stuck saying, "I'm so sorry. I don't know how to interpret this"—something I hate to have to say when I know how important every visit is.

Same thing with imaging reports—your provider wants to actually see your mammogram reports, not just hear that your ob/gyn said it was normal. Make sure the doctor has a copy of that report in front of them. Also, if there's a supplement that you want to discuss with your provider, send a picture of the label or send a link to the supplement ahead of time because that allows the doctor to look it up and create an informed opinion.

- **THINK THROUGH ANY DIFFICULTIES** you're having implementing your plan. Are you able to swallow all the pills? Is something too complicated? Are you experiencing side effects from any medications or supplements? An appointment is a chance to troubleshoot.

- **SEND ANY RESEARCH ARTICLES IN ADVANCE.** If there's a research article or a news article that you read recently that refers to a research article, send it ahead of time. And bring a printed copy to leave behind, just in case they didn't have time to read it in advance. It's hard to track down an exact study when all you have to go on are vague details. That makes it hard for them to give you an opinion about it.

- **SET GOALS FOR YOUR VISIT.** Are there certain treatments or approaches you want to discuss? Do you need clarity around a certain subject? Would you like to make changes to your prescriptions or supplements? Think about what would be most helpful to you as you come out of that next visit. You also want to think about your long-term goals—perhaps those include changes in a MoCA score or behavior, or there's a certain milestone you'd like to see achieved. You want to be committed to making positive changes without getting attached to specific outcomes, because there is some unpredictability in how each person responds to a protocol. Let's say your goal is to get steadier on your feet and stronger in your lower body so that your fall risk is lower—that can mean it's time to talk about a referral to physical therapy and maybe supplementing with testosterone and/or estrogen to contribute to muscle development or bone strength.

- **SHARE YOUR GOALS FOR THE VISIT** with your provider in the beginning of the appointment. There are some patient visits during which we start reviewing the labs and I don't realize that they have a list of concerns they'd like to address until our last five minutes together. The doctor will have an agenda for your visit, too, but it's your appointment. Sharing your agenda early on will help your provider manage the available time more efficiently.

- **GO OVER THE TIMELINE OF YOUR SUBSEQUENT VISITS.** When will you meet again? How will you measure outcomes? When will you repeat labs? When will you take another MoCA or other cognitive assessment test?

- LEAVE WITH A PLAN. You want to walk out of the office with any referrals you need for other specialists or procedures, an appointment for a follow-up visit, prescriptions for any labs or new meds, as well as a plan for your next steps (do you need to get someone to come check for mold, make an appointment with a biological dentist, or find a dance class, for example?). A lot of your prescriptions may come from different pharmacies because, just like doctors, pharmacies specialize, too. If you're getting hormones from one pharmacy, gut meds from another pharmacy, and supplements from an online source, make sure you leave with all the information that you need to get those prescriptions filled so you can get them started right away.

  Once you're home, you want to get organized so you can put the plan into practice. This may mean putting some aspects of your treatment plan on your calendar. Plan out your days reviewing what's best to do or take in the morning, at midday, and at night. You will want to be able to update your daily and weekly schedule so that the activities and priorities you discuss have a place in your days.
- TAKE NOTES. There's a lot to cover in these appointments—make sure you're writing things down while you're in the room so that you can remember them later. Don't assume you'll remember—even if you bring support people with you, there are details that can slip through the cracks if you don't write them down.

MOST HELPFUL LABS FOR ASSESSING COGNITIVE RISK

This represents the labs I most typically request for my patients. I've separated them into things you can request from a primary care physician (and hopefully have covered by insurance), and things you likely have to ask a functional medicine, naturopathic, or Bredesen-trained physician for (and, thus, will probably require you to pay out of pocket).

If you're working with your primary care physician, you can share this list with them and then say, "I understand you may not always order these, but I've read about the literature that outlines the modifiable risk factors that are known to contribute to Alzheimer's. I'm willing to do the work to change those things, and I'd love for you to help me to order the labs so that we can track my changes over time."

Remember that although it is very helpful to be able to quantify the factors that influence your brain health so that you can see where you're starting from and measure progress along the way (and even sometimes identify an underlying cause, like the buildup of a toxin such as mercury), lifestyle is still the most powerful lever you have. After all, labs primarily capture downstream effects—the results of the choices you make. When you're struggling with or seeking to ward off cognitive decline, you want your focus to be on the upstream causes—all those components of brain health that I outlined in Chapter 1, including diet, exercise, sleep, toxic exposure, infectious burden, and nutrient status.

If you are limited to only what your primary care provider can order for you, or what Medicare or Medicaid covers, get what tests you can and then double down on the lifestyle factors—exercise, diet, meditation, sleep, and environment.

Labs you can ask your primary care doctor to request (and will likely be covered by insurance):

» Heavy metals tests (for lead, mercury, and arsenic)
» Complete blood count (CBC)
» Vitamin D
» Thyroid hormone panel
» Hormone testing (for estrogen, progesterone, testosterone)
» Omega-3s
» B vitamins
» H-CRP
» Sleep study (can be done at home and is covered by insurance)

» MoCA score
» MRI of the brain
» EEG
» Infection tests for Lyme and herpes

If you do have the privilege of working with a functional medicine doctor, naturopath, or Bredesen-trained provider, these are the panels to ask for:

» Full male panel/full female panel
» Hemoglobin A1C
» Fasting insulin
» Homocysteine
» Mycotoxins
» Chemical toxins
» Heavy metal toxins
» Antioxidant status
» Mineral status—particularly magnesium, zinc, and copper
» Mitochondrial function
» Methylation status
» Microbiome and gut status testing (stool)
» Cortisol testing (salivary and urine)

Again, while some are covered by Medicare and insurance, some of them will likely be out of pocket—in my clinic a full panel costs about $2,500. Keep in mind that the full suite of labs includes a thorough evaluation of potential risk factors that might put you on the path to dementia. Dr. Bredesen calls this full workup a "cognsoscopy," and compares it to the now-routine colonoscopy that identifies risk for colon cancer. Just as everyone should have a colonoscopy at age fifty, everyone should also have a cognoscopy. I get that it feels like a significant investment, but remember, these labs cost a fraction of the amount of money and effort that it costs to treat and care for someone with dementia. If you know about these risk factors now, you can do something about them right away.

A Key Thing to Discuss with Your Provider: Bioidentical Hormone Therapy

It's a natural progression in life that our reproductive hormones decline as we age. While that makes sense from a reproductive standpoint—we don't necessarily want to be having children when we may not live long enough to raise them to adulthood—it's not great for brain health.

Most people don't realize how hormones, such as estrogen, progesterone, and testosterone, influence brain health. They do so by sending signals to the brain that support the formation of new neurons and connections between neurons. Think back to puberty, when your hormones were raging but you were also learning new things and building new skills every day. It wasn't just that you had the energy of youth—you also had a rising tide of hormones to support your cognition.

My background as a naturopathic physician taught me that menopause and andropause (the decline in reproductive hormones that men experience) are natural transitions. But then I learned in my dementia training how beneficial the practice known as hormone therapy (HT) or menopause hormonal therapy (MHT) can be for the brain, and started to see how much better people feel on it. Luckily, we can take these hormones in the form of pills, patches, or creams and support our cognition—and so much more, including our bone health, muscle mass, and heart health. In my practice I exclusively use bioidentical hormones, or those that are biochemically identical to the hormones produced naturally in your body, as opposed to chemicals that are similar but not identical as is typically used in conventional HT, including forms of birth control. Bioidentical hormone therapy is abbreviated BHT, and that is how I will refer to it in this chapter.

BHT isn't without its controversies. Yes, there are risks that need to be carefully weighed with a hormone-savvy doctor, but in my experience the benefits largely outweigh the risks, especially for women without a personal or family history of breast cancer, and who have a personal or family risk of osteoporosis or dementia.

Women have been taking supplemental estrogen as a remedy for menopausal symptoms at least since the early 1940s when a synthetic estrogen was granted FDA approval. Despite decades of precedent, this practice screeched to a halt in the early 2000s as the result of one poorly designed—and poorly reported upon—study.

The Women's Health Initiative (WHI) study was a large-scale study funded by the National Institutes of Health that was designed to assess the benefit of hormone replacement therapy on postmenopausal women. In 2002, the NIH halted the study because it found a small but still significant increase in risk of heart disease and breast cancer in women taking hormones. The media picked up the story and ran with it. Worse, that small increase in risk was reported as if it were much scarier than it truly was—it went from 2.33 people per 100 getting breast cancer to 2.95 people per 100, yet the media reported that as an increase in risk of 26 percent. While it's true that 2.95 is 26 percent higher than 2.33, it doesn't accurately convey the danger. (Consider that smoking increases cancer risk by 2,600 percent.)

Beyond the reporting, there were major issues with the study design: The majority of the women in the study were sixty and above, meaning they were farther out from menopause and simply farther along their aging journey, and aging itself is a major risk factor for disease. Also, the women in the study were taking synthetic estrogen in pill form, something I advise against—you want to take bioidentical hormones, which means the label needs to say "estradiol" and "progesterone," as anything else is chemically different from the hormones that your body naturally manufactures. And taking estrogen orally—as the women in the study did—means your liver has to metabolize it, and during that process the liver will produce clotting agents that can contribute to the risk of stroke and aneurysm. When you take estrogen via a transdermal patch, which is common today, you bypass the liver and, thus, the formation of the clotting agents.

Today, the pendulum is swinging back toward HT. Multiple randomized, placebo-controlled studies have found that HT administered in women under the age of sixty significantly reduces the risk of all-cause mortality and cardiovascular disease. A large-scale Finnish study followed nearly five hundred thousand women on some form of HT for fifteen years and found a significant reduction in breast cancer risk compared to the rest of the similarly aged population. A 2021 British study that compared approximately 105,000 women on HT with two hundred thousand women who did not use HT found that taking hormones reduced the risk of all-cause mortality by 9 percent.

There are certain precautions we now take. Most importantly, today we are able to prescribe bioidentical hormones, which, as their name suggests, are chemically identical to the hormones our bodies manufacture, and not some close look-alike that may bind with the same receptors but have a different chemical structure and, thus, different effects on the body. And we can now prescribe those hormones to be administered via the skin with either patches or creams.

That said, BHT isn't risk-free. One risk factor to BHT is that, while it doesn't cause cancer, if you have a cancer that is estrogen or progesterone receptor-positive—such as breast, uterine, ovarian, or endometrial cancer—it can cause that cancer to grow. So you want to make sure cancer isn't present before you start treatment, and then stay current on your screenings to ensure that an undetectable cancer hasn't grown. I require all clients to do breast imaging once a year to mitigate the risk of BHT.

The risks of BHT are different depending on your age and menopausal status. For women who are still perimenopausal (meaning, it's been less than a year since their most recent period, although their cycles have become erratic and they are likely experiencing symptoms such as hot flashes, mood changes, vaginal dryness, and sleep disturbances) or who have been in menopause for fewer than ten years, the risks of HT are lower than for women who are more than ten years out from menopause.

If you are a candidate for BHT, supplementing with bioidentical forms of estrogen, progesterone, and testosterone can help with the following:

- Signaling the brain to create new neurons and neuronal connections and strengthen the neurons and neural pathways that already exist (estrogen)
- Cueing bones to maintain their density and integrity, reducing the risk of osteopenia, osteoporosis, and debilitating fractures (estrogen and progesterone)
- Keeping cholesterol in check (estrogen)
- Maintaining muscle mass and preventing frailty and falls (testosterone)

- Reducing inflammation by soaking up free radicals (estrogen)
- Maintaining or restoring libido, helping us get that all-important sense of physical connection (testosterone and estrogen)
- Lowering risk of uterine cancer, promoting more restful sleep, and supporting mental and emotional health (progesterone)

While everything on this list is vitally important, it's really the brain benefits of BHT that I'm focused on. Neuroscientist Lisa Mosconi, PhD, author of the book *The XX Brain: The Groundbreaking Science Empowering Women to Maximize Cognitive Health and Prevent Alzheimer's Disease* describes the crucial role estrogen plays in women's brain health in an interview on NPR's *TED Radio Hour* program: "At the cellular level, estrogen literally pushes neurons to burn glucose to make energy. If your estrogen is high, your brain energy is high. When your estrogen declines, though, your neurons start slowing down and age faster," she said. Supplementing with estradiol can help prevent this hormone-related decline. "My work in particular has shown that Alzheimer's disease starts earlier in women's brains than men's brains, specifically in midlife and even more specifically during the transition to menopause." What I take from this insight is that the sooner you start taking BHT, the better for your brain—assuming you have undergone a detailed health history and risk assessment with a hormone-savvy doctor.

Deciding whether to do BHT and in what doses is a very individualized decision that you should make in collaboration with a doctor who is well versed in BHT. (Many doctors, particularly those trained after 2002, when the Women's Health Initiative Study came out, were taught that BHT is almost never a safe idea, and this continues to be their framework.) Hormone replacement therapy requires balance—you don't want too little or too much. You want the amount that's just right for you, and that may take some trial and error. For example, women whose testosterone levels get too high can develop acne, start to grow facial hair, and/or experience aggression. Granted, it takes a lot to get these side effects, but you do want to be working with a hormone-savvy doctor—generally a functional medicine physician, a naturopath, or a Bredesen-trained provider who will be able to steer you toward the proper dose for you that provides plenty of benefit while still mitigating any potential risks.

In my practice, I put women who pass the risk assessment analysis, no matter their age—even in their eighties—on BHT. They tend to get pep in their step, their mood lifts, their cognition improves. If you already have dementia or mild cognitive impairment, or have a close relative who does, and/or you're a caregiver for someone who does, yet you've never had cancer or heart disease and don't have a family history of either, the upside of BHT is often high enough to be worth the risk. And remember, we monitor that risk with yearly mammograms and blood work.

Honestly, the risk that the WHI found wasn't any higher than taking birth control pills—and the potential benefit of BHT is that you don't have to suffer through menopausal symptoms, and you make it less likely that you get osteoporosis or dementia. If dementia is a reality or a likely reality for you, it's at least worth it to have the conversation with a doctor. Just remember that it can't be had in fifteen minutes, so you have to talk to someone other than your PCP or even your ob/gyn.

The hormones that you could choose to replace include these:

- Estrogen—technically, estrogen is an umbrella term for a few different hormones. Estradiol is the form of estrogen women in their reproductive years make when they are not pregnant, and is also the form you want to take as hormone therapy as it is bioidentical to the version your ovaries once made (unlike Premarin, a conjugated estrogen, for example, which is derived from horse urine and not bioidentical). I recommend my patients use an estradiol transdermal patch or use a compounded bioidentical cream for two reasons: (1) it's one less pill to take, and (2) absorbing it through the skin means it doesn't need to be metabolized by the liver, a process that can create clotting agents that can contribute to the risk of blood clots.

- Progesterone—balances the effect of estrogen and also prevents the lining of the uterus from ripening, lowering the risk of endometrial cancer (which is a risk for women who replace estrogen without also taking progesterone). Progesterone is also a relaxant—I advise my female patients to take it just before bed as it helps them sleep. It's also good for mood. While you can apply it as a cream, I recommend taking it orally if you have any issues with sleep or mood. If you sleep well, for some women it is simpler to combine their estradiol and progesterone into one cream to apply once daily.

- Testosterone—although primarily considered a male hormone, women make it, too. For both sexes, it helps with energy levels, brain signaling, libido, and muscle building, which helps reduce the risk of falling, general frailty, and losing too much weight on a ketogenic diet.
- Pregnenolone and DHEA—DHEA is a precursor to testosterone, cortisol, or estrogen. And pregnenolone is a precursor to progesterone as well as DHEA. I often prescribe DHEA and testosterone to men, in amounts that are much higher than what I would give women. While they are both available over the counter, it's really easy to get the dosing wrong—and potential side effects include acne and hair loss. Resist the temptation to dose yourself, and work with a trained provider to get the dosing right for you.

Working with a Biological Dentist

As I covered in Chapter 1, your oral health has a strong influence on the rest of the body, especially the brain. The three primary avenues by which what's happening in your mouth impact your brain are (1) mercury, (2) bacteria, and (3) airway obstruction or sleep apnea. A biological dentist is trained to take into consideration the connection between your oral health and the impact of any dental issue or procedure on the rest of your body, including your brain.

Let's start with mercury. Despite being considered the most toxic heavy metal, mercury has been used for over 150 years in the silver amalgams used to fill cavities. If you have these old-school fillings, mercury vapor is released each time you chew your food or brush or grind your teeth. Mercury is a potent neurotoxin, and mercury toxicity is associated with depression, headaches, inability to focus, memory issues, dizziness, as well as a lowered immune system. Unfortunately, having the silver fillings removed and replaced with a white composite material (that, in addition to not containing heavy metals, also looks much nicer) releases mercury vapor in large amounts. This is why you want to use what's known as a biological or holistic dentist—a doctor of dentistry who is committed to always seeking the safest and least-toxic way to administer oral care. Biological dentists follow a careful protocol for the removal of mercury fillings that includes using a dental dam (so that you don't inadvertently swallow mercury) and an oxygen mask (so that you don't inhale its vapors). They can also advise you on how to assist your body in detoxing any mercury that has accumulated in your system over the years with nutrition and binding supplements.

As I've covered, the oral bacteria *P. gingivalis* (found in the plaque that forms on your teeth and responsible for the inflammation of the gums known as gingivitis, and an underlying cause of more serious periodontal disease) has been found in the brains of Alzheimer's patients. For this reason, if you have any regular bleeding of the gums or toothaches, don't wait until your next regularly scheduled teeth cleaning to get it checked out— book an appointment with a biological or holistic dentist who will seek to treat your whole-body health in a way that reduces risk of harm to your other bodily systems.

As for sleep apnea, it can be caused by airway obstruction that can have a variety of triggers, such as mouth breathing (which can trigger swollen tonsils and throat tissue), tongue placement, and jaw alignment. A biological dentist may be able to help remedy these root causes with oral devices and even tongue exercises that can diminish sleep apnea without the use of the typical treatment—continuous positive airway pressure (CPAP) machines. (Although CPAP machines are often effective and covered by insurance—a sleep medicine physician can help you determine if you need one and prescribe one for you.)

It is true that biological dentists tend to charge more, and that they are less likely to be covered by dental insurance. Again, consider the costs of providing long-term care later that you can mitigate now by removing a primary source of neurological damage. I've seen too many patients who have had their old silver fillings removed and replaced and enjoyed a noticeable uptick in not just their cognitive function but also their resilience to infections to discount the benefit of making an investment in your oral health. (See the Resources section for information on how to find a biological or holistic dentist near you.)

Boosting Your Nutritional Baseline with Supplements

I am a big believer in the power of supplements to address nutritional deficiencies and to support your body's natural chemical processes, including detoxification. Nearly every patient I see leaves with a list of recommended supplements. Even though supplements are something you can do on your own, it is a good idea to also have a trained healthcare provider who knows everything you're taking so that they can keep an eye on potential interactions and guide you on proper dosages.

In order to make taking your pills more doable and less overwhelming, I highly recommend using a pillbox—the bigger the better. (See the Resources section for the specific one I recommend.) You don't want to open the cabinet and wonder, "Wait, which one? How many? Have I already taken this today?"

This means that you only need to deal with all your pills once a week—or every two weeks, if your pillbox is big enough. I recommend setting aside an hour or so on a Saturday morning or afternoon to get all your bottles out and set them up in a group to the left of where you're sitting. Then, as you populate each day with a supplement, move the bottle over to your right so that you don't accidentally double up on any supplement. Be hyper-organized about this for an hour and then you don't have to think about it again for another week or two.

Of course, you'll need to refer to your list of supplements and medications that has been updated since your most recent doctor's appointment.

As you go through the week and realize that you're having a hard time remembering to take a specific supplement or medication—perhaps because you need to take it two hours before your midday meal, and that time typically blows right past you without your realizing it—set a reminder on your phone or watch. Hopefully after a while it just becomes a habit and you won't even need to hear the alarm go off—you'll have already taken it.

If swallowing pills is an issue, or if you or your care partner has pill fatigue, try one of these strategies:

- Talk to your provider to see if you can find powders instead of capsules or tablets, or if there's a version that has an easier-to-swallow coating, or if a particular medication is crushable. (Some things need to get through the GI tract before they're broken down and, therefore, cannot be crushed.)
- If the pill is small enough, or if it's a powder, you can try putting it in food. A high-fat plain yogurt is ketogenic diet–friendly, as is an avocado chocolate pudding or chia pudding.
- If the pill must be swallowed, try either placing it right behind the two bottom front teeth, or lower your chin toward your chest after you've put the pill in your mouth but before you swallow the water. Both of these techniques help propel the pill to the back of the throat and into the esophagus.
- If you're taking pills with a meal, take them after you've started eating, or even after you've finished eating, so that you or your loved one doesn't fill up on water and lose their appetite.

There are five specific supplements or categories of supplements that I recommend to just about everyone, although I, of course, recommend working with your healthcare provider to discuss dosages and possible interactions with any medications you may be taking.

Nootropics

"Nootropic" is a fancy word for a substance that supports cognitive function. There are many nootropic (*no-uh-TROPE-ic*) supplements on the market—see the Resources section for a few of my favorites. These supplements typically include a blend of vitamins (such as B vitamins), fats (particularly omega-3s), amino acids (such as L-theanine, a relaxant found in black and green tea leaves), herbs (such as ginkgo biloba, lion's mane, and curcumin), and perhaps caffeine. My personal experience with nootropics, as well as that of my patients, friends, and colleagues, is that they help with focus, mental clarity, mood, and better-quality sleep at night. It can give you a level up on days that you haven't gotten enough sleep or eaten well. I take them on days I'm giving talks or when I have a lot of work to get through and need to be on all day—they help me power through, feel productive, and sleep better at night.

One caveat: If you are on mood-stabilizing psychiatric medications, discuss adding nootropics with you provider first, because some nutrients and herbs can interact with prescribed medications in a potentially dangerous way. (Be sure to show your provider the ingredient list for the particular supplement you're considering.)

DOSAGE: Follow dosing instructions on the label. For people already experiencing cognitive decline of any severity, I recommend taking several capsules (again, following label instructions) four to five days a week for six months. From there, or if your goal is merely prevention, take on an as-needed basis.

Vitamin D with K

These fat-soluble vitamins have roles all over the body—particularly in maintaining bone health, but they are also directly related to cognitive function. Vitamin D helps maintain calcium balance within your cells, and when calcium accumulates in the neurons, it can foster neuronal dysfunction. Although we don't fully understand the connection between D and cognitive functions, when people have enough vitamin D, it appears to prevent cognitive decline. Vitamin K works with D to direct calcium into the bones. Like vitamin D, having higher levels of circulating vitamin K is associated with better cognitive function.

DOSAGE: Aim for 5,000 IUs of vitamin D and 90 mcg of K2 (if you are considering taking vitamin K, talk with your provider to determine an appropriate amount as it can interact with some blood-thinning medications).

Omega-3s

Omega-3 essential fatty acids are anti-inflammatory—and are believed to help reduce neuroinflammation and heart disease risk (and what's good for the heart is also good for the brain). In addition, when there are ample omega-3s on hand in the bloodstream, they become incorporated into cellular membranes throughout the body, including brain cells. Once there, they enable those membranes to stay pliable and well functioning. Higher levels of omega-3s in the blood are associated with a bigger hippocampus, a stronger ability to use logical reasoning, and—in people with at least one APOE4 allele—healthier microvasculature.

Again, I'm including some of my favorite brands of omega-3 supplements in the Resources section. No matter what kind you buy, you want to store them in the fridge so that they don't become rancid—in which case they become harmful to your cells, not helpful.

DOSAGE: Aim for 4 to 5 grams combined of EPA and DHA (two forms of omega-3s that are typically listed separately on the supplement label—you'll have to add them up to determine how many supplements add up to 4 or 5 grams).

Probiotics

There is a strong documented link between gut health and brain health. Your friendly gut bacteria help digest your food, making the nutrients more bio-available so that you can assimilate more of them. They also manufacture neurotransmitters, playing a crucial role in mood and mindset—which we know, thanks to Dr. Becca Levy's research, which I covered in Chapter 2, have a huge influence on our dementia risk. Equally as important, good gut bugs reduce inflammation and help our nervous systems get out of defend-and-attack mode. Also, you need the good bacteria to fight infectious actors such as *C. diff* and *H. pylori*, which are associated with cognitive issues, before they have a chance to take hold. At a very causal level they help us maintain balance in the gut, which is where all health or disease starts, and have a bowel movement every day, which reduces our toxic load.

I recommend several different brands in the Resources section—I also advise mixing up the blends you take because getting a variety of bacterial strains helps promote diversity and longevity, two hallmarks of a healthy microbiome.

DOSAGE: Aim for 100 billion live units (also known as colony-forming units, or CFUs) per day, taken with food—this is the dosage that I've seen really move the needle with my patients. I also encourage lots of fermented foods, such as kimchi, sauerkraut, unsweetened kefir, and miso soup.

Digestive Enzymes

As you age, your levels of hydrochloric acid—which helps break down your food so that you can access and assimilate the nutrients within it—decline. Taking digestive enzymes in supplement form can counteract this decline and help your body adjust to a healthier diet.

There are different types of digestive enzyme supplements, and different enzymes help break down different categories of foods. For example, lipase helps break down fats, protease targets proteins, and lactase breaks down the naturally occurring sugar called lactose in dairy products. Hydrochloric acid helps digest everything, but it can aggravate acid reflux if you have it. Ideally, you'd work with a provider who can steer you toward a digestive enzyme that will help you digest your food and assimilate nutrients in a meaningful way, as well as help with bloat, indigestion, and nutrient depletion.

DOSAGE: One or two tablets or chewable pills—without hydrochloric acid—taken at the start of a meal is helpful and safe for most people.

Connection over Correction

The idea of using loving communication doesn't apply just to your relationship with your care partner, it's also helpful in your relationship with your doctors. I recommend approaching all interactions with your doctor with a spirit of collaboration.

After all, doctors are trained to meet patients where they're at. As a doctor, I ascribe to that philosophy. I also encourage you, as a patient, to meet your doctors where they're at. Keep in mind that many of them weren't trained in the modifiable risk factors for dementia, because we've only recently started talking about them. *The Lancet* published its first list in 2017, and it can take decades for science to trickle down enough to impact what happens in doctors' offices. Most conventionally trained physicians have very little training in nutrition, or hormone therapy, or supplementation.

It helps to approach your relationship with your doctors with the mindset that everyone's doing their best with the information they have. While you may have differing approaches and priorities, you and your doctor form a team. You want to collaborate with them. The best way to do that is by being polite, sincere, and respectful, and to remember that they are part of a bigger system that isn't yet set up to focus on prevention when it comes to cognitive health.

Even though from our perspective what you may be asking them feels like common sense, it's still cutting edge in the traditional medical paradigm. As such, you increase your odds for having a successful partnership by asking them for things that are in their wheelhouse. For a traditional primary care doctor, that means standard labs and referrals to specialists, such as a sleep clinic, if you suspect sleep apnea, or to a provider certified in menopausal medicine, if you're looking to start bioidentical hormone therapy. Keep sharing what you're learning, and as they see you make progress, you may even inspire them to get more training.

Remember, although we are starting to see studies that demonstrate the brain health benefits of stacking lifestyle interventions, it takes years for literature to translate into clinical practice. Resist the urge to go in reminding them you know more than they do. Rather, go in with a plan, look for ways you can collaborate, ask what tests they can run through your insurance, and be grateful for whatever they can provide. Doctors are sometimes just sadly misinformed and now you have up-to-date empowering info that has a track record of bringing about results.

In those office visits, if you are there with your loved one who is experiencing some amount of cognitive decline, you may find that you remember things differently, or that they don't think their cognitive issues are that big of a deal. It could get combative at times. It might be best for your relationship if you were to have a separate conversation with the doctor. For many of my patients, I discuss the treatment plan primarily with the caregiver—it can make things simpler, so the person struggling with dementia isn't so focused on feeling defensive or out of control.

You may also need to have difficult conversations with other family members or loved ones about the time and expense of working with the types of providers I've outlined in this chapter. In my experience, it's very helpful to do a little research so that you can use some real numbers to help determine whether the investment in care is worth it. Find out how much assisted-living and memory-care facilities cost in your area. (Keep in mind that there is generally a base rate that then goes up if you need one-on-one care—get numbers for all the options.) Research how much it costs to pay for live-in care. Get a picture of the real costs of care per month and then compare that to spending $15,000 to $20,000 with a mix of providers over the course of the next year—that's the expected cost I share with potential patients. I know that's a big number, and that there is such a thing as reality—if the money's not there, it's not there. And yet the investment you make in partnering with one or more providers has the potential to save you so much later. I think you'll find that spending that $15,000 to $20,000 now equals what you would spend in only two or three months for twenty-four-hour care, whether at home or in a facility. (If you have long-term-care insurance, it can cost less to live in memory care or assisted living. If you have that safety net, that may be what makes the most sense for you.) There are so many emotions at play when deciding how to care for a loved one; I have found that attaching some numbers can help clarify things about what is possible and what is not. This gives you a clearer idea about the choices you have to make. Even if all you do is delay the need for someone to go into memory care, you could easily recoup the money you spend now.

Again, I'll close with the message that the most powerful interventions you can make with regard to your cognitive health are the choices you make every day about what to eat, how much to move, when to go to bed, and how to spend your time. If you do the cost-benefit analysis and decide that now is not the time to work with a healthcare provider, you still have multiple significant tools at your disposal. If you do decide to forgo working with a provider at this time, my one suggestion is that you do some thinking about when you will revisit this decision. Will it be a particular milestone, such as a certain MoCA score, or a specific symptom? Or will it perhaps be a set date in the future—perhaps three, six, or, at most, twelve months from now? Put some parameters on it, because although reversal is possible, prevention is a much easier lift.

To watch a summary video of this chapter and download the
Reversing Alzheimer's workbook go to ReversingAlzheimersBook.com.

Reflection questions:

- Does it make sense to schedule an appointment with any healthcare providers at this time?
- Do you have the bandwidth to devote the time and energy to making these appointments? How much time and energy are you willing and able to commit?
- Do you have the financial resources to devote to these appointments? How much money are you willing and able to commit?
- If you're ready to work with a healthcare provider, what research do you need to do? (For example: Do you need to search for a local Bredesen-trained provider, health coach, or biological dentist? Is there someone you can ask for referrals?)
- On a scale of 1 to 10, how urgent is it that you seek out care from a healthcare provider?
- On a scale of 1 to 10, how motivated are you to set aside the time toward partnering with a healthcare provider?
- Is there a member of your family with whom you need to share this chapter and get their support to move forward?

Looking Forward

CHAPTER 12

A Glimpse into the Near Future

Now that you've been introduced to—and have hopefully started implementing—the new Alzheimer's toolkit, I hope that you're starting to envision a different future for your loved one, yourself, your patients, and even the world. As Dr. Becca Levy's research, which I shared in Chapter 2, has demonstrated, having a positive view of what's to come has a big positive influence on health in general and dementia in particular.

I also know that it's not always easy to maintain hope. For those moments when you need something in addition to the tools you've just learned about in order to stay hopeful, in this chapter I'm offering a glimpse of the treatments that are becoming available, and a peek ahead into the not-so-distant future at what will be possible for our collective brain health as we as individuals, the medical community, and society in general adopt a more preventive approach to brain health.

Cutting-Edge Treatments

I think of these as things to layer into your Reversing Alzheimer's protocol if or when you have the resources and bandwidth, based on how much you stand to benefit from them. They each have their upsides and their down-sides, which I've listed below. I've also included information on how to decide if this might be something to devote money and time toward.

I've listed these treatments in order of where I think they are in terms of readiness, starting with the most established and ending with the most speculative. Things are changing quickly in this space—by the time this book has been printed, there will likely be new developments. To hear about the latest science and potential treatments, sign up for my newsletter at drheathersandison.com.

Red Light Therapy

Red light therapy, also known as photobiomodulation (PBM), which I also cover in Chapter 8 as a potential health-boosting activity, uses red or near-infrared light to stimulate healing processes in the body, and has an impressive and growing body of research that demonstrates benefits for brain health.

This part of the light spectrum approximates the light emitted at sunrise and sunset. From an evolutionary perspective, this part of the light spectrum helps calibrate your circadian rhythm, which plays a role in regulating multiple systems of the body. It also boosts the function of mitochondria, helping them produce more energy in the form of ATP with fewer resources, in part by enhancing function of the cytochrome c oxygenase enzyme, which shuttles electrons into the mitochondria. It increases blood flow to the brain and the removal of waste products through the stimulation of the flow of lymphatic fluid; reduces neuroinflammation and swelling; promotes the formation of new blood vessels and synapses; and raises levels of brain-derived neurotrophic factor (BDNF) and antioxidants.

Studies have found benefits of PBM in both animal and human experiments on traumatic brain injury, stroke, and dementia. Research out of Harvard Medical School and the University of California at San Francisco has found that wearing a transcranial photobiomodulation device (which looks like a helmet) at home creates a decrease in symptoms of cognitive decline, angry outbursts, and anxiety, and an increase in sleep and cognitive function.

Although the research is compelling, the reason I decided to invest in red light therapy devices and make their use a priority for Marama residents is because I had patients telling me how much benefit they got out of using these devices. One of the first residents who used the cranial device had very high anxiety, needed a lot of one-on-one care, and would sometimes wake up in the mornings with an impaired ability to speak. After twenty minutes of using the device, she would come back to her baseline. Of course, there are so many variables at play—including diet, exercise, activities, and community—that you can't isolate just one as being the cause of benefit. But my strong suspicion is that red light helps our residents. It's also very low risk—the only potential downsides are the cost of the device and the time you spend using them. (See the Resources section for the red light devices we use at Marama.)

UPSIDES: Very low risk, strong body of research, and my clinical experience points to important brain benefits.

DOWNSIDES: Cost of purchasing the device (although you can share red light devices with other people in your household or even a neighboring household, reducing the investment) and time spent using it (it appears to work best with consistent use of about twenty minutes five to six days per week, although you can do other things while using it, like cook, meditate, or read).

YOU'RE A GOOD CANDIDATE IF: Red light therapy has a broad application and benefit, whether you're actively experiencing cognitive decline or not. As I mentioned, many of our twenty-something staff members at Marama have used our red light devices and report that it helps them feel less anxious. You do not need to be actively experiencing memory loss to benefit.

Plasmapheresis

Also known as "young blood," or "therapeutic plasma exchange," plasmapheresis is essentially a transfusion of only a portion of the blood—the plasma, which carries everything that's not blood cells, including exosomes, cytokines (immune molecules that when present in large amounts can trigger dangerous levels of inflammation), and nutrients.

This treatment was inspired by animal studies that paired old mice with young mice in a practice known as parabiosis, where the animals' circulatory systems are combined so that their blood is commingled. Parabiosis has a long history—it first emerged in the late eighteenth century, then had a resurgence in the 1950s, and then in the early 2000s researchers from Harvard and Stanford began using it with mice, finding that the practice helped the older mice renew their liver cells, heal from injury, and even grow new neurons in the hippocampus. In 2023, a similar study found that giving old mice blood from young mice extended their life spans by 6 to 9 percent, or the equivalent of six years in humans.

The question is the mode of benefit—is it getting rid of certain components in the blood of older animals that's helpful, or is it that there are certain components in the blood of younger animals that's beneficial? The answer is likely both—inflammatory molecules, toxins, and perhaps infectious molecules present in old blood are reduced, and signaling molecules in young blood that can stimulate growth and repair are increased.

Of course, results found in animal studies don't directly translate into similar effectiveness or safety in humans. But two big clinical trials have shown a reduction in the rate of cognitive decline in patients with dementia after plasma exchange. One trial showed a 60 percent reduction in cognitive decline after fourteen months and improvement in language and processing speed; another showed improved cognitive function in patients with mild Alzheimer's. Compare that to the latest FDA approved medications for Alzheimer's, and plasmapheresis looks more than twice as effective at slowing the rate of progression (which was 27 percent for lecanemab).

Some clinics provide plasmapheresis—it currently costs about $5,000. When researching a place to have the procedures, there are variables to consider. Most importantly, after the plasma is removed, what is it replaced with? Is it plasma that comes from donors? Or is it something else? Some clinics replace plasma with albumin, a transport protein made in the liver that is present in plasma. Sometimes they use a substitute solution, such as saline and/or a combination of nutrients, such as vitamin C, minerals, B vitamins, and amino acids. My preference is rehydration, amino acids, vitamins, and minerals, if that option is available to you.

I've had patients who have done plasmapheresis. These patients had high levels of inflammation and toxins, and they experienced relief of symptoms ranging from pain, sensitivities to foods, and anxiety.

A more affordable option, if you are in prevention mode and are relatively healthy, is to donate your plasma through your local blood center or the American Red Cross—or even sell it to biotech companies. Donating plasma cues the body to create more, meaning it's *hormetic* (a beneficial stressor). The drawback to donating plasma is it's a fairly involved process, and many people won't be eligible. It can take four to five hours and requires a high-gauge needle.

The simplest approximation is to donate blood, which also has a hormetic effect—as you get rid of the old blood, you send signals to create new blood, including new plasma.

One big benefit of donating plasma or blood is that you're saving people's lives. Yet it's not without risk—if you have any depletion status, such as low iron or any deficiency, you can really throw things off.

UPSIDES: Can reduce inflammation and toxicity (although it doesn't remove the trigger); doesn't need to be done continuously over a long period of time to maintain benefit—you may want to do a series of treatments in the beginning and then shift into doing it at a longer interval, such as once a year, as regular maintenance; donating plasma or blood helps saves others' lives.

DOWNSIDES: Not specific to brain; will work better for some patients than for others (I hypothesize it works best for people for whom inflammation or toxicity is a contributing factor to a decline in cognition); when plasma is replaced with albumin, some patients experience uncomfortable and systemic swelling for a short period of time afterward; if you are donating plasma or blood, you may trigger a deficiency (such as anemia or dehydration).

YOU'RE A GOOD CANDIDATE IF: For plasmapheresis, if you are dealing with toxicity and/or inflammation, and you are also following the protocol and taking steps to address the sources of that toxicity and/or inflammation. For donating plasma or blood, if you are in prevention mode and looking for a low-risk way to stimulate your body to build its resistance and potentially reduce levels of harmful components that you may have in circulation, and if you work with your doctor to keep your eye on any potential nutrient deficiencies, such as iron.

Stem Cell Therapy

Stem cells are cells that have the potential to grow into a range of different types of cells. They're crucial for the repair of our tissues. While adults do have stem cells, they decline as we age. Stem cell therapies provide patients with an infusion of new stem cells in hopes of giving the body the building blocks it needs to repair itself. There is evidence that mesenchymal stem cells have the potential to increase the growth of new hippocampal nerves, and some studies of animal models have shown improvement in memory and learning ability after treatment.

Although stem cell therapy holds a lot of promise and is already used for many purposes, including dementia, it's a mixed bag. I have a patient with severe Alzheimer's who's had several rounds of stem cell treatments, and each time she gets a massive boost. I have another patient, with a MoCA score of 22, who experienced no change after investing in stem cell treatment.

Stem cell therapy is also very expensive. One treatment generally costs between $10,000 and $30,000. As of this writing, the cost for 5 million stem cells is $3,000. Dosing goes up to 50 million cells, and in general the more cells you use, the better likelihood of the treatment working.

I start thinking about stem cells when we've tried everything else—BHT, a ketogenic diet, reducing and remediating toxic exposures, exercising, and meditating—and still the patient isn't getting better. Of course, financial resources also come into play.

Beyond the fact that sometimes they don't seem to provide any benefit, there's also an argument that stem cell treatments could trigger inflammation, which certainly gives me pause. Also, stem cell treatments don't specifically target the brain—they are placed via catheter into the cerebrospinal fluid or into the blood, and can go anywhere from there. Suffice it to say, I don't have a ton of confidence that you're going to see a dramatic result—although some people do.

It's important to know that there is no FDA-approved stem cell treatment, although there is promising research on the effectiveness of stem cell treatment for dementia that has been conducted on animals. The dearth of research on humans is largely because stem cells are very political in the United States—some stem cells can come from either the blood found in the umbilical cord when babies are born, or from embryos—and it's not easy to get approval to study them from internal review boards (IRBs).

If, despite all these factors, you are interested in stem cell therapy, the variables you need to take into account are the number of cells you're receiving and where they're coming from—are they your own or someone else's? If they're your own, they typically come from either your bone or fat tissue, so there's little danger of your body rejecting them. But, the older you are, the lower quantity and quality of stem cells you'll tend to have. Your own stem cells will also have to be modified in order to become pluripotent, or able to grow into multiple different types of cells. If they are someone else's, you may have to take immunosuppressive drugs so that your body doesn't register them as invaders and attack them. You also need to consider if they are from an adult (which have to be modified in order to become pluripotent), from cord blood (which is inherently pluripotent), or from an embryo (which raises huge ethical questions and legal hurdles).

In the United States, there are complex regulations of human cells as biologic medications that require FDA approval for use unless they are specifically deemed minimally manipulated. Because of that law and the lack of FDA approval, if you want to use your own stem cells, you have to leave the country to go to places like Mexico, Panama, and, before the war broke out, Ukraine, where companies will take and store your stem cells and grow them into different types of cells.

UPSIDES: A small portion of my dementia patients who try them experience a dramatic boost in their cognitive function.

DOWNSIDES: Very expensive, not well researched in humans, ethical considerations if using embryonic stem cells, may require additional cost of international travel, possibility of flu-like symptoms after treatment.

YOU'RE A GOOD CANDIDATE IF: You've been diligent about implementing the protocol and you're not experiencing improvements in your cognition, *and* you have financial resources to spare. Again, results are hit or miss. At this stage, I consider stem cells to be a Hail Mary option. I'm looking forward to more research and specificity being applied to stem cells and dementia.

Peptides

Peptides are signaling molecules that are composed of chains of amino acids roped together, like pearls on a string. Your body is designed to make peptides out of amino acids, although they can also be made in a lab and then injected. For example, the best-known peptide is insulin. Its function is to allow glucose to move from your bloodstream into your cells, where it can be turned into energy. If you are basically healthy, your body will make plenty of insulin. But if you have type 1 diabetes, your body no longer has the ability to create insulin, so you take it in an injectable medicine form.

Specific peptides have specific functions. If your system is not creating the peptides that signal the brain to create new neurons and synapses, you can attempt to spur neurogenesis and synaptogenesis by injecting the relevant peptides.

Taking peptides isn't habit-forming, and yet more peptides are not always better. You still want to keep your system balanced, and you want to avoid having too much or too little of any one thing. (For example, if you have too much insulin, you can develop insulin resistance, which can have negative inflammatory effects.) That said, there are safe and effective doses of peptides.

Four primary peptides that target the brain:

- Cerebrolysin. This is the heavy-hitter peptide product for brain health—it's a blend of peptides that stimulates neurogenesis and promotes the growth of axons (the branches of neurons that connect to the axons of other neurons). It makes your neurons stronger and more resilient. It's also anti-inflammatory and works to prevent amyloid proteins from stacking up on top of one another and forming amyloid plaques. Research has found that Cerebrolysin aids in recovery after stroke and traumatic brain injury.
- Selank. This peptide blend modulates the nervous system, nourishes the brain, and helps to curb anxiety. From a nootrophic perspective, it helps

with the balance of neurotransmitters, elevates BDNF, and promotes memory, cognition, focus, and attention. What I've seen with my patients is that Selank is most effective in the early stages of mild cognitive impairment. They initially get a little boost from them and then they plateau, so we stop using them. But I still think it's a very worthwhile tool, because it can help you regain the clarity and focus to implement other parts of the program. You do need a prescription for Selank.

- Semax. Like Selank, Semax helps increase the level of BDNF and promotes memory, cognition, focus, and attention. Semax is more helpful as an antidepressant than an anxiolytic (as Selank is). Semax is more readily available in the United States than Cerebrolysin, although it can still take some searching to find a pharmacy that can fill the prescription.

- Dihexa. In animal studies, this peptide reduces neuroinflammation and restores spatial learning and cognitive function. It also enhances the connections between neurons and is sevenfold more potent than BDNF. This peptide can be administered in capsule form, without the need for an injection. Since we don't have human studies on Dihexa, we don't know enough about potential side effects like irritability, mood swings, anxiety, nausea, and insomnia. Long-term use is potentially related to an increase in cancer risk, and there is the risk of withdrawal.

I think that we are just scratching the surface of peptide use and that they will continue to become better studied and more widely available.

UPSIDES: Cognitive benefits of varying intensity and duration at a fraction of the cost of stem cell treatments—hundreds of dollars per treatment versus several thousands of dollars per treatment.

DOWNSIDES: Cerebrolysin must be injected and costs the most. It can be hard to find in the United States (it's more popular, and accessible, in Europe), so you have to work with a doctor who really knows how to source them. One avenue can be to get them by participating in a clinical trial. Selank and Semax are easier to track down, less expensive, and can be taken intranasally, but they don't seem to have as big an impact. The struggle is finding doctors who are knowledgeable and then finding consistent sourcing.

YOU'RE A GOOD CANDIDATE IF: You are working with a provider who understands peptide mechanisms, sourcing, and dosing well. They aren't a silver bullet, but if you can get them, they have the potential to augment the new Alzheimer's toolkit.

Exosomes

Exosomes are vesicles—little packets of information that are smaller than cells and more complex than peptides—that contain a lot of signaling information. Some exosomes contain signals that cue the growth of neurons and neuronal connections. They are extracted from the plasma around stem cells—I think of them as "stem cells light." They don't have the politics, cost, or potential for rejection and inflammation. On the downside, they aren't as foundational as stem cells: If stem cells are seeds that can grow into neurons, exosomes are fertilizer.

There are helpful exosomes and harmful exosomes. Some are involved in the pathology of Alzheimer's as they can cue the development of toxic proteins like amyloid and tau. Although not yet available to the general public, looking at the exosomes you have in your body can help diagnose specific types of dementia.

Similar to stem cells, I've used exosomes in my practice when a patient has tried multiple elements of the protocol but hasn't significantly improved, and they have the resources to spend on a speculative treatment—although no one has yet reported a profound benefit the way some patients who have tried stem cell treatments have.

Although exosomes have promise, I don't think they are reliably helpful yet because they are still very general and not necessarily targeted to supporting cognitive function. As the research accelerates, I hope that we will be able to get more specific about the exosomes we choose to help with neurodegenerative disease. In the meantime, I suspect they'll be used more for diagnostics—drawing blood or cerebrospinal fluid and looking at the exosomes to see what they're transporting, whether it's tau, beta amyloid, Lewy bodies, or vesicles associated with Parkinson's. We'll be able to open up that package and see what's going on. This insight could help us personalize treatment, both by defining the pathology and by identifying if there's deficiency that we could rectify. Looking a little further out, my hope is that we might be able to use exosomes to target neurogenesis in specific parts of the brain, such as the hippocampus or the frontal temporal region.

UPSIDE: Much more affordable than stem cell treatments, with similar aims.

DOWNSIDES: Not targeted to the brain, more moderate effects. More expensive than peptides; however, peptides are used over weeks and months, whereas exosomes are typically administered by IV in intervals of up to twelve weeks.

Psychedelics

There has been a resurgence of research in psychedelics, such as psilocybin and LSD. The majority of therapeutic focus has been on mental health disorders, like anxiety, depression, and PTSD; however, the proposed mechanisms of benefit include the stimulation of the growth of new neurons, new connections between neurons and a reduction in neuroinflammation—all of which would point to promise as an Alzheimer's therapeutic. While most psychedelic drugs are still illegal, psilocybin and 3,4-methylenedioxy-methamphetamine (MDMA) have been granted breakthrough therapy designation by the FDA (meaning they are legal to use in an approved research setting), and multiple states have passed legislation that makes psilocybin, and sometimes MDMA, legal. Many highly regarded academic institutions have established programs in the study of psychedelics, including Johns Hopkins, Massachusetts General Hospital, and the University of California, Berkeley. And in 2023, the FDA issued draft guidance for the study of psychedelics, an important milestone in the approval process.

If you are interested in psychedelics as a potential therapeutic for dementia, I recommend searching the list of current and future clinical trials for an opportunity near you. You can do this at https://www.alzheimers.gov/clinical-trials. For example, as I write this, researchers at Johns Hopkins University are recruiting for a clinical trial that will evaluate psilocybin as a potential aid for depression in early Alzheimer's disease.

Vaccines

There are no Alzheimer's-specific vaccines available at this moment, although there are companies who are working on them.

As we understand, there are multiple pathways that can result in dementia. While that fact makes it tricky to create one vaccine that addresses all possible pathways (especially since dementia is not strictly an infectious disease, which is what vaccines are historically best suited to prevent), there are some vaccines in the works that could help block one or more pathways.

One potential vaccine currently in the development pipeline aims to prevent the formation of amyloid plaques. While this seems like a helpful outcome, as we understand amyloid plaques now, they appear to be a protective mechanism against harmful agents, such as *P. gingivalis*. While there is such a thing as too many amyloid plaques, just as there is such a thing as too much inflammation (another protective mechanism that can get out of hand), if we completely impair our body's ability to form them, we may be making our brains even more vulnerable. And since the presence of amyloid plaques doesn't necessarily correspond to a decline in cognitive function, we may not be getting improvement in cognition, either. While I am keeping a watchful eye on this development, I am not holding out a lot of hope, either.

A vaccine that I would love to see in the not-so-distant future would target Lyme disease, the increasingly common tick-borne disease that promotes inflammation and can negatively impact cognition. There is also a vaccine in the works for *P. gingivalis*, the oral bacteria that can travel throughout the body and has been found in the plaques of Alzheimer's patients. We already have a lot of individual power to keep the spread of *P. gingivalis* at bay by brushing, flossing, and oil pulling daily—although some people aren't able to commit to these practices every day, so a potential vaccine may be even more helpful for them.

Any new vaccines take time to develop and then to test in clinical trials. I can't counsel waiting on any vaccine to protect you or your loved one's brain.

WHAT YOU CAN DO NOW: Get your flu, pneumonia (if you are over sixty-five), and shingles (if you are over fifty) vaccines. Why? We know that herpes viruses, especially herpes simplex type 1 (which triggers cold sores) and herpes zoster (which causes chicken pox and shingles), are associated with Alzheimer's. These viruses can lie dormant for months and years at a time, and stressful events, including getting the flu and pneumonia, can reawaken them. Plus, both flu and pneumonia can knock you out for weeks and, in some cases, be deadly. While not life-threatening, shingles can be extremely painful, and its residual effects can linger for months. That's enough of a reason to get the shingles vaccine. But science has also found that the shingles vaccine is associated with a 15 percent reduction in the risk of developing both Alzheimer's and Parkinson's. Although 15 percent isn't a big number, when it comes to blocking a potential pathway to dementia, I'll take every reduction in risk I can get, particularly when it comes from something with relatively little risk or expense. Flu and pneumonia vaccines are annual; the shingles vaccine requires two doses every five years.

A New Vision of Aging

When I envision the future of aging, there are two pervasive themes: (1) As the global population skews older, we're going to have both more people who require dementia care and fewer younger people around to provide that care. This is the doomsday theme. (2) As we learn more about the pathways that lead to dementia, we have more power than ever to reverse it, delay it, or even prevent it from happening in the first place. This is the hopeful theme.

As the global population skews older, we'll have more and more people living with dementia—from the current 55 million to an estimated 78 million people worldwide by 2030, according to World Health estimates. That means we'll need more people to care for people with dementia, and as the demand for care increases, the supply of younger people who can provide that care won't be able to keep up with demand. It may soon come to pass that only the wealthiest among us will be able to hire caregivers. It worries me. Who's going to take care of the rest of us?

While I am heartened by certain developments in elder care, such as

Marama, which aims to return its residents to independent living, and Alzheimer's villages, where residents are able to live autonomously while also receiving the care they need (described in the box below), my main takeaway is this: We each have to do what we can to take responsibility for extending the number of years that our cognition stays strong. We have to do everything we can to make sure we age well and age gracefully so that we, at the very least, delay becoming the ones who need care—and perhaps prevent ourselves from experiencing the kind of decline that requires daily assistance altogether. We've been taught to prepare for retirement by investing in our 401(k)s. We need to do the same kind of preparation for our physical health—not just our financial health.

DEMENTIA VILLAGES CREATE NEW POSSIBILITIES FOR LIVING WITH ALZHEIMER'S

European countries—particularly the Netherlands and France— have pioneered so-called Alzheimer's villages. These planned communities function as their own small towns, with homes that house groups of people with dementia. Residents are allowed and encouraged to live autonomously—no set daily schedules, no locked doors, and access to staples of daily life such as a grocery store, restaurants, and a salon that are staffed by people who are trained in dementia care. Doctors, nurses, and psychologists live on-site and visit patients in their homes. The outside world is welcomed in so there isn't an "out-of-sight, out-of-mind" situation. Europe's socialized healthcare and government funding makes living in these villages much more affordable than they likely would be in the States, where families would be required to pay much higher fees. But there is an Alzheimer's village in development in Holmdel, New Jersey. There are also dementia villages in Bellmere, Australia; Baerum, Norway; and Langley, British Columbia. Of course, we'd need a lot more dementia villages to match demand, but they are an exciting and humane step in the right direction.

This personal investment in our physical health has a huge potential payoff. With a combination of feeding ourselves a more brain-friendly diet, getting more movement, reducing our stress, pursuing activities that stimulate us and help us socialize, treating any infections, we not only help to keep dementia (1) a rarity and (2) reversible in the instances where it does develop, we also enrich our lives in the present. Taking that sailing class (or whichever activity you decide to pursue) not only teaches you new skills, it also introduces you to new people, gets you outside, and gives you a sense of purpose so that you can boost your skills enough to go on a longer sailing trip. Taking up strength training can not only build your muscles and signal your brain to keep making new neurons and synapses, it can also introduce you to a new community, reduce your fall risk, and help you stay mobile so that you can spend your later years doing what calls to you. All these interventions are win-win-win, for you, for your family (since they will be less likely to have to figure out how to care for you once you can no longer care for yourself), and society at large (since you will be a more active participant and require fewer resources).

That's the individual side. Of course, any problem of such a big scope requires a collective response. It will take a concerted, collaborative effort between the research community, pharmaceutical companies, government, Medicare, insurance companies, medical professionals, the food industry, and the business world to avoid the fate of having 78 million people living with dementia. It will take a moonshot. But we are finally starting to get on the right path.

Although the FDA-approved pharmaceutical treatments that I covered in Chapter 2 are still too focused on reducing amyloid plaques as opposed to improving cognition, and carry too many risks at too high a cost, in my hopeful vision of the future, these drugs evolve to the point where we can use them to safely and confidently clean up existing pathophysiological changes, such as plaques and tangles. We'll still need to minimize the many possible triggers of dementia and support the brain by feeding it the nutrients and giving it the signals (via exercise, activities, and relaxation practices) that will keep the brain strong and cognition sharp as we age. But the thought of the combination of reducing the triggers and repairing existing damage is very exciting. As I've said, the brain is a complex organ, Alzheimer's is a complex disease, and any treatment that addresses this disease also needs to be complex. I hope that there will be medications—whether prescription drugs or some of the other therapies I outlined earlier in this chapter—that will be part of the solution.

The challenge before us, when it comes to diminishing the prevalence and severity of dementia, is enormous, but there are opportunities within it. If you are entrepreneurial, consider establishing retreat centers where people can come immerse themselves in the diet and lifestyle that supports brain span and really dial in those new habits. I also forecast a growing market for health coaches. We all need support to change old habits and adopt new ones.

My biggest vision for the future is that memory-care facilities as we know them today are a thing of the past. As we age, we get to stay in our communities, helping to raise the next generation, showing up at community board meetings, being mentors, and helping to dream up creative solutions to the world's many challenges. We get to stay intertwined in the lives of our loved ones, not siloed away.

This isn't just some starry-eyed, unrealistic dream I have. I've seen what's possible when you start taking the steps that lead away from dementia and toward brain health. This possibility is embodied powerfully by one of our study participants, Larry, who had a MoCA score of 15 when the trial began. He was struggling to communicate and having difficulty cooking for himself. In his work as a handyman, Larry would often end up creating a bigger problem for his clients than initially existed. He was declining to the point that his adult daughter was in the process of selling her home in the Midwest and moving her husband and kids back to California so that she could be his caretaker.

By the time Larry's daughter arrived six months after the trial started—and Larry had been following the Reversing Alzheimer's protocol, including remediating his house for mold—his cognition had recovered to the point that he no longer needed care. In fact, he was helping his daughter—driving the kids around, working on their house, and running errands for her while she was at work. Even though it turned out Larry's daughter didn't need to move nearby in order to care for her dad, she was so grateful to have him integrated into her life, and for her kids to grow up knowing their granddad as the sweet soul he is.

This is an incredible story of recovering cognition, but imagine if you didn't have to decline that dramatically in the first place, or live in fear that you would. That is the future that's possible. It's not radical. It's within reach. All it takes is one small step, and then another, and then another—a journey you have already begun by reading this book. Thank you for being one of the pioneers in changing our current dementia reality for the better.

Recipes

KETO OATMEAL

A warm bowl of oatmeal in the morning is incredibly comforting—and pretty high-carb. This keto version keeps the carbs low but delivers plenty of filling protein, fiber, and good fats from the mixture of seeds. It's also creamy and sweet-tasting, just the way you want oatmeal to be.

Note: The small amount of blueberries used here likely won't knock you out of ketosis, but measure your ketones an hour after eating the first time you prepare it to see how your body reacts. (If your ketones go below .7 mmol, try either adding fewer berries, or skipping them altogether.)

Serves 2
Prep time: 2 minutes
Cook time: 6 minutes

Ingredients:

2 cups unsweetened almond milk, coconut milk, whole dairy milk, or water
1 teaspoon vanilla extract
½ teaspoon ground cinnamon
½ cup hemp seed hearts
½ cup flaxseed meal

½ cup chia seeds
1 to 2 tablespoons of monk fruit sweetener, to taste
¼ cup fresh blueberries (optional)
1 tablespoon sliced almonds (optional)
1 tablespoon unsweetened coconut flakes (optional)

Instructions:

1. Place a saucepan on medium-high heat. Add the unsweetened almond milk, vanilla extract, and cinnamon and stir.
2. Add the hemp seed hearts, flaxseed meal, and chia seeds. Turn down the heat on the stove to medium. Stir to combine.
3. Stir in the monk fruit.
4. Keep the mixture uncovered on medium heat until the oatmeal thickens, about five minutes.
5. Serve in a bowl and top with blueberries, almonds, and/or coconut flakes, if using.

MINI KETO FRITTATAS

Eggs are so nutrient-dense I consider them a perfect food. From a brain health perspective, I love eggs because they are a great source of choline—an essential nutrient that the body uses to create acetylcholine, a neurotransmitter associated with memory—and multiple amino acids that play a role in mood. They are also so easy to prepare, reliably tasty, and so versatile. (They are also a common allergen—I myself am allergic to them. If you suffer from migraines, an egg allergy may be a hidden trigger.) This recipe is something you can make on Sunday to have as a quick and satisfying breakfast or snack at the ready for the rest of the workweek. Use the ingredients listed, or improvise based on what you have in the fridge, swapping in cilantro, dill, or Swiss chard for the parsley and spinach, or leftover sautéed zucchini or mushrooms instead of red peppers.

Serves 6
Prep time: 10 minutes
Cook time: 15 to 20 minutes

Ingredients:

Cooking spray or butter for greasing the muffin tin
6 large eggs
¼ cup heavy cream or full-fat coconut milk
Salt and pepper to taste
½ cup shredded cheddar cheese (or any other cheese you prefer)

¼ cup bell peppers (red, green, or a mix of colors), diced
¼ cup cooked bacon or sausage, diced (optional)
¼ cup tomatoes, diced
2 tablespoons fresh parsley or spinach or a mix of the two, chopped (optional)

Instructions:

1. Preheat your oven to 375°F.
2. Grease a 12-cup muffin tin with cooking spray or butter.
3. In a medium-sized bowl, whisk together the eggs and heavy cream or coconut milk until well combined. Season with salt and pepper to taste.
4. Add the shredded cheese, diced bell peppers, diced bacon or sausage (if using), diced tomatoes, and chopped parsley and/or spinach (if using) to the egg mixture. Stir everything together until the ingredients are evenly distributed.
5. Pour the egg mixture into the greased muffin tin, dividing it equally among the cups.
6. Bake the mini frittatas in the preheated oven for 15 to 20 minutes, or until they are set and slightly golden on top. You can check for doneness by inserting a toothpick into the center of one frittata—if it comes out clean, they're ready.
7. Remove the muffin tin from the oven and let the frittatas cool for a few minutes.
8. Once cooled, use a knife or a small spatula to gently loosen the edges of the frittatas from the muffin tin. Carefully lift them out and place them on a plate.

continued

9. Enjoy your mini keto frittatas warm or let them cool completely before storing them in an airtight container in the refrigerator for a quick grab-and-go keto snack or breakfast option. (They'll stay fresh up to four days.)

BERRY-CREAM PARFAIT

These parfaits are in the breakfast section, but they also make a refreshing snack and a tasty dessert that can satisfy a craving for sweets without knocking you out of ketosis. And if you, like me, are one of the many people who are allergic to eggs, this can be one of your go-to, no-cook breakfasts. Make sure you don't go overboard with the berries; having too many may knock you out of ketosis—particularly when you are following a ketogenic diet for the first time and your body is relearning how to make the switch to burning fat. As with the Keto Oatmeal, test your ketones an hour after eating to assess how the berries impacted your blood sugar. It's worth the effort because berries are loaded with phytonutrients known as polyphenols, which are anti-inflammatory and promote circulation throughout the body, including the brain.

Serves 2
Prep time: 2 minutes
Cook time: 6 minutes (plus 15 minutes of cooling time)

Ingredients:

½ cup shredded, unsweetened coconut
2 tablespoons coconut oil
⅛ teaspoon ground cinnamon
⅛ teaspoon ground cardamom
⅛ teaspoon sea salt

¼ cup fresh, washed blueberries
¼ cup fresh, washed raspberries
¾ cup unsweetened almond, coconut, or whole-milk yogurt
¾ cup coconut cream

Instructions:

1. Preheat the oven to 300°F.
2. Line a roasting tray with parchment paper. In a medium bowl, toss the coconut with the oil, cinnamon, cardamom, and salt.
3. Bake for 3 minutes then mix and bake for another 3 minutes, or until light golden and aromatic.
4. Let the coconut cool to room temperature for about 15 minutes.
5. In two wide-rimmed glasses, layer in a spoonful of the berries, then yogurt, and then coconut cream; top with the toasted coconut mixture.

NOTE: You can toast the coconut in advance and then store in an airtight container in the pantry up to two weeks or in the refrigerator up to one month.

EMPTY-THE-FRIDGE SCRAMBLE

At Marama, we tend to follow recipes, but in my house, I do a lot of winging it—using whatever's on hand in a basic template to whip up something fresh, tasty, and home-cooked in just a couple of minutes. This is my attempt to codify the instructions for the breakfast my daughter and I eat most often. It's a great way to use up leftovers and nourish yourself in one fell swoop. Serve with half of a small sliced avocado on the side, or a tablespoon or two of kimchi or sauerkraut, if you like.

Ingredients:

1 tablespoon avocado oil
1 clove garlic
½ to 1 cup chopped nonstarchy veggies
  from your fridge or pantry, such as:
½ onion
½ medium zucchini
½ cup mushrooms
½ large tomato, or a small handful
  of cherry tomatoes, or even a few
  sundried tomatoes

2 eggs, scrambled, or 4 ounces of
  tofu, crumbled (soft, medium, or firm,
  depending on your preference)
Salt and pepper to taste
Large handful of leafy greens
½ to 1 teaspoon spice, such as turmeric,
  chili powder, or paprika (optional)
1 tablespoon fresh herbs, such as basil,
  cilantro, or parsley, chopped (optional)

Instructions:

1. Heat olive oil in a well-seasoned cast-iron skillet on low-medium heat while chopping veggies into bite-sized pieces.
2. Sauté the garlic and onion until soft, about 4 minutes, then add the zucchini, mushrooms, and other veggies and sauté until lightly browned, 5 to 6 minutes.
3. Add the eggs or tofu and scramble with veggies until cooked through, about 2 minutes. Season with salt and pepper to taste.
4. Add the leafy greens and mix until wilted, about 1 minute.
5. Add the optional herbs and spices and stir until mixed thoroughly.
6. Remove pan from heat and serve.

Lunch

EGG SALAD LETTUCE WRAPS

These quick-to-assemble wraps are tasty, filling, and don't require utensils to eat. I suggest using avocado oil or olive oil mayonnaise if you can because those are healthier fats than the soybean, canola, or safflower oils most mayonnaises use (as the omega-9 fat, known as oleic acid, that olive and avocado oil contain are less inflammatory than the omega-6 fats found in soy, canola, and safflower oils).

Serves 2
Prep time: 5 minutes
Cook time: n/a (unless you're hard-boiling the eggs first, then 15 minutes)

Ingredients:

4 hard-boiled eggs, chopped
2 tablespoons mayonnaise (you can use a keto-friendly mayo or make your own)
1 tablespoon Dijon mustard
¼ cup diced celery
2 tablespoons chopped green onions
Salt and pepper to taste
Large lettuce leaves (such as romaine or butter lettuce) for wrapping

Instructions:

1. In a medium-sized bowl, combine the chopped hard-boiled eggs, mayonnaise, and Dijon mustard.
2. Add the diced celery and chopped green onions to the bowl. Mix everything together until the ingredients are well combined.
3. Taste the egg salad and season with salt and pepper to your liking. Adjust the amount of mayo or mustard if you prefer a creamier or tangier flavor.
4. Lay the large lettuce leaves flat on a clean surface.
5. Spoon the egg salad onto each lettuce leaf, dividing it equally among the leaves.
6. Carefully roll up the lettuce leaves to create a wrap, making sure the egg salad is secured inside.
7. Serve the keto egg salad lettuce wraps immediately.

INGREDIENT NOTE: You can buy preboiled eggs at the grocery store. Or, to boil your own, set eggs in a pot of cold water. Place pot on burner, cover, and turn to medium-high to bring water to a boil. Once water is at a full boil, turn heat down to medium-low and set a timer for 13 minutes. When timer goes off, immerse eggs in bowl of ice water. Allow to cool completely in ice bath before peeling.

SHRIMP SCAMPI WITH ZOODLES

This recipe sounds fancy—and thus, labor-intensive—but it is a lot easier and faster than you might think, and it is so tasty that it may make you feel like you're dining out. The zoodles are a great base for this dish and so many other things—think of them as your new pasta.

Serves 4
Prep time: 15 minutes
Cook time: 10 to 12 minutes

Ingredients:

4 tablespoons unsalted butter
4 cloves garlic, minced
¼ teaspoon red pepper flakes (optional)
1 pound (450 g) large shrimp, peeled and deveined

3 to 4 medium zucchinis, spiralized into zoodles, or a 16-ounce package of precut zoodles
Zest and juice of 1 lemon
Salt and pepper to taste
2 tablespoons chopped fresh parsley
Grated parmesan cheese (optional)

Instructions:

1. In a large skillet, melt 2 tablespoons of butter over medium heat.
2. Add the minced garlic and red pepper flakes (if using) to the skillet. Sauté for about 1 minute until the garlic becomes fragrant.
3. Add the shrimp to the skillet and cook for 2 to 3 minutes on each side until they turn pink and opaque.
4. Once the shrimp are cooked, empty them into a bowl and set aside.
5. In the same skillet, melt the remaining 2 tablespoons of butter.
6. Add the zucchini noodles (zoodles) to the skillet. Cook, stirring occasionally, until they are slightly softened but still have a bit of crunch, 2 to 3 minutes.
7. Turn off the heat, add the lemon zest and lemon juice to the pan, and season with salt and pepper to taste.
8. Return the cooked shrimp to the skillet with the zoodles and toss everything together to evenly distribute the lemon-butter sauce.
9. Stir in the chopped parsley and sprinkle with grated parmesan cheese, if using.

CREAMY BROCCOLI SOUP

This rich and satisfying soup is a favorite at Marama, and a great way to convert keto skeptics.

Serves 4 as a meal, 6 as an appetizer or side dish
Prep time: 10 minutes
Cook time: 1 hour 20 minutes

Ingredients:

1½ sticks (12 tablespoons) butter
2 tablespoons extra-virgin olive oil
1 medium yellow or white onion, diced
2 medium carrots, peeled and diced
5 stalks of celery, trimmed and diced
½ tablespoon garlic, minced
1 large or 2 small broccoli stalks, peeled and chopped
3 bay leaves

½ tablespoon dried thyme
32 ounces boxed chicken or vegetable broth
10 ounces baby spinach, chopped
1½ cups heavy cream
1 large or 2 small broccoli crowns, chopped
1 tablespoon sea salt
1 teaspoon ground black pepper

Instructions:

1. Place soup pot on medium heat and melt the butter; add the olive oil while butter is melting.
2. Sauté the onions, carrots, celery, garlic, broccoli stalks, bay leaves, and thyme until vegetables are softened, about 15 minutes.
3. Add the chicken broth and bring to a boil, about 3 minutes.
4. Turn the heat down to a simmer and let cook for about 45 minutes until the stalks soften and the flavors meld.
5. Take out the bay leaves and add the spinach, then use a handheld blender to puree until the soup turns bright green and smooth. (To use a traditional blender, work in two batches and leave the lid slightly ajar so that steam can escape, then return the soup to the pot.)
6. Add the heavy cream and the chopped broccoli crowns and simmer until crowns are soft, about 20 minutes.
7. Season with salt and pepper.

CANNED SALMON SALAD

This recipe makes a quick and tasty lunch out of ingredients you likely already have on hand, and is a cost-effective way to eat wild salmon, which is the quintessential brain food because it's packed with healthy fats and protein. (Make sure the label on the can says "wild," and take care to remove any remaining skin and bones before you start mixing the salmon.) Serve in a keto wrap, on keto bread, wrapped in lettuce leaves, or on top of a bed of greens drizzled with a little olive oil and fresh lemon juice.

Serves 2
Prep time: 10 minutes
Cook time: n/a

Ingredients:

One 6- to 8-ounce can of salmon, drained and flaked

2 to 3 tablespoons avocado oil or olive oil mayonnaise

1 to 2 teaspoons Dijon mustard

1 to 2 tablespoons red onion, diced

1 to 2 stalks of celery, diced

1 to 2 tablespoons fresh dill, chopped (or 1 teaspoon dried dill)

Salt and pepper to taste

Juice from ½ lemon (optional)

1 to 2 tablespoons capers (optional)

Lettuce leaves or mixed greens for serving

Instructions:

1. Drain the salmon and flake it into a medium mixing bowl, removing any skin or bones.
2. Add the mayonnaise, Dijon mustard, red onion, celery, and dill; stir to combine.
3. Season with salt and pepper to taste, then add the lemon juice and/or capers, if using. Stir to combine.

Dinner

ONCE-A-WEEK DINNER

I am a big believer in having go-to meals—things you can make without much thought that become part of your weekly routine. This is the recipe for my once-a-week dinner. To keep it interesting, I use different spice blends to season the finished dish (my current favorites are the Green Goddess, Chili Lime, and Multipurpose Umami Seasoning Blends from Trader Joe's). I hope that this recipe will help make your weeks a little easier and lot tastier, too. For a little extra fat, fiber, and flavor, serve with avocado slices sprinkled with sea salt, or for probiotics, serve with a kimchi or sauerkraut.

Serves 2 to 3
Prep time: 15 minutes
Cook time: 25 minutes

Ingredients:

2 tablespoons avocado oil or ghee, divided

4 to 6 organic boneless, skinless, chicken thighs

1 medium-sized head of broccoli or cauliflower, chopped into bite-sized florets

1 tablespoon olive oil

3 big handfuls of leafy greens, such as spinach, kale, Swiss chard, or collards, roughly chopped

Salt and pepper to taste

Avocado, kimchi, and/or sauerkraut (optional, for serving)

Instructions:

1. Heat one tablespoon avocado oil or ghee in a stainless steel or cast-iron skill over medium-high heat until hot but not smoking.
2. Add the chicken thighs to the pan, flipping every 3 to 4 minutes until cooked, 20 to 25 minutes total. Once cooked, add the optional seasonings to taste.
3. While the chicken is cooking, place the broccoli or cauliflower florets in a mixing bowl and stir in one tablespoon of ghee or avocado oil. Season with salt and pepper to taste.
4. Place the broccoli/cauliflower in an air fryer and cook until browned, 10 to 12 minutes. (If you don't have an air fryer, roast in a 400°F oven or toaster oven for 20 minutes.)
5. While the chicken and broccoli/cauliflower cook, heat 1 tablespoon olive oil in a separate sauté pan on low-medium heat until warm, 1 to 2 minutes, then add leafy greens and cook, stirring frequently, until soft, 2 to 5 minutes (collards will take longer than other greens).
6. To serve, place 1 to 2 of the sliced chicken thighs, 1 cup of broccoli/cauliflower, and a large helping of leafy greens on a plate.
7. Add the optional sides of avocado, kimchi, or sauerkraut.

EGG ROLL IN A BOWL

Satisfy any craving for Chinese takeout and get a big helping of cabbage (a cruciferous vegetable with anti-cancer and anti-inflammatory properties as well as a lot of fiber, vitamin C, and B vitamins) with this quick and tasty stir-fry. A longtime Marama favorite.

Serves 4
Prep time: 10 minutes
Cook time: 8 minutes

Ingredients:

1 tablespoon avocado oil or ghee
1 pound ground beef or pork
1 clove garlic, minced
½ large green cabbage, cored and shredded
¼ cup liquid aminos or tamari (gluten-free soy sauce)

1 teaspoon fresh ginger, grated
1 egg
Sriracha (to taste)
1 tablespoon sesame oil
2 tablespoons sliced green onions

Instructions:

1. Heat one tablespoon avocado oil or ghee in a large stainless steel or cast-iron skillet over medium heat until hot but not smoking.
2. Add the pork or beef to the pan and cook, stirring frequently, until no longer pink, about 3 minutes.
3. Add garlic and sauté for 30 seconds.
4. Add the shredded cabbage, liquid aminos, ginger and sauté until cabbage softens slightly, about 3 minutes. Add one tablespoon water as needed to prevent cabbage from burning.
5. Reduce heat to low and push contents of the skillet to the sides to make a well for the egg. Crack the egg into the center of the hot pan and scramble until egg is fully cooked, about 1 minute. Turn off the heat.
6. Stir in the sriracha, if using, and drizzle with sesame oil.
7. Place serving into a bowl and garnish with chopped green onion.

SALMON SALAD

You've got to love a 10-minute, brain-health-friendly, ketogenic meal that makes the most of fresh, wild salmon. You can even cook it in the toaster oven. You'll likely have some salmon left over, meaning you can eat it for lunch the next day on a bed of cauliflower rice (with a little soy sauce and sriracha for an Asian flair), or made into the salmon version of tuna salad, or over another bed of greens.

Serves: Customizable
Prep time: 5 to 10 minutes
Cook time: 20 minutes

Ingredients:

½ pound wild salmon per person

2 large handfuls butter lettuce, washed and torn into bite-sized pieces, per person

1 tablespoon extra-virgin olive oil per person

Lemon juice, to taste

Pitted and sliced black olives, to taste

Red onion, thinly sliced, to taste

Capers, to taste (optional)

Salt and pepper, to taste

Preparation

1. Preheat the oven to 350°F.
2. Place salmon on baking sheet and coat each piece with ¼ tablespoon olive oil and salt and pepper to taste.
3. Bake for 12 to 20 minutes depending on the thickness of the salmon and you're preferred level of doneness.
4. Remove salmon from oven, squeeze with a little fresh lemon juice, if desired, and let cool while you prepare the salad.
5. Arrange lettuce on plate and then add olive oil, more fresh lemon juice, salt, pepper, olives, red onion, and capers to taste. Place salmon on top of salad and serve.

CAULIFLOWER CRUST PIZZA

Pizza is one of those reliable comfort foods that may seem like it's off limits if you're following a ketogenic diet, but there are multiple ways to scratch that itch without knocking yourself out of ketosis. I suggest using it as an opportunity to load up on healthy fats and phytonutrients, too, by opting for pesto instead of tomato sauce. But if you want that red sauce experience, be sure to buy or make a tomato sauce with no added sugars (if purchasing prepared tomato sauce, be sure to choose one that comes in a glass jar; tomatoes are acidic, they can cause the lining of a can to leach into the sauce, and you don't want your pizza to come with a side of chemicals). And if you want to skip the step of making your own crust, there are brands that make keto-friendly cauliflower pizza crusts, including Outer Aisle, Cali'flour Foods, and Kbosh Artisan Keto.

Serves: 2
Prep time: 20 minutes
Cook time: 24 minutes

Ingredients:

For the crust:
1 medium-sized cauliflower head, cut into small florets
1 large egg
1 cup mozzarella cheese, shredded
1 teaspoon dried oregano
½ teaspoon garlic powder
Salt and pepper to taste

For the pizza toppings:
¼ to ½ cup no-sugar-added tomato sauce or pesto
1 cup shredded mozzarella cheese
Your favorite keto-friendly pizza toppings (e.g., pepperoni, cooked sausage, sliced bell peppers, mushrooms, spinach)

Instructions:

1. Preheat your oven to 425°F. Line a baking sheet with parchment paper and set aside.
2. Rinse the cauliflower head and remove the leaves and stem. Cut the cauliflower into small florets.
3. Using a food processor, pulse the cauliflower florets until they resemble rice-like grains. You may need to do this in batches.
4. Transfer the cauliflower rice to a microwave-safe bowl and microwave on high for 4 to 5 minutes, or until softened.
5. Let the cauliflower cool for a few minutes, then place it in a clean kitchen towel or cheesecloth. Squeeze out as much moisture as possible.
6. In a mixing bowl, combine the drained cauliflower rice, egg, shredded mozzarella cheese, dried oregano, garlic powder, salt, and pepper. Mix everything until well combined.

continued

7. Transfer the cauliflower mixture to the prepared baking sheet. Use your hands to press and shape it into a thin and even pizza crust, about 8 inches across and ¼ inch thick.

8. Bake the cauliflower crust in the preheated oven for 15 to 20 minutes, or until it turns golden brown and starts to crisp up.

9. Remove the cauliflower crust from the oven and let it cool slightly, about 2 minutes.

10. Spread a thin layer of pesto or tomato sauce over the crust, leaving a small border around the edges for the crust.

11. Sprinkle the shredded mozzarella cheese over the sauce.

12. Add your favorite toppings on top of the cheese.

13. Return the pizza to the oven and bake for an additional 10 to 12 minutes, or until the cheese is melted and bubbly and the toppings are heated through.

14. Slice and serve.

15. Let the pizza cool for 3 to 5 minutes before slicing and serving.

Snacks/Dessert

ROASTED NUTS

Not only is this recipe a crowd favorite, it's a great activity to do together if you're caring for someone with dementia—they can help spoon out and then mix the nuts. There are two caveats to keep in mind: because they are salty, you want to serve them with a glass of spring water, and because they are so tasty, it's easy to eat a lot of them and have the moderate carb content of nuts add up to the point that it kicks you out of ketosis. To help keep them fresh and reduce the possibility of eating too many in one sitting, store half the completed recipe in a mason jar in the freezer. Use whole, raw, organic nuts whenever possible.

Serves 12
Prep time: 5 minutes
Cook time: 15 minutes

Ingredients:

12 Brazil nuts
¼ cup almonds
¼ cup macadamia nuts
¼ cup pistachios

¼ cup pecans
¼ cup walnuts
1 tablespoon coconut oil
½ tablespoon sea salt

Instructions:

1. Preheat the oven to 350°F.
2. In a medium bowl toss together all the nuts with the coconut oil and sea salt.
3. Roast in a single layer on a sheet pan for 15 minutes, or until light brown.
4. Remove from oven and let cool in the pan until room temperature—serve right away or store in an airtight glass container in a dark cupboard for up to two weeks. (Store them in the freezer if you want them to last longer—they'll stay good up to a year.)

BROWNIE FAT BOMBS

Sometimes you just want something chocolate-y and delicious. With this recipe you can satisfy that craving and stay in ketosis. Even better, this recipe makes a large amount, so you'll have plenty of treats on hand for several days.

Serves 24
Prep time: 10 minutes
Refrigeration time: 1 hour (to freeze the fat bombs before serving)

continued

Ingredients:

2 ounces dark chocolate
1 cup nut butter of your choice (I love
  almond butter)
⅔ cup cocoa powder

4 to 5 tablespoons of monk fruit
¼ teaspoon salt
2 tablespoons coconut oil

Instructions:

1. Place chocolate in a microwave-safe bowl and microwave until chocolate is melted.
2. Blend nut butter, cocoa powder, monk fruit, salt, and coconut oil in blender or food processor.
3. Add melted chocolate and blend everything together.
4. Use an ice-cream scoop to scoop ingredients into a silicone candy mold or silicone ice cube tray (they'll likely stick to a standard ice cube tray).
5. Place the fat bombs in the freezer to set for 1 hour.
6. Pull out however many fat bombs you need 15 minutes before serving to let them thaw.

Note: Store fat bombs in an airtight glass container in the freezer—they'll last about a month.

CARDAMOM ALMOND BUTTER FAT BOMBS

A fat bomb is just what it sounds like–a delivery system for healthy fats. Fat bombs can counteract a craving for sweets, tide you over until the next meal when eaten as a snack, or act as a decadent-feeling dessert. I love this recipe because the almond butter also delivers protein and fiber, and the cardamom adds a subtle sweetness. If you find you don't like the taste of cardamom, or don't want to buy a new spice, you can substitute cinnamon, or omit spice altogether.

Serves 12
Prep time: 5 minutes
Refrigerator time: 1 hour (to freeze the fat bombs before serving)

Ingredients:

½ cup almond butter (unsweetened, no
  added oils)
¼ cup coconut oil (virgin, unrefined)
¼ cup unsalted butter or ghee
1 teaspoon ground cardamom
½ teaspoon vanilla extract

A pinch of salt, if using unsalted almond
  butter
Up to 1 tablespoon allulose or monk fruit
  sweetener, to taste

Instructions:

1. In a microwave-safe bowl or in a pan on the stovetop over low heat, melt the coconut oil and unsalted butter or ghee together until fully liquid, about 1 minute in the microwave and 1 to 2 minutes on the stove. Be careful not to overheat.
2. In a separate bowl, combine the almond butter, ground cardamom, vanilla extract, and salt, if using.
3. Add the melted oil and butter mixture to the bowl with the almond butter mixture. Stir until everything is well combined and smooth.
4. Taste the mixture and add your preferred sweetener, if desired.
5. Pour the mixture into a silicone candy molds or an ice cube tray.
6. Place the molds or tray in the freezer and let the fat bombs set for 1 hour.
7. Once the fat bombs are solid, pop them out of the molds or tray and store them in an airtight container in the freezer, where they'll keep for about a month.

GRANDMOTHER'S DILL DIP

This was my grandmother's recipe, which she served at happy hour during family vacations at the lake. It makes a great spread for wraps in addition to being a dip. Herbs in general are about more than flavor, they are also medicine. Dill aids with digestion and inflammation and is an antibacterial; it's also a good source of vitamins C, A, K, and iron. Parsley is an excellent source of vitamins A and K as well as the antioxidants known as flavones. It's a powerful diuretic that can help lower blood pressure.

Serves 4
Prep time: 10 minutes
Refrigeration time: 2 hours (in order to allow flavors to meld)

Ingredients:

1 cup full-fat plain yogurt
1 cup avocado oil mayonnaise (I use
  Veganaise)
2 tablespoons fresh dill weed, or
  1 tablespoon dried dill

1 tablespoon onion powder
2 tablespoons diced parsley, or
  1 tablespoon dried parsley
1 teaspoon sea salt

Instructions:

1. Add all ingredients to a small bowl and stir well to combine.
2. Cover and refrigerate for 2 hours or more, to allow the flavors to meld.
3. Serve with assorted vegetables for dipping.

KETO CELEBRATION CAKE

Sometimes you want to celebrate in a big way, whether it's someone's birthday, a holiday, or an important milestone. This delicious recipe gives you a perfect way to celebrate while still staying in ketosis.

Ingredients:

For cake:
3¾ cup almond flour
1½ cup cocoa powder
1½ cup monk fruit sweetener
1½ tablespoon baking powder

12 eggs
¾ cup melted butter
1 cup unsweetened almond milk
1½ teaspoons vanilla extract

For frosting:
3 cups powdered monk fruit sweetener
½ cup butter, room temperature
1 teaspoon vanilla extract

½ cup cocoa powder
1 to 2 tablespoons milk of choice

Instructions:

For the cake:
1. Preheat the oven to 325°F.
2. In a medium-sized bowl, whisk together the dry ingredients.
3. In another bowl, beat the eggs, butter, milk, and vanilla extract until smooth. Gently add dry ingredients and mix well.
4. Bake for 27 to 30 minutes.

For the frosting:
1. Mix the powdered monk fruit sweetener and butter until fully combined.
2. Add the vanilla extract and cocoa powder and stir until combined.
3. Add the milk until frosting reaches the desired texture, then set aside.
4. Once the cake has cooled to room temperature, spread the frosting.

CREAMY KETO LEMON POPSICLES

I have a few lemon trees in my backyard and often have lemons coming out of my ears during the hottest months. In my quest to put all the lemons to good use I found this refreshing recipe and enjoyed it so much I had to share it.

Makes: 12 popsicles
Prep Time: 10 minutes

Freeze Time: 6 hours

Ingredients:

1 tablespoon finely grated lemon zest
¼ cup freshly squeezed lemon juice
 (about 2 lemons)
1 cup allulose or monk fruit sweetener

⅛ teaspoon fine sea salt
1½ cups heavy cream
½ cup whole milk

Instructions:

1. Whisk together lemon juice, lemon zest, salt, and sweetener.
2. Gradually add milk and cream to mixture while whisking constantly. Whisk until sweetener dissolves completely. This usually takes 2 to 3 minutes.
3. Pour the mixture into your popsicle molds and allow to freeze for 6 hours or overnight.

Resources

As more and more people age and are at risk for developing dementia, creative, novel solutions are arising. I'll be keeping my community up-to-date through an email newsletter. Join the community at drheathersandison.com.

Websites

ReversingAlzheimersBook.com

Because the list of suppliers and supplies is evolving, I will be continually updating resources, tips, and supportive tools for those looking to optimize brain health for themselves and their loved ones on this website. Sign up for my email list to stay in the loop as we learn and share more.

MaramaExperience.com

The website of the Marama senior-living facilities, where residents are immersed in the Reversing Alzheimer's protocol and where our goal is to return our residents to independent living.

Reversingalzheimersathome.com

The online home of the virtual group coaching programs I lead that walk you through the Reversing Alzheimer's protocol.

Solcere.com

The website of my medical clinic in Encinitas, California, where my staff and I work with patients one-on-one.

Apollohealthco.com

This is Dr. Bredesen's website, where he offers information on the full Bredesen protocol, and has online cognitive assessments, cognitive games, ways to track your progress and also to gain access to Bredesen-trained health coaches and healthcare providers. It's packed with information and tools; it does have a monthly fee.

PacificNeuroScienceInstitute.org

Dr. Bredesen is also affiliated with the Brain Health Center at the Pacific Neuroscience Institute directed by my friend, Dr. David Merrill. The Pacific Neuroscience Center is on the cutting edge of everything from Parkinson's and Alzheimer's to psychedelic-assisted therapies and dual-task exercise. At Marama we are learning from Dr. Merrill, Dr. Karen Miller, Ryan Glatt, candidate, and Molly Ropozo, to apply their cutting-edge research and techniques in a residential setting.

Keto-mojo.com

This website of the company that makes my favorite ketone- and glucose-testing device, the Keto-Mojo, is packed with information about getting into and staying in ketosis, recipes, testing tips, and more.

youtube.com/watch?v=jfKEAiwrgeY&t=20s

This is the YouTube video we play each day at Marama to guide our residents through the Kirtan Kriya meditation.

challengehound.com; theconqueror.events

These apps gamify getting more movement by letting you set up your own virtual challenge or join an existing one. Possible challenges include walking the length of Ireland or the Appalachian Trail. Get your friends and family to participate in a walking, running, or cycling challenge, and you can stay connected while also inspiring one another to get active.

Support Groups

Free: My team and I run a Reverse Alzheimer's at Home Facebook group, available at https://www.facebook.com/groups/740726920550907

Paid: You can also gain access to community via Dr. Bredesen's ReCODE Program membership (available at apollohealthco.com) and/or through the Reversing Alzheimer's at Home group coaching program that I run four times a year. Sign up to be informed of the next session at drheathersandison.com.

Products

Air purifier

GC Multigas Air Purifier by IQ Air

This air purifier covers twelve hundred square feet and removes gases, chemicals, viruses, volatile organic chemicals, tobacco smoke, and mycotoxins from the air. It's very quiet, and you have to change the filter only every two and a half years. We have one on each floor in the hallways at Marama.

Contrast oxygen therapy device

Adaptive Contrast System by LiveO2

This is the contrast oxygen therapy device we use at Marama. Full disclosure—LiveO2 has sponsored my Reversing Alzheimer's Summit in the past, although I don't use the product because they paid me to; I started using the product because I believed in it, and we developed a business relationship as a result. (I do not receive a commission if you purchase one.)

Water purifier

AquaTru countertop reverse osmosis water filtration system

This reverse osmosis filter requires no plumbing or installation—just find a spot for it on your counter and plug it in. It also wastes less water than most under-the-counter reverse osmosis systems.

Mattresses

Eco Organic Mattress by Avocado

These are the mattresses we use at Marama and that my daughter and I sleep on. While their customer service hasn't been anything to write home about, they are the best mattress at the best price.

Samina Sleep System

The Samina Sleep System is top of the line when it comes to mattresses and bedding. Created by a German physician, their products do not compromise quality at any step. They are designed to inhibit the growth of mold and have no chemicals that will off-gas when new.

Nontoxic Personal Care Brands

Dr. Bronner's

EO Products

Honest Company

Ilia Makeup

Nontoxic Home Care Brands

BioKleen

Branch Basics

Seventh Generation

Pillbox

Weekly Pill Organizer, 2X-Large Push Button Compartments, 4 Times a Day by Ezy Dose

This pill organizer lets you divide your daily supplements and medications into four separate doses. Sort pills on Sunday afternoon and make it that much easier to stay on track with your supplements during the week. It also helps you keep track of what you've taken and what you haven't.

Red Light Therapy Devices

Neuro Duo by Vielight

The Neuro Gamma model is designed to induce gamma brain waves, which are associated with focus, memory, and concentration. They also have a Neuro Alpha model that is designed to stimulate alpha brain waves, which promote mental calmness and lower stress. At Marama, we have the Neuro Duo model, which offers both gamma and alpha waves. For boosting cognition, the Neuro Gamma is likely all you need. As of this writing, these devices are nearly $2,000. To bring the cost down, you could go in on the device with a neighbor. Or you can buy only the intranasal piece for about $400—start there and see if it feels worth it to invest in the full Neuro Gamma or Neuro Duo model.

Solo Red Light by Joovv

This red light and near-infrared light-emitting device is big enough to cover half your body in one sitting—you can also add additional panels over time. We have multiple Solo lights built into a wall in the casita at Marama—our residents spend up to twenty minutes in front of them per day.

Saunas

Higher Dose Infrared Sauna Blanket

This is the sauna blanket I have at home. I use it for ten minutes after I work out for increased circulation, and for a longer session of thirty to forty minutes once a week.

Sunlighten Saunas

If you are looking for a larger wood sauna for your home, Sunlighten has gone to great lengths to create a thoughtful, well-designed solution for you and your loved ones.

Supplements

The trusted supplement brands I recommend most often are:

Integrative Therapeutics

Neurohacker Collective

Orthomolecular

Priority One

Pure Encapsulations

Xymogen

Specific supplements I recommend include:

Relaxation/Sleep Support

RelaxMax by Xymogen

If you drink a glass of wine or a beer with dinner to help you wind down, I recommend a scoop of this powder dissolved in a glass of water as an alternative (you can even drink it in a wineglass!). It provides magnesium and amino acids, including inositol, GABA, taurine, and theanine to promote relaxation, neurotransmitter balance, glial cell function, and mood.

Seriphos by InterPlexus

This supplement contains phosphorylated serine with a blend of calcium and magnesium to help quiet the stress response and invite deeper sleep.

Exogenous Ketones

For reasons I don't quite understand, the companies that make and sell exogenous ketones are always changing. While I can't recommend a specific supplement, I can tell you that there are two kinds: ketone esters and ketone salts. Ketone esters are more concentrated and more expensive (as much as $150 per serving). They also have a very strong (and I think, unpleasant) taste. Athletes tend to use them as they will typically shoot your ketone levels up significantly. Ketone salts are more affordable ($2 to $5 per serving) and have a more pleasant taste, as well as a more moderate effect on ketone levels. I recommend using ketone esters to help you get into ketosis or to jump-start brain healing over the short-term. Ketone salts you can use longer term, as more of an everyday aid in staying in ketosis once you're there.

Immune Boosting

IgG 2000 GWP by Xymogen

This powder contains an immunoglobulin (also known as an antibody) concentrate derived from whey peptides that also provides protein and growth factors to support immune function, gut health, and tissue repair.

Biotic Extra by Priority One

This blend contains arabinogalactan—a naturally derived polysaccharide—mushroom extracts, garlic, vitamin C, zinc, goldenseal, and garlic—all ingredients selected for their track record of boosting immunity.

Minerals

Perfect Minerals by AquaTru or Concentrace Trace Mineral Drops by Trace Minerals

These liquid supplements add minerals back into reverse-osmosis filtered water.

Nootropics

Qualia Mind or Qualia Mind Caffeine Free by Neurohacker Collective

I take four Qualia Mind whenever I have a big day ahead of me and I need to be "on," and I believe it helps me think more clearly and creatively. Surprisingly, I also sleep better at night. It does contain caffeine—if you'd like a cognitive boost without the stimulation of caffeine, there is also a caffeine-free version.

Omega-3 Fatty Acids

EcoSmart Omega-3 by Carlson, Omega MonoPure by Xymogen, and Ultimate Omega by Nordic Naturals

Omega-3 fatty acids are crucial for brain health, as they are incorporated into brain cell membranes and contribute to reducing inflammation, including neuroinflammation, which is a hallmark of dementia. You do want to take care when choosing omega-3 supplements that they have been purified and are environmentally friendly—these three options pass those tests.

Probiotics

Once Daily by Garden of Life, Ortho Biotic by Ortho Molecular Products, ProbioMax by Xymogen, Ther-Biotic Complete or Vital 10 by Klaire Labs, Akkermansia by Pendulum

Because I recommend mixing up the strains of probiotics you take, I'm sharing a few different probiotic supplements. When you run out of one, try another.

Labs

These are the labs I rely on:

Diagnostic Solutions Laboratory (diagnosticsolutionslab.com)

Genova Diagnostics (gdx.net)

Life Extension (lifeextension.com/lab-testing)

Quest Labs (questhealth.com)

Quicksilver Scientific (quicksilverscientific.com)

RealTime Laboratories (realtimelab.com)

Ulta Labs (ultalabtests.com)

Activities

Grouper Health

Grouperhealth.com

The large body of evidence showing social engagement improves health outcomes has inspired health insurance companies to cover your club fees for clubs like bowling, bridge, golf, and even your fishing license. Talk to your insurance provider to see if you can get reimbursed for any fees you may have for your chosen activities.

American Contract Bridge League

acbl.org

Find a local bridge teacher or club for real-world play. Or you can hone your skills by playing progressively more challenging versions of bridge online.

Brain HQ

Brainhq.com

This brain-training service regularly assesses your changes over time, and adjusts to get harder the better you get at it.

Bridge Base Online

bridgebase.com

This online bridge community allows you to play unlimited games of the classic card game for free.

Buzztime Games

buzztime.com

This gaming network lets you join in trivia, arcade, or sports-betting games in participating pubs and restaurants.

Providers

To find a Bredesen-trained doctor or health coach in your area (note that the list of providers is behind a paywall):

Apollohealthco.com

To see a self-curated list of healthcare practitioners who specialize in working with patients who have one or two APOE4 alleles:
wiki.apoe4.info/wiki/ApoE4-Aware_Healthcare_Practitioners

To find a certified functional medicine provider, visit the site of the Institute for Functional Medicine:
ifm.org/find-a-practitioner

To find a naturopathic doctor, visit the site of the American Association of Naturopathic Physicians:
naturopathic.org/search

To find a medical doctor certified in menopause medicine, visit the site of the Menopause Society and look for the "find a practitioner" link:
menopause.org

To find a biological dentist, visit the sites of the International Academy of Biological Dentistry & Medicine and the International Academy of Oral Medicine & Toxicology:
iabdm.org/location
iaomt.org/for-patients/search

To find an Egoscue-trained physical therapist, visit the website of the Egoscue Method:
egoscue.com/therapy

Environmental Specialists

Mary Cordaro, Inc., RestCon Environmental and John Banta
marycordaro.com; restconenvironmental.co; johncbanta.com
These are two environmental hygienists I have referred many patients to for help testing and remediating their home environments for mold and other pollutants.

Online Cognitive Assessment Tools

CNS Vital Signs
cnsvs.com
This is a similar but different assessment to the MoCA that you can do at home.

MoCA Cognition
mocacognition.com/training-certification
The organization that developed the MoCA assessment offers a reasonable training certification program so that you can assess your loved one's cognition without having to pay a provider or get an appointment each time.

Books

Cognitive Health

The Alzheimer's Antidote: Using a Low-Carb, High-Fat Diet to Fight Alzheimer's Disease, Memory Loss, and Cognitive Decline, by Amy Berger

The End of Alzheimer's: The First Program to Prevent and Reverse Cognitive Decline, by Dale E. Bredesen, MD

The End of Alzheimer's Program: The First Protocol to Enhance Cognition and Reverse Decline at Any Age, by Dale E. Bredesen, MD

The First Survivors of Alzheimer's: How Patients Recovered Life and Hope in Their Own Words, by Dale E. Bredesen, MD

The Neurogenesis Diet & Lifestyle: Upgrade Your Brain, Upgrade Your Life, by Brant Cortright, PhD

The XX Brain: The Groundbreaking Science Empowering Women to Maximize Cognitive Health and Prevent Alzheimer's Disease, by Lisa Mosconi, PhD

Grain Brain: The Surprising Truth about Wheat, Carbs, and Sugar—Your Brain's Silent Killers, by Dr. David Perlmutter, MD

Brain Maker: The Power of Gut Microbes to Heal and Protect Your Brain—for Life, by Dr. David Perlmutter, MD

Cookbooks

Ketotarian: The (Mostly) Plant-Based Plan to Burn Fat, Boost Your Energy, Crush Your Cravings, and Calm Inflammation: A Cookbook, by Dr. Will Cole

Essential Ketogenic Mediterranean Diet Cookbook: 100 Low-Carb, Heart-Healthy Recipes for Lasting Weight Loss, by Molly Devine

Dementia Care

Learning to Speak Alzheimer's, by Joanne Koeing Coste

Positive Caregiving: Caring for Older Loved Ones Using the Power of Positive Emotions, by Sarah Teten Kanter, PhD

The 36-Hour Day: A Family Guide for People Who Have Alzheimer Disease and Other Dementias, by Nancy L. Mace, MA, and Peter V. Rabins, MPH

Creative Engagement: A Handbook of Activities for People with Dementia, by Rachael Wonderlin

Understanding the Changing Brain: A Positive Approach to Dementia Care, by Teepa Snow

Teepa Snow also has a wonderful YouTube channel and TikTok account (@teepasnow) with great educational videos

Pain Management

Pain Free: A Revolutionary Method for Stopping Chronic Pain, by Pete Egoscue

Toxins

Toxic: Heal Your Body from Mold Toxicity, Lyme Disease, Multiple Chemical Sensitivities, and Chronic Environmental Illness, by Neil Nathan, MD

Keto-Friendly Food Lists

This list was originally created and inspired by Dr. Jenna Jorgensen, ND, and Dr. Bonnie Nedrow, ND, who turned me from a keto skeptic to a proponent after sharing healing stories of their patients. It has evolved as I have learned more over the years.

Phase 1 Foods

Raw or Cooked Greens

Alfalfa sprouts	Dandelion greens	Parsley
Arugula	Endive	Purslane
Bok choy	Escarole	Radicchio
Cabbage	Kale	Radishes
Cardoon	Kelp	Sauerkraut (cabbage-based)
Chard	Lettuce	
Chicory	Mesclun	Sorrel
Cilantro	Mixed greens	Spinach
Collard greens	Mustard greens	Watercress

Aboveground Veggies

Asparagus	Celery	Mushrooms
Avocado	Chayote	Nopales
Broccoli	Chives	Onions, green
Broccoli rabe	Cucumber	Summer squash, crookneck
Brussels sprouts	Fennel	
Cabbage (any type)	Green beans	Zucchini
Cauliflower	Kelp noodles	

These veggies are all slightly higher in carbs than greens are; you may need to limit them if you are struggling to get your blood ketone levels >1.0.

Fruits

Blueberries	Lemon	Lime

Fats

Avocados	Coconut oil	Olive oil
Butter	Flax oil	Olives
Coconut milk	Ghee	Sesame oil

Nuts & Seeds

Almonds	Macadamia nuts	Pecans

Dairy (grass-fed, organic, hormone-free)

Blue cheese	Feta	Whey protein powder
Brie	Goat cheese	Whole-milk cheddar
Cream	Sour cream	Whole-milk mozzarella
Cream cheese	Triple cream cheese	

Animal Proteins (grass-fed, organic, hormone-free)

Bacon	Goat	quail)
Beef	Lamb	Venison
Bison	Pork	
Eggs	Poultry (turkey, chicken,	

Be very cautious with processed meat, such as bacon and sausage; these products may contain sugar even though they claim zero carbs.

Vegetarian Proteins

Hemp protein powder (carb-free)	Pumpkin seed protein powder	Whey protein powder, non-denatured

If you are vegetarian, add category two nuts and seeds to your diet right away to ensure adequate protein.

Fish

Anchovies	Mussels	Shrimp
Atlantic mackerel	Salmon, wild	
Herring	Sardines	

Beverages

Club soda	Tea, black	Water (okay to add lemon, lime, mint, etc. for flavor)
Coffee (okay to add MCT oil, coconut oil, butter, or other fat)	Tea, green	
	Tea, herbal, unsweetened	

Sweeteners and Treats

Allulose—1:1 substitute for granulated cane sugar	Monk fruit—liquid is preferable to granulated because granulated contains erythritol which has been linked to blood clots	Stevia
Cardamom		Vanilla
Cinnamon		Xylitol
Cocoa powder		

Herbs and Spices

Basil	Cloves	Horseradish
Capers	Garlic	Mint
Cilantro	Ginger	Rosemary

All herbs and spices are okay to use on the ketogenic diet—just be careful to avoid premixed spices and sauces that contain sugar.

Sauces

Mustard	Vinegar (unsweetened rice vinegar is zero carb, others are variable)	Wasabi
Soy sauce		
Tabasco		

Phase 2 Foods

Fruit

Apples	Clementine	Plums
Blackberries	Honeydew melon	Raspberries
Cantaloupe	Kiwi	Strawberries
Cherries	Persimmon	Watermelon

Vegetables

Artichokes	Leeks	Shallots
Beet greens	Mung bean sprouts	Snow peas
Celery root	Okra	Squash, spaghetti
Daikon radish	Onions	Tomatillo
Eggplant	Peppers	Tomato
Jicama	Pumpkin	Turnip
Kelp	Rutabaga	Wakame
Kohlrabi	Scallions	

Nuts and Seeds

Brazil nuts	Coconut butter	Tahini
Cashews	Hazelnuts	

Dairy

Gouda	Parmesan

Vegetarian Protein

Lentils	Tempeh	Tofu

Phase 3 Foods

Fruits

Apricots	Nectarines	Pears
Grapefruit	Orange	Pineapple
Grapes	Papaya	Tangerine
Mango	Peaches	

Root Veggies

Beets	Jerusalem artichokes	Yams
Carrots	Parsnips	
Cassava	Sweet potatoes	

Aboveground Veggies

Acorn squash	Butternut squash	Corn

Nuts and Seeds

Coconut Water

Grains

Buckwheat	Quinoa
Millet	Whole-grain rice

Beans

Black	Garbanzo	Pinto
Black-eyed peas	Kidney	

PROTEIN AND FAT CONTENT OF PROTEIN-RICH FOODS

Animal protein			
FOOD	SERVING	PROTEIN	FAT
Ground beef, 10% fat	4 ounces	21 grams	7 grams
Wild salmon	4 ounces	24 grams	8 grams
Chicken breast	4 ounces	26 grams	1.5 grams
Chicken thighs, skin	4 ounces	19 grams	19 grams
Turkey, dark	4 ounces	23 grams	11 grams
Lamb	4 ounces	16.5 grams	23 grams
Bison	4 ounces	17 grams	4 grams
Bacon	1 slice	3 grams	3 grams

Vegetarian protein			
Egg	1 egg	6 grams	5 grams
Coconut yogurt, plain	1 cup	1 gram	6 grams
Chia seeds	2½ tbsp	5 grams	9 grams
Tofu	1 cup	16 grams	9 grams
Greek yogurt, plain	1 cup	20 grams	12 grams
Hemp seeds	1 tbsp	3 grams	4 grams

A Month of Keto Meals

This month of meals is adapted directly from our monthly menu at Marama, customized to the recipes included in this book and the realities of home cooking (meaning, acknowledging that there will be leftovers and you don't have a full-time chef). I share this to help you see that eating keto is doable and that there is plenty of variety. Of course, you can keep your meal options simpler than this and eat Keto Oatmeal, every day if that's your preference (I often take this approach). But if you start to get bored or burned out on the same foods, refer to this meal plan to get some new ideas.

If you are vegetarian, check out *The Ketotarian Cookbook* by Dr. Will Cole for an entire cookbook dedicated to a vegetarian keto diet. If you are vegan, it is possible to be vegan and keto; however, work with a nutritionist, health coach, or healthcare provider to ensure you are not developing nutritional deficiencies. I don't recommend a vegan keto diet for more than two weeks.

Week 1

	BREAKFAST	LUNCH	SNACK	DINNER
MONDAY	Mini Frittatas	Creamy Broccoli Soup	Cucumber slices and celery sticks with Dill Dip	Egg Roll in a Bowl
TUESDAY	Keto Oatmeal	Easy Shrimp Scampi with Zoodles	Leftover Mini Frittata	Once-a-Week Dinner
WEDNESDAY	Empty-the-Fridge Scramble	Spinach and goat cheese salad with leftover sautéed chicken	Roasted Nuts	Baked salmon with roasted asparagus (serve with leftover Dill Dip)
THURSDAY	Leftover Keto Oatmeal	Egg Salad Lettuce Cups	Brownie Fat Bomb	Cauliflower Crust Pizza
FRIDAY	Berry-Cream Parfait	Leftover Cauliflower Crust Pizza	Brie and flaxseed crackers	Red curry chicken over cauliflower rice
SATURDAY	Keto waffles with whipped cream	Smoked salmon and cream cheese roll-ups served with a simple green salad	Deviled eggs	Keto-friendly chili
SUNDAY	Cheesy omelet	Chicken-salad-stuffed avocado half with flaxseed crackers	Brownie Fat Bomb	Carnitas burrito bowl with cauliflower rice

Week 2

	BREAKFAST	LUNCH	SNACK	DINNER
MONDAY	Scrambled eggs and bacon	Cauliflower Crust Pizza	Roasted Nuts	Creamy Broccoli Soup
TUESDAY	Berry-Cream Parfait	Arugula and romaine salad with feta, red onion, and smoked salmon	Hard-boiled egg sprinkled with Everything But the Bagel seasoning	Once-a-Week Dinner
WEDNESDAY	Keto Oatmeal	Turkey and cheese roll-ups	Cottage cheese with berries	Zoodles with Bolognese sauce

THURSDAY	Empty-the-Fridge Scramble	Canned Salmon Salad Wrap	Cardamom Fat Bomb	Roasted chicken wings with air-fried cauliflower florets
FRIDAY	Leftover Keto Oatmeal	Shrimp Scampi with Zoodles	Cardamom Fat Bomb	Cheeseburger with a keto bun
SATURDAY	Berry-Cream Parfait	Taco salad bowl (with leftover hamburger meat) with guacamole and salsa	Olives and cheese cubes	Salmon Salad
SUNDAY	Avocado and bacon omelets	Creamy Broccoli Soup	Keto Celebration Cake	Veggie lasagna (use thin sliced zucchini instead of noodles)

Week 3

MONDAY	Mini Frittatas	Leftover lasagna	Cucumber	Chicken fajitas
TUESDAY	Berry-Cream Parfait	Canned Salmon Salad wrap	Leftover Mini Frittata	Shrimp stir-fry with fried cauliflower rice
WEDNESDAY	Scrambled eggs and bacon	Coconut-lime soup (also known as Tom Kha soup) with leftover shrimp	Cucumber and celery sticks served with Dill Dip	Roasted salmon and roasted Brussels sprouts served with pesto
THURSDAY	Berry-Cream Parfait	Creamy Broccoli Soup	Cottage cheese and berries	Once-a-Week Dinner
FRIDAY	Empty-the-Fridge Scramble	Smoked salmon and cream cheese roll-ups served with leftover Dill Dip	Olives and cheese cubes	Steak burrito bowl with cauliflower rice
SATURDAY	Keto waffles with whipped cream and blueberries	Spinach salad with leftover steak	Leftover Creamy Broccoli Soup	Cauliflower Crust Pizza
SUNDAY	Cheesy omelet with avocado	Leftover Cauliflower Crust Pizza	Brownie Fat Bomb	Egg Roll in a Bowl

Week 4				
MONDAY	Keto Oatmeal	Egg Salad Lettuce Cups	Cottage cheese and berries	Carnitas burrito bowl with cauliflower rice
TUESDAY	Fried egg(s) with leftover carnitas and salsa	Turkey and cheese roll-ups	Deviled eggs	Once-a-Week Dinner
WEDNESDAY	Keto Oatmeal	Chicken Caesar Salad	Olives and cheese cubes	Zoodles with Bolognese sauce
THURSDAY	Mini Frittatas	Arugula and romaine salad with feta, red onion, and smoked salmon	Beef jerky	Keto teriyaki chicken bowls
FRIDAY	Berry-Cream-Parfait	Philly cheese steak bowl	Leftover Mini Frittata	Salmon Salad
SATURDAY	Keto Oatmeal	Chicken-salad-stuffed avocado half with flaxseed crackers	Beef jerky	Creamy Broccoli Soup
SUNDAY	Cheesy omelet with avocado	Leftover Creamy Broccoli Soup	Brownie Fat Bomb	Cheeseburger on a keto bun

Sample Daily Schedule

When it comes to protecting cognitive function, you need a mix of predictability and novelty. So while having a basic schedule is vital for helping you know that you have designated time for each piece of the protocol, you also have a lot of leeway in choosing which activities you'll do during those appointed times.

This basic template is the one we follow at Marama and reserves time for all the categories of activities covered in this book.

There are also things that will happen on a weekly basis, such as time for appointments and errands. I recommend choosing a regular time for those things to happen and blocking them out on your calendar so they don't throw off your routine or become an excuse not to get in the meals and activities that support your brain health.

8 a.m.	Breakfast
9 a.m.	Walk
10:30 a.m.	Cognition-enhancing activity
12:00 p.m.	Lunch
1:30 p.m.	Creative activity
2:30 p.m.	Snack
3 p.m.	Exercise
6 p.m.	Dinner
7 p.m.	Games
8 p.m.	Bedtime routine
9 p.m.	Bed

If you are in prevention mode and not actively caregiving a loved one with cognitive decline, your schedule doesn't need to be as granular, but you can still establish a basic rhythm to your days that helps you carve out time for taking care of yourself.

7 a.m.	Morning routine
8 a.m.	Breakfast
9 a.m. to 12 p.m.	Work
12 p.m.	Lunch
12:30 p.m.	Walk
1 p.m. to 5 p.m.	Work
6 p.m.	Dinner
7 p.m.	After-dinner activity
9:30 p.m.	Bedtime routine
10:30 p.m.	Bed

No- or Low-Cost Cognitive Health Interventions

Remember many of the most impactful and effective things you can do to prevent or reverse dementia cost nothing (or very little). Weaving these things into your daily life will do more than help your cognition—they will also enrich your life in ways that may surprise you.

To help you stay focused on these powerful changes, I've created this list inspired by Barbara, a coaching client, who called it her Daily Dozen. These are no- or low-cost interventions. If you ever feel overwhelmed, refer to this list and find something on here to add or recommit to.

Barbara's Daily Dozen:

1. Reach out to a loved one outside of our immediate family unit
2. Pray or meditate
3. Get outside
4. Brush and floss teeth twice a day
5. De-clutter
6. Cook a meal and sit down to eat
7. Exercise
8. Garden
9. Open doors and windows for an hour
10. Do one act of kindness
11. Read for at least twenty minutes
12. Go to bed earlier

Additional Ideas:

Giving blood

Socializing

Taking your shoes off indoors

Turning the TV off

Volunteering

Performing acts of kindness

Choosing whole foods over the processed foods

Replacing old household and personal care products for less toxic ones
when you run out

Progress Tracker

| Date | | | |

Hours of Sleep [ ]

Quality of Sleep   Excellent   Good   Average   Fair   Terrible

Fasting Ketones [ ]

Breakfast [ ]   ☐ Supplements

Ketones 1–2 hours later [ ]

Lunch [ ]   ☐ Supplements

Ketones 1–2 hours later [ ]

Dinner [ ]   ☐ Supplements

Ketones 1–2 hours later [ ]

Exercise Type and Amount [ ]

Water intake Oz [ ]

Symptoms   anxious   relaxed   energetic   fatigued   forgetful   engaged

Bowel Movement Today [ ]

Activities   time outside   brain stimulation   creativity   relaxation   connection   self-care

Other Observations [ ]

Energy   Low ———— High   1 2 3 4 5 6 7 8 9 10

Stress   Low ———— High   1 2 3 4 5 6 7 8 9 10

ACKNOWLEDGMENTS

The process of writing this book was one of the most fun, collaborative, and creative experiences of my life. I have never felt this book is "mine." This book belongs to my patients and their tireless caregivers. It is about and for the many people whose lives have intersected with mine as patients, coaching clients, Marama residents, and those who care about them. My privilege has been to witness their journeys and provide an account of them here.

The team of hardworking individuals who support Solcere and Marama are an endless source of inspiration and crucial to the successes shared in this book, including Karrie Shotts, our director of operations at Marama, Dr. Stephanie Lund, ND at Solcere, Tyler Walsh, our incredible and dedicated health coach, Barbara Zerbe and Lee Busch who have helped tirelessly to get the word out, Pam Hohman who captains the Solcere ship, as well as Mira Aguilar, her first mate. The entire team at Marama who helped us get through Covid and beyond including but not limited to Garrett Bick, Leigha Brown, Dana Connolly, Victoria Dyckman, Shawnta Foster, Montana "Rose" Hammond, Alexis Kopcak, Chef Gil Manipon, Monica Navarrete, Joana Oducayen, Jane Resendiz, Harley Zenns, and Elsa Zeray.

Thank you to Greg Erickson for passionately believing in Marama and me from the moment I mentioned the concept. Thank you to Jim and Holly Miller, John and Marci Cavanaugh, Bill and Candi Miholich, and Greg Williams for your partnership and support through the unexpected challenges of Covid. Marama would not exist without you all. Extra thanks to Marci Cavanaugh for making Marama feel like home. Marama is beautiful because of your great eye, hard work, and attention to detail.

Along with the privilege of working with these pioneers I also had the incredible fortune of meeting my literary agent Stephanie Tade who guided me in creating the all-star team who have made this book what it is. I had no idea a writing collaborator as skilled, fun, kind, easy to work with, and efficient as Kate Hanley existed. I am grateful beyond words to my colleague Dr. Kara Fitzgerald for introducing me to both Stephanie and Kate.

It is a dream come true to work for the talented and seasoned team at HarperCollins led by our editors Karen Rinaldi and Rachel Kambury.

Dr. Dale Bredesen paved the path that led me to my life's purpose. He is a critically important thought leader and it is an honor to join him in his quest to make Alzheimer's both rare and optional. For that alone I am grateful beyond measure. I am consistently humbled by Dr. Bredesen and Lance Kelly at Apollo for their support, collaboration, and encouragement.

Daniel Schmachtenberger, Sanjiv Sidhu, and Chandra Pai your kindness, friendship, mentorship, support, encouragement, and essentially adult parenting profoundly shifted my worldview and impacted who I have become and any positive impact I have been able to make.

Thank you to the Helfgott Research team including Dr. Ryan Bradley, ND, MPH, Dr. Nini Callan, ND, Dr. John Phipps, PhD, and Dr. Ram Rao, PhD, from the Apollo team who were essential to publishing our research findings. Thank you to James Walton for the funding that made the research and so much else possible.

Thank you to my friends and family for understanding every time I needed to prioritize "The Book" and especially to Chuck, my loving partner, for reading every word from start to finish with insightful perspective and a careful eye.

Mom, you've jumped on a plane countless times to roll your sleeves up and contribute to my latest project. You've provided a model of caring for others, the grit to get things done, unmatched resourcefulness, plus the love and support to last a lifetime. Thank you.

GLOSSARY

Acetylcholine: a neurotransmitter that influences memory, learning, attention, and muscle movement. Donepezil, a common Alzheimer's medication, prevents the breakdown of acetylcholine.

Amygdala: the almond-shaped area of the brain that is adjacent to the hippocampus and is generally thought to be responsible for emotions, particularly those related to fear, anger, and trauma. The amygdala also plays a role in memory.

Beta-amyloid plaques: misfolded proteins that accumulate in the brain in response to infections, toxins, sleep deprivation, and other stressors. Some researchers suggest they are the cause of Alzheimer's disease; however, pharmaceuticals targeting beta-amyloid plaques have thus far failed to provide meaningful improvements in cognition.

Brain waves: an electrical impulse in the brain driven by the activity of neurons, the cells that make up brain tissue. There are five primary brain waves—delta, theta, alpha, beta, and gamma. Each type of brain wave is associated with different brain states, from sleeping to highly alert. Theta brain waves are most associated with memory.

Dopamine: an excitatory neurotransmitter that influences memory, movement, pleasure/reward, motivation, focus, and attention. Deficient dopamine levels are associated with Parkinson's disease. Dopamine is broken down to make two other neurotransmitters, epinephrine, and norepinephrine.

Glial cells: these cells are the supportive network of cells for neurons in the brain. Their work is to hold neurons in place, clean up dead cells and toxic buildup, insulate neurons from one another, and facilitate the delivery of oxygen and other nutrients to the neurons.

Hippocampus: the area of the brain deep in the temporal lobe responsible for learning, memory, and understanding where we are in space. The hippocampus and amygdala work together in connecting memories with emotion. This part of the brain typically shrinks as a patient progresses through Alzheimer's disease.

Ketones: the small, acidic chemical compounds made from fats and used as fuel by cells when you are in the metabolic state of ketosis. They are an alternative to using sugar or glucose for fuel. They can be supplemented as pills or powders when you are in the process of getting into ketosis.

Microglia: these are immune cells and scavenger cells that work in the brain to maintain neural networks, regulate repair of damaged neurons, and respond to infections. Even in a healthy brain, microglial cells are constantly on alert to quickly respond when the need arises.

Neurons: the fundamental cells of the nervous system that send electrical nerve impulses and neurotransmitters in the brain and spinal cord (central nervous system) and out to every organ and to the tips of our fingers and toes (peripheral nervous system) for communication between body parts. They receive sensory input from the outside world (smells, sounds, sights, touch, taste), send signals to move, and are responsible for how we feel and what we think.

Neuroplasticity: the ability of the brain to change by rewiring connections between neurons. This allows us to think differently and learn new skills as we age.

Neurotransmitter: a chemical substance neurons use to communicate. The seven main neurotransmitters are acetylcholine, dopamine, gamma-aminobutyric acid (GABA), glutamate, histamine, norepinephrine, and serotonin. Neurotransmitters directly impact how we think, learn, remember, and feel. We can have too little or too many of them, and nutrients like amino acids, minerals, and vitamins impact how many we make and how quickly we break them down.

Prefrontal cortex: this is the part of the brain, right behind the forehead, that is responsible for what makes us human—our personalities, decision-making, complex cognitive processes, verbal ability, and how we interact socially. This part of the brain is often affected in those suffering with Alzheimer's disease.

Tau proteins: when working properly, these are responsible for maintaining neuronal structure. When diseased, they are chemically altered in a process called phosphorylation that leads to accumulation and deposition in a way that inhibits neuronal function, particularly in areas of the brain associated with memory and cognitive function.

NOTES

Introduction: Hope for Alzheimer's

xv 64 percent of all Americans: SNWS Staff. (September 6, 2021). More than 60% of people polled are afraid of this happening when they get older. SWNS Digital. https://swnsdigital.com/us/2020/11/more-than-60-of-people-are-afraid-of-this -happening-when-they-get-older/

xv 11.2 million by 2040: Alzheimer's Association. (2022). 2022 Alzheimer's Disease Facts and Figures. https://www.alz.org/media/Documents/alzheimers-facts-and -figures.pdf

Chapter 1: The Truth About Brain Health

12 Ketones are the preferred source of fuel: Cunnane, S. C., Courchesne-Loyer, A., Vandenberghe, C., St-Pierre, V., Fortier, M., Hennebelle, M., Croteau, E., Bocti, C., Fulop, T., & Castellano, C. A. (2016). Can ketones help rescue brain fuel supply in later life? Implications for cognitive health during aging and the treatment of Alzheimer's disease. *Frontiers in Molecular Neuroscience*, *9*, 53. https://doi.org/10.3389/fnmol .2016.00053; Croteau, E., Castellano, C. A., Fortier, M., Bocti, C., Fulop, T., Paquet, N., & Cunnane, S. C. (2018). A cross-sectional comparison of brain glucose and ketone metabolism in cognitively healthy older adults, mild cognitive impairment and early Alzheimer's disease. *Experimental Gerontology*, *107*, 18–26. https://doi.org/10.1016/j.exger .2017.07.004; Roy, M., Fortier, M., Rheault, F., Edde, M., Croteau, E., Castellano, C. A., Langlois, F., St-Pierre, V., Cuenoud, B., Bocti, C., Fulop, T., Descoteaux, M., & Cunnane, S. C. (2021). A ketogenic supplement improves white matter energy supply and processing speed in mild cognitive impairment. *Alzheimer's & Dementia (New York, N.Y.)*, *7*(1), e12217. https://doi.org/10.1002/trc2.12217; Fortier, M., Castellano, C. A., Croteau, E., Langlois, F., Bocti, C., St-Pierre, V., Vandenberghe, C., Bernier, M., Roy, M., Descoteaux, M., Whittingstall, K., Lepage, M., Turcotte, É. E., Fulop, T., & Cunnane, S. C. (2019). A ketogenic drink improves brain energy and some measures of cognition in mild cognitive impairment. *Alzheimer's & Dementia: The Journal of the Alzheimer's Association*, *15*(5), 625–634. https://doi.org/10.1016/j.jalz.2018.12.017

14 elevated levels of the stress hormone cortisol: Ouanes, S., & Popp, J. (2019). High cortisol and the risk of dementia and Alzheimer's disease: A review of the literature. *Frontiers in Aging Neuroscience*, *11*, 43. https://doi.org/10.3389/fnagi.2019.00043

17 will further affect the brain: Wyss-Coray, T., & Rogers, J. (2012). Inflammation in Alzheimer disease: A brief review of the basic science and clinical literature. *Cold Spring Harbor Perspectives in Medicine*, *2*(1), a006346. https://doi.org/10.1101/cshperspect .a006346

17 some infections are associated: Gosztyla, M. L., Brothers, H. M., & Robinson, S. R. (2018). Alzheimer's amyloid-β is an antimicrobial peptide: A review of the evidence. *Journal of Alzheimer's Disease: JAD*, *62*(4), 1495–1506. https://doi.org/10.3233/JAD -171133

17 threefold risk of dementia: Lopatko Lindman, K., Hemmingsson, E. S., Weidung, B., Brännström, J., Josefsson, M., Olsson, J., Elgh, F., Nordström, P., & Lövheim, H. (2021). Herpesvirus infections, antiviral treatment, and the risk of dementia: A registry-based cohort study in Sweden. *Alzheimer's & Dementia (New York, N.Y.)*, *7*(1), e12119. https://doi.org/10.1002/trc2.12119

18 has been shown to reduce dementia risk: Tzeng, N. S., Chung, C. H., Lin, F. H., Chiang, C. P., Yeh, C. B., Huang, S. Y., Lu, R. B., Chang, H. A., Kao, Y. C., Yeh, H. W., Chiang, W. S., Chou, Y. C., Tsao, C. H., Wu, Y. F., & Chien, W. C. (2018). Anti-herpetic medications and reduced risk of dementia in patients with herpes simplex virus infections: A nationwide, population-based cohort study in Taiwan. *Neurotherapeutics*, *15*, 417–429. https://doi.org/10.1007/s13311-018-0611-x

18 found in the brains of Alzheimer's patients: Costa, M., de Araújo, I., da Rocha Alves, L., da Silva, R. L., Dos Santos Calderon, P., Borges, B., de Aquino Martins, A., de Vasconcelos Gurgel, B. C., & Lins, R. (2021). Relationship of Porphyromonas gingivalis and Alzheimer's disease: A systematic review of pre-clinical studies. *Clinical Oral Investigations*, *25*(3), 797–806. https://doi.org/10.1007/s00784-020-03764-w, PMID: 33469718

18 lead to misfolded amyloid proteins: ibid.

19 negatively affecting the brain: Miklossy, J., Khalili, K., Gern, L., Ericson, R. L., Darekar, P., Bolle, L., Hurlimann, J., & Paster, B. J. (2004). Borrelia burgdorferi persists in the brain in chronic Lyme neuroborreliosis and may be associated with Alzheimer disease. *Journal of Alzheimer's Disease: JAD*, *6*(6), 639–681. https://doi .org/10.3233/jad-2004-6608; Wormser, G. P., Marques, A., Pavia, C. S., Schwartz, I., Feder, H. M., & Pachner, A. R. (2022). Lack of convincing evidence that Borrelia burgdorferi infection causes either Alzheimer disease or Lewy body dementia. *Clinical Infectious Diseases: An Official Publication of the Infectious Diseases Society of America*, *75*(2), 342–346. https://doi.org/10.1093/cid/ciab993

19 elevated risk of early onset cognitive decline: Liu, Y. H., Chen, Y., Wang, Q. H., Wang, L. R., Jiang, L., Yang, Y., Chen, X., Li, Y., Cen, Y., Xu, C., Zhu, J., Li, W., Wang, Y. R., Zhang, L. L., Liu, J., Xu, Z. Q., & Wang, Y. J. (2022). One-year trajectory of cognitive changes in older survivors of COVID-19 in Wuhan, China: A longitudinal cohort study. *JAMA Neurology*, *79*(5), 509–517. https://doi.org/10.1001/jamaneurol.2022.0461

20 link between reproductive hormones and cognitive health: Uchoa, M. F., Moser, V. A., & Pike, C. J. (2016). Interactions between inflammation, sex steroids, and Alzheimer's disease risk factors. *Frontiers in Neuroendocrinology*, *43*, 60–82. https://doi .org/10.1016/j.yfrne.2016.09.001; Trova, S., Bovetti, S., Bonzano, S., De Marchis, S., & Peretto, P. (2021). Sex steroids and the shaping of the peripubertal brain: The sexual-dimorphic set-up of adult neurogenesis. *International Journal of Molecular Sciences*, *22*(15), 7984. https://doi.org/10.3390/ijms22157984

20 bioidentical hormone replacement . . . appears to be safer: Cagnacci, A., & Venier, M. (2019). The controversial history of hormone replacement therapy. *Medicina (Kaunas, Lithuania)*, *55*(9), 602. https://doi.org/10.3390/medicina55090602

22 correlated to the size of your hippocampus: Erickson, K. I., Prakash, R. S., Voss, M. W., Chaddock, L., Heo, S., McLaren, M., Pence, B. D., et al. (2010). Brain-derived neurotrophic factor is associated with age-related decline in hippocampal volume. *Journal of Neuroscience, 30*(15), 5368–5375. https://doi.org/10.1523/JNEUROSCI .6251-09.2010

23 eating one-half cup a day: Krikorian, R., Skelton, M. R., Summer, S. S., Shidler, M. D., & Sullivan, P. G. (2022). Blueberry supplementation in midlife for dementia risk reduction. *Nutrients, 14*(8), 1619. https://doi.org/10.3390/nu14081619

Chapter 2: How Have We Gotten It So Wrong?

27 only 2 percent of people: Braak, H., Thal, D. R., Ghebremedhin, E., & Del Tredici, K. (2011). Stages of the pathologic process in Alzheimer disease: Age categories from 1 to 100 years. *Journal of Neuropathology & Experimental Neurology, 70*(11), 960–969. https://doi.org/10.1097/NEN.0b013e318232a379

27 only 10 percent of people sixty-five and older experience measurable cognitive impairments: Jansen, W. J., Ossenkoppele, R., Knol, D. L., Tijms, B. M., Scheltens, P., Verhey, F. R., Visser, P. J., & the Amyloid Biomarker Study Group. (2015). Prevalence of cerebral amyloid pathology in persons without dementia: A meta-analysis. *JAMA, 313*(19),1924–38. https://doi.org/10.1001/jama.2015.4668; Braak, H., et al. (2011). Stages of the pathologic process in Alzheimer disease. *Journal of Neuropathology & Experimental Neurology, 70*(11), 960–969. Garrett, M. (2018). A critique of the 2018 National Institute on Aging's research framework: Toward a biological definition of Alzheimer's disease. *Current Opinion in Neurobiology, 9*(2), 49–58.

30 Percentage of population with this genotype: Liu, C. C., Liu, C. C., Kanekiyo, T., Xu, H., & Bu, G. (2013). Apolipoprotein E and Alzheimer disease: Risk, mechanisms and therapy. *Nature Reviews. Neurology, 9*(2), 106–118. https://doi.org/10.1038 /nrneurol.2012.263

30 Lifetime risk of dementia: Verghese, P. B., Castellano, J. M., & Holtzman, D. M. (2011). Apolipoprotein E in Alzheimer's disease and other neurological disorders. *The Lancet: Neurology, 10*(3), 241–252. https://doi.org/10.1016/S1474 -4422(10)70325-2

30 developing a positive attitude about aging: Levy, B. R., Slade, M. D., Pietrzak, R. H., Ferrucci, L. (2018). Positive age beliefs protect against dementia even among elders with high-risk gene. *PLOS One, 13*(2), e0191004. https://doi.org/10.1371/journal .pone.0191004

31 much more common senile dementia: Katzman, R. (1976). Editorial: The prevalence and malignancy of Alzheimer disease. A major killer. *Archives of Neurology, 33*(4), 217–218. https://doi.org/10.1001/archneur.1976.00500040001001

31 spent on Alzheimer's disease research: Herrup, K. (2021). *How Not to Study a Disease* (Cambridge, Massachusetts: MIT Press), 107.

32 half of cases with senile dementia: Tomlinson, B. E., Blessed, G., & Roth, M. (1970). Observations on the brains of demented old people. *Journal of the Neurological Sciences*, *11*(3), 205–242. https://doi.org/10.1016/0022-510x(70)90063-8

32 only ten that had absolutely no plaques or tangles: Braak, H., et al. (2011). Stages of the pathologic process in Alzheimer disease. *Journal of Neuropathology & Experimental Neurology*, *70*(11), 960–969. Aizenstein, H. J., Nebes, R. D., Saxton, J. A., Price, J. C., Mathis, C. A., Tsopelas, N. D., Ziolko, S. K., James, J. A., Snitz, B. E., Houck, P. R., Bi, W., Cohen, A. D., Lopresti, B. J., DeKosky, S. T., Halligan, E. M., & Klunk, W. E. (2008). Frequent amyloid deposition without significant cognitive impairment among the elderly. *Archives of Neurology*, *65*(11), 1509–1517. https://doi.org/10.1001/archneur.65.11.1509

33 99.6 percent of the research on pharmaceutical interventions for Alzheimer's has failed: Cummings, J. (2018). Lessons learned from Alzheimer disease: clinical trials with negative outcomes. *Clinical and Translational Science*, *11*(2), 147–152. https://doi.org/10.1111/cts.12491

33 some seminal Alzheimer's research appears to have been falsified: Piller, C. (2022). Blots on a field? *Science*, *377*(6604), 358–363. https://doi.org/10.1126/science.add9993

34 the paper in question: Piller, C. (2022). Whistleblower finds possible misconduct in his own papers. *Science, 378*(6621), 694–695. https://doi.org/10.1126/science.adf8360

34 majority of data collected showed there was no benefit at all: Walsh, S., Merrick, R., Milne, R., Brayne, C. (2021) Aducanumab for Alzheimer's disease? *BMJ*, *374*, n1682. https://doi.org/10.1136/bmj.n1682; Sevigny, J., Chiao, P., Bussière, T., Weinreb, P. H., Williams, L., Maier, M., Dunstan, R., Salloway, S., Chen, T., Ling, Y., O'Gorman, J., Qian, F., Arastu, M., Li, M., Chollate, S., Brennan, M. S., Quintero-Monzon, O., Scannevin, R. H., Arnold, H. M. . . . Sandrock, A. (2016). The antibody aducanumab reduces Aβ plaques in Alzheimer's disease. *Nature, 537*(7618), 50–56. https://doi.org/10.1038/nature19323. Update in: (2017)/ *Nature, 546*(7659), 564; Alexander, G. C., Emerson, S., Kesselheim, A. S. (2021). Evaluation of aducanumab for Alzheimer disease: Scientific evidence and regulatory review involving efficacy, safety, and futility. *JAMA*, *325*(17), 1717–1718. https://doi.org/10.1001/jama.2021.3854

34 "probably the worst drug approval decision in recent US history": Mahase, E. (2021). Three FDA advisory panel members resign over approval of Alzheimer's drug. *BMJ*, *373*, n1503. https://doi.org/10.1136/bmj.n1503

35 actually makes cognition worse: Kennedy, R. E., Cutter, G. R., Fowler, M. E., Schneider, L. S. (2018). Association of concomitant use of cholinesterase inhibitors or memantine with cognitive decline in Alzheimer clinical trials: A meta-analysis. *JAMA Network Open, 1*(7): e184080. https://doi.org/10.1001/jamanetworkopen.2018.4080

37 risk factors listed by *The Lancet* 2020 report include: Livingston, G., Huntley, J., Sommerlad, A., Ames, D., Ballard, C., Banerjee, S., Brayne, C., Burns, A., Cohen-Mansfield, J., Cooper, C., Costafreda, S. G., Dias, A., Fox, N., Gitlin, L. N., Howard, R., Kales, H. C., Kivimäki, M., Larson, E. B., Ogunniyi, A., Orgeta, V. . . .

Mukadam, N. (2020). Dementia prevention, intervention, and care: 2020 report of the Lancet Commission. *Lancet, 396*(10248), 413–446. https://doi.org/10.1016/S0140-6736(20)30367-6

38 One French study: Schwarzinger, M., Pollock, B. G., Hasan, O. S. M., Dufouil, C., Rehm, J., & QalyDays Study Group (2018). Contribution of alcohol use disorders to the burden of dementia in France 2008–13: A nationwide retrospective cohort study. *The Lancet: Public Health, 3*(3), e124–e132. https://doi.org/10.1016/S2468-2667(18)30022-7

39 people with the lowest levels of physical activity: Yan, S., Fu, W., Wang, C., Mao, J., Liu, B., Zou, L., & Lv, C. (2020). Correction: Association between sedentary behavior and the risk of dementia: A systematic review and meta-analysis. *Translational Psychiatry, 10.* https://doi.org/10.1038/s41398-020-0799-5; Wang, S., Liu, H.-Y., Cheng, Y.-C., & Su, C.-H. (2021). Exercise dosage in reducing the risk of dementia development: Mode, duration, and intensity—a narrative review. *International Journal of Environmental Research and Public Health, 18*(24), 13331. https://doi.org/10.3390/ijerph182413331

39 depressive episodes in the first half of life: Byers, A. L., & Yaffe, K. (2011). Depression and risk of developing dementia. *Nature Reviews Neurology, 7*(6), 323–331. https://doi.org/10.1038/nrneurol.2011.60; Barnes, D. E., Yaffe, K., Byers, A. L., McCormick, M., Schaefer, C., & Whitmer, R. A. (2012). Midlife vs late-life depressive symptoms and risk of dementia: Differential effects for Alzheimer disease and vascular dementia. *Archives of General Psychiatry, 69*(5), 493–498. https://doi.org/10.1001/archgenpsychiatry.2011.1481

41 250 to 600 percent greater than the general population: Norton, M. C., Smith, K. R., Østbye, T., Tschanz, J. T., Corcoran, C., Schwartz, S., Piercy, K. W., Rabins, P. V., Steffens, D. C., Skoog, I., Breitner, J. C., Welsh-Bohmer, K. A., & Cache County Investigators (2010). Greater risk of dementia when spouse has dementia? The Cache County study. *Journal of the American Geriatrics Society, 58*(5), 895–900. https://doi.org/10.1111/j.1532-5415.2010.02806.x

42 published her grievances in *The Lancet: Neurology* in 2020: Hellmuth, J. H. (2020). Can we trust *The End of Alzheimer's? The Lancet: Neurology, 19*(5), 389–390.

43 Bredesen published a case series: Bredesen, D. E. (2014). Reversal of cognitive decline: A novel therapeutic program. *Aging, 6*(9), 707–717. https://doi.org/10.18632/aging.100690

43 another case series . . . on ten participants: Bredesen, D. E., Amos, E. C., Canick, J., Ackerley, M., Raji, C., Fiala, M., & Ahdidan, J. (2016). Reversal of cognitive decline in Alzheimer's disease. *Aging, 8*(6), 1250–1258. https://doi.org/10.18632/aging.100981

43 another case series of one hundred dementia patients: Bredesen, D. E., Sharlin, K., Jenkins, D., Okuno, M., Youngberg, W. S., Cohen, S., Stefani, A., Brown, R. L., Conger, S., Tanio, C. P., Hathaway, A., Kogan, M., Hagedorn, D. K., Amos, E. C., Amos, A., Bergman, N., Diamond, C. A., Lawrence, J., Rusk, I. N. . . . Braud, M. (2018). Reversal of cognitive decline: 100 patients. *Journal of Alzheimer's Disease & Parkinsonism, 8*(5). http://dx.doi.org/10.4172/2161-0460.1000450

Chapter 3: Unpack the New Alzheimer's Toolkit

52 over 20 percent of energy expenditure each day: Du, F., Zhu, X. H., Zhang, Y., Friedman, M., Zhang, N., Ugurbil, K., & Chen, W. (2008). Tightly coupled brain activity and cerebral ATP metabolic rate. *Proceedings of the National Academy of Sciences of the United States of America*, *105*(17), 6409–6414. https://doi.org/10.1073/pnas.0710766105

53 they help the brain perform better: Cunnane, S. C., Courchesne-Loyer, A., Vandenberghe, C., St-Pierre, V., Fortier, M., Hennebelle, M., Croteau, E., Bocti, C., Fulop, T., & Castellano, C.-A. (2016). Can ketones help rescue brain fuel supply in later life? Implications for cognitive health during aging and the treatment of Alzheimer's disease. *Frontiers in Molecular Neuroscience*, *53*. https://doi.org/10.3389%2Ffnmol.2016.00053

55 moderate exercise mobilizes immune stem cells: Nieman, D. C., & Wentz, L. M. (2019). The compelling link between physical activity and the body's defense system. *Journal of Sport and Health Science*, *8*(3), 201–217. https://doi.org/10.1016/j.jshs.2018.09.009

55 demonstrated neuroprotective functions: Rody, T., De Amorim, J. A., & De Felice, F. G. (2022). The emerging neuroprotective roles of exerkines in Alzheimer's disease. *Frontiers in Aging Neuroscience*, *14*, 965190. https://doi.org/10.3389/fnagi.2022.965190

61 people in their thirties and forties have more amyloid plaques after just one night of sleep deprivation: Shokri-Kojori, E., Wang, G. J., Wiers, C. E., Demiral, S. B., Guo, M., Kim, S. W., Lindgren, E., Ramirez, V., Zehra, A., Freeman, C., Miller, G., Manza, P., Srivastava, T., De Santi, S., Tomasi, D., Benveniste, H., Volkow, N. D. (2018). β-Amyloid accumulation in the human brain after one night of sleep deprivation. *Proceedings of the National Academy of Sciences of the United States of America*, *115*(17), 4483–4488. https://doi.org/10.1073/pnas

65 the better the outcomes we can achieve over time: Jia, J., Zhao, T., Liu, Z., Liang, Y., Li, F., Li, Y., Liu, W., Li, F., Shi, S., Zhou, C., Yang, H., Liao, Z., Li, Y., Zhao, H., Zhang, J., Zhang, K., Kan, M., Yang, S., Li, H., Liu, Z. . . . Cummings, J. (2023). Association between healthy lifestyle and memory decline in older adults: 10 year, population based, prospective cohort study. *BMJ*, *380*, e072691. https://doi.org/10.1136/bmj-2022-072691

Chapter 4: Set the Stage with a Doable Plan

66 the risk of developing dementia fell by 6 percent: Gregory, A. (2023). Seven healthy habits may help cut dementia risk, study says. *The Guardian*. https://www.theguardian.com/society/2023/feb/27/seven-healthy-habits-may-help-cut-dementia-risk-study-says

67 true even for the participants who carried an APOE4 gene: Jia, J., Zhao, T., Liu, Z., Liang, Y., Li, F., Li, Y., Liu, W., Li, F., Shi, S., Zhou, C., Yang, H., Liao, Z., Li, Y., Zhao, H., Zhang, J., Zhang, K., Kan, M., Yang, S., Li, H., Liu, Z. . . . Cummings, J. (2023). Association between healthy lifestyle and memory decline in older adults: 10

year, population based, prospective cohort study. *BMJ, 380*, e072691. https://doi.org/10.1136/bmj-2022-072691

Chapter 5: Get Organized with Daily Routines

91 The average American spends two and a half hours a day watching TV: Statista. (2023). Average Daily Time Spent Watching TV in the United States from 2019 to 2024 (in minutes). https://www.statista.com/statistics/186833/average-television-use-per-person-in-the-us-since-2002/

93 good brain health is linked to good oral health: Yamaguchi, S., Murakami, T., Satoh, M., Komiyama, T., Ohi, T., Miyoshi, Y., Endo, K., Hiratsuka, T., Hara, A., Tatsumi, Y., Totsune, T., Asayama, K., Kikuya, M., Nomura, K., Hozawa, A., Metoki, H., Imai, Y., Watanabe, M., Ohkubo, T., & Hattori, Y. (2023). Associations of dental health with the progression of hippocampal atrophy in community-dwelling individuals: The Ohasama study. *Neurology, 101*(10), e1056–e1068. https://doi.org/10.1212/WNL.0000000000207579

96 A form of inositol: Tanaka, K., Takenaka, S., & Yoshida, K. (2015). *Scyllo*-inositol, a therapeutic agent for Alzheimer's disease. *Journal of Clinical Neurology, 2*(4), 1040.

96 a trial in Israel: Barak, Y., Levine, J., Glasman, A., Elizur, A., & Belmaker, R. H. (1996). Inositol treatment of Alzheimer's disease: A double blind, cross-over placebo controlled trial. *Progress in Neuro-psychopharmacology & Biological Psychiatry, 20*(4), 729–735.

97 associated with cognitive decline: Ferreira, P., Ferreira, A. R., Barreto, B., & Fernandes, L. (2022). Is there a link between the use of benzodiazepines and related drugs and dementia? A systematic review of reviews. *European Geriatric Medicine, 13*(1), 19–32. https://doi.org/10.1007/s41999-021-00553-w

97 medications with similar risks include Ambien and Lunesta: Leng, Y., Stone, K. L., & Yaffe, K. (2023). Race differences in the association between sleep medication use and risk of dementia. *Journal of Alzheimer's Disease: JAD, 91*(3), 1133–1139. https://doi.org/10.3233/JAD-221006

97 they reduce the important neurotransmitter acetylcholine: Risacher, S. L., McDonald, B. C., Tallman, E. F., West, J. D., Farlow, M. R., Unverzagt, F. W., Gao, S., Boustani, M., Crane, P. K., Petersen, R. C., Jack, C. R., Jr, Jagust, W. J., Aisen, P. S., Weiner, M. W., Saykin, A. J., & Alzheimer's Disease Neuroimaging Initiative, (2016). Association between anticholinergic medication use and cognition, brain metabolism, and brain atrophy in cognitively normal older adults. *JAMA Neurology, 73*(6), 721–732. https://doi.org/10.1001/jamaneurol.2016.0580; Gray, S. L., Anderson, M. L., Dublin, S., Hanlon, J. T., Hubbard, R., Walker, R., Yu, O., Crane, P. K., & Larson, E. B. (2015). Cumulative use of strong anticholinergics and incident dementia: A prospective cohort study. *JAMA Internal Medicine, 175*(3), 401–407. https://doi.org/10.1001/jamainternmed.2014.7663; Coupland, C. A. C., Hill, T., Dening, T., Morriss, R., Moore, M., & Hippisley-Cox, J. (2019). Anticholinergic drug exposure and the risk of dementia: A nested case-control study. *JAMA Internal Medicine, 179*(8), 1084–1093. https://doi.org/10.1001/jamainternmed.2019.0677

101   two and a quarter of those hours are spent on social media: Flynn, J. (2023). 18
        Average Screen Time Statistics [2023]: How Much Screen Time Is Too Much?
        Zippia. https://www.zippia.com/advice/average-screen-time-statistics/

104   has been found to reduce the stress and burden of caregiving, as well as reduce the
        incidence of using dysfunctional strategies: Lloyd, J., Muers, J., Patterson, T. G., &
        Marczak, M. (2019). Self-compassion, coping strategies, and caregiver burden in
        caregivers of people with dementia. *Clinical Gerontologist*, *42*(1), 47–59. https://doi
        .org/10.1080/07317115.2018.1461162

Chapter 6: Move the Body to Strengthen the Mind

108   walking ten thousand steps a day reduces your risk of dementia by 50 percent:
        Del Pozo Cruz, B., Ahmadi, M., Naismith, S. L., & Stamatakis, E. (2022). Association of
        daily step count and intensity with incident dementia in 78,430 adults living in the UK.
        JAMA Neurology, *79*(10), 1059–1063. https://doi.org/10.1001/jamaneurol.2022.2672

110   compared to people who did not exercise: Ahlskog, J. E., Geda, Y. E., Graff-Radford, N. R.,
        & Petersen, R. C. (2011). Physical exercise as a preventive or disease-modifying treatment
        of dementia and brain aging. *Mayo Clinic Proceedings*, *86*(9), 876–884. https://doi.org/10
        .4065/mcp.2011.0252

110   helping to keep good genes turned on and bad genes turned off: Magliulo, L., Bondi, D.,
        Pini, N., Marramiero, L., & Di Filippo, E. S. (2022). The wonder exerkines-novel
        insights: A critical state-of-the-art review. *Molecular and Cellular Biochemistry*, *477*(1),
        105–113. https://doi.org/10.1007/s11010-021-04264-5

112   positive epigenetic changes that reverse these typical age-related trends: Grazioli, E.,
        Dimauro, I., Mercatelli, N., Wang, G., Pitsiladis, Y., Di Luigi, L., & Caporossi, D.
        (2017). Physical activity in the prevention of human diseases: Role of epigenetic
        modifications. *BMC Genomics*, *18*(Suppl 8), 802. https://doi.org/10.1186/s12864
        -017-4193-5; Sanchis-Gomar, F., Garcia-Gimenez, J. L., Perez-Quilis, C., Gomez-
        Cabrera, M. C., Pallardo, F. V., & Lippi, G. (2012). Physical exercise as an epigenetic
        modulator: Eustress, the "positive stress" as an effector of gene expression. *Journal
        of Strength and Conditioning Research*, *26*(12), 3469–3472. https://doi.org/10.1519;
        Dimauro, I., Paronetto, M. P., & Caporossi, D. (2020). Exercise, redox homeostasis
        and the epigenetic landscape. *Redox Biology*, *35*, 101477. https://doi.org/10.1016/j
        .redox.2020.101477

112   promotes healthy expression of the gene that codes for BDNF: Gomez-Pinilla, F.,
        Zhuang, Y., Feng, J., Ying, Z., & Fan, G. (2011). Exercise impacts brain-derived
        neurotrophic factor plasticity by engaging mechanisms of epigenetic regulation. *The
        European Journal of Neuroscience*, *33*(3), 383–390. https://doi.org/10.1111/j
        .1460-9568.2010.07508.x; Liu, P. Z., & Nusslock, R. (2018). Exercise-mediated
        neurogenesis in the hippocampus via BDNF. *Frontiers in Neuroscience*, *12*, 52. https://
        doi.org/10.3389/fnins.2018.00052

120   helps people who have had a stroke or a traumatic brain injury recover their
        faculties: Beck, E. N., Intzandt, B. N., & Almeida, Q. J. (2018). Can dual task

walking improve in Parkinson's disease after external focus of attention exercise? A single blind randomized controlled trial. *Neurorehabilitation and Neural Repair*, *32*(1), 18–33. https://doi.org/10.1177/1545968317746782; Zheng, Y., Meng, Z., Zhi, X., & Liang, Z. (2021). Dual-task training to improve cognitive impairment and walking function in Parkinson's disease patients: A brief review. *Sports Medicine and Health Science*, *3*(4), 202–206. https://doi.org/10.1016/j.smhs .2021.10.003; Yang, Y. R., Wang, R. Y., Chen, Y. C., & Kao, M. J. (2007). Dual-task exercise improves walking ability in chronic stroke: a randomized controlled trial. *Archives of Physical Medicine and Rehabilitation, 88*(10), 1236–1240. https:// doi.org/10.1016/j.apmr.2007.06.762

120 help healthy older adults improve their gait, balance, and walking speed and reduce the risk of falls: Varela-Vásquez, L. A., Minobes-Molina, E., & Jerez-Roig, J. (2020). Dual-task exercises in older adults: A structured review of current literature. *Journal of Frailty, Sarcopenia and Falls*, *5*(2), 31–37. https://doi.org/10.22540/JFSF-05-031

120 small to moderate improvements in cognitive function: Karssemeijer, E. G. A., Aaronson, J. A., Bossers, W. J., Smits, T., Olde Rikkert, M. G. M., & Kessels, R. P. C. (2017). Positive effects of combined cognitive and physical exercise training on cognitive function in older adults with mild cognitive impairment or dementia: A meta-analysis. *Ageing Research Reviews*, *40*, 75–83. https://doi.org/10.1016/j.arr .2017.09.003

Chapter 7: Feed the Brain

133 ketone uptake in the brain increases when glucose consumption decreases: Cunnane, S. C., Courchesne-Loyer, A., Vandenberghe, C., St-Pierre, V., Fortier, M., Hennebelle, M., Croteau, E., Bocti, C., Fulop, T., & Castellano, C. A. (2016). Can ketones help rescue brain fuel supply in later life? Implications for cognitive health during aging and the treatment of Alzheimer's disease. *Frontiers in Molecular Neuroscience*, *9*, 53. https://doi.org/10.3389/fnmol.2016.00053

135 statistical and clinically significant improvement on the cognitive assessment at the end of the trial: Sheffler, J. L., Arjmandi, B., Quinn, J., Hajcak, G., Vied, C., Akhavan, N., & Naar, S. (2022). Feasibility of an MI-CBT ketogenic adherence program for older adults with mild cognitive impairment. *Pilot and Feasibility Studies*, *8*(1), 16. https://doi.org /10.1186/s40814-022-00970-z

135 a placebo to the control group: Cunnane, S. (2022). Brain energy rescue with ketones improves cognitive outcomes in MCI. *Alzheimer's & Dementia, 18*(S4), e059627. https://doi.org/10.1002/alz.059627

135 tested the ketogenic diet on participants diagnosed with Alzheimer's disease: Phillips, M. C. L., Deprez, L. M., Mortimer, G. M. N., Murtagh, D. K. J., McCoy, S., Mylchreest, R., Gilbertson, L. J., Clark, K. M., Simpson, P. V., McManus, E. J., Oh, J. E., Yadavaraj, S., King, V. M., Pillai, A., Romero-Ferrando, B., Brinkhuis, M., Copeland, B. M., Samad, S., Liao, S., & Schepel, J. A. C. (2021). Randomized crossover trial of a modified ketogenic diet in Alzheimer's disease. *Alzheimer's Research & Therapy*, *13*(1), 51. https://doi.org/10.1186/s13195-021-00783-x

143 linked to increased rates of cancer, diabetes, and heart disease: Harvard T.H. Chan
School of Public Health. Are all processed meats equally bad for health? Retrieved
February 9, 2023, from https://www.hsph.harvard.edu/news/hsph-in-the-news/are
-all-processed-meats-equally-bad-for-health/

150 highly processed foods increase your risk of developing dementia: Gomes Gonçalves, N.,
Vidal Ferreira, N., Khandpur, N., Martinez Steele, E., Bertazzi Levy, R., Andrade
Lotufo, P., Bensenor, I. M., Caramelli, P., Alvim de Matos, S. M., Marchioni, D. M.,
& Suemoto, C. K. (2023). Association between consumption of ultraprocessed foods
and cognitive decline. *JAMA Neurology, 80*(2), 142–150. https://doi.org/10.1001
/jamaneurol.2022.4397

163 allows for up to five servings of pastries and sweets a week: Harvard T. H. Chan
School of Public Health. (Reviewed 2023). Diet review: MIND diet. https://www
.hsph.harvard.edu/nutritionsource/healthy-weight/diet-reviews/mind-diet/

163 no difference in effectiveness than a slightly calorie-restricted diet: Barnes, L. L.,
Dhana, K., Liu, X., Carey, V. J., Ventrelle, J., Johnson, K., Hollings, C. S., Bishop, L.,
Laranjo, N., Stubbs, B. J., Reilly, X., Agarwal, P., Zhang, S., Grodstein, F., Tangney, C. C.,
Holland, T. M., Aggarwal, N. T., Arfanakis, K., Morris, M. C., & Sacks, F. M.
(2023). Trial of the MIND diet for prevention of cognitive decline in older persons.
The New England Journal of Medicine, 389(7), 602–611. https://doi.org/10.1056
/NEJMoa2302368

165 diets high in refined carbohydrates can negatively impact cognitive function
in a variety of ways: Hawkins, M. A. W., Keirns, N. G., & Helms, Z. (2018).
Carbohydrates and cognitive function. *Current Opinion in Clinical Nutrition &
Metabolic Care, 21*(4), 302–307. https://doi.org/10.1097/mco.0000000000000471

Chapter 8: Foster Cognition with Activities

168 as well as a slower rate of cognitive decline: Yates, L. A., Ziser, S., Spector, A., &
Orrell, M. (2016). Cognitive leisure activities and future risk of cognitive impairment
and dementia: systematic review and meta-analysis. *International Psychogeriatrics,
28*(11), 1791–1806. https://doi.org/10.1017/S1041610216001137

168 the lower their risk of cognitive impairment: Hansdottir, H., Jonsdottir, M. K.,
Fisher, D. E., Eiriksdottir, G., Jonsson, P. V., & Gudnason, V. (2022). Creativity,
leisure activities, social engagement and cognitive impairment: the AGES-Reykjavík
study. *Aging Clinical and Experimental Research, 34*(5), 1027–1035. https://doi.org
/10.1007/s40520-021-02036-1

168 able to access more resources for processing and retaining information: Shukla, A.
(2018, updated 2020). Why fun, curiosity & engagement improves learning: mood,
senses, neurons, arousal, cognition. *Cognition Today.* https://cognitiontoday.com/why
-fun-improves-learning-mood-senses-neurons-arousal-cognition/#:~:text=Research%20
shows%20that%20having%20fun,the%20other%20for%20focused%20attention

174 as harmful to your health as smoking fifteen cigarettes a day: Holt-Lunstad, J.,
Smith, T. B., Baker, M., Harris, T., & Stephenson, D. (2015). Loneliness and social
isolation as risk factors for mortality: A meta-analytic review. *Perspectives on*

Psychological Science: A Journal of the Association for Psychological Science, *10*(2), 227–237. https://doi.org/10.1177/1745691614568352

174 significantly associated with premature death, cardiovascular disease, elevated cortisol, an upregulation of inflammatory genes, depression, and yes, dementia: Bhatti, A. B., & Haq, A. U. (2017). The pathophysiology of perceived social isolation: Effects on health and mortality. *Cureus, 9*(1). e994. https://doi.org/10.7759/cureus.994

174 the better your health outcomes—such as blood pressure, inflammation, and cognitive function—tend to be: Holt-Lunstad, J., Robles, T. F., & Sbarra, D. A. (2017). Advancing social connection as a public health priority in the United States. *American Psychologist, 72*(6), 517–530. https://doi.org/10.1037/amp0000103

177 lower or decrease blood pressure: Bai, Z., Chang, J., Chen, C., Li, P., Yang, K., & Chi, I. (2015). Investigating the effect of transcendental meditation on blood pressure: A systematic review and meta-analysis. *Journal of Human Hypertension, 29*(11), 653–662. https://doi.org/10.1038/jhh.2015.6

177 inflammation: Rosenkranz, M. A., Davidson, R. J., Maccoon, D. G., Sheridan, J. F., Kalin, N. H., & Lutz, A. (2013). A comparison of mindfulness-based stress reduction and an active control in modulation of neurogenic inflammation. *Brain, Behavior, and Immunity, 27*(1), 174–184. https://doi.org/10.1016/j.bbi.2012.10.013

177 the perception of pain: Rod, K. (2015). Observing the effects of mindfulness-based meditation on anxiety and depression in chronic pain patients. *Psychiatria Danubina, 27*(Suppl 1), S209–S211.

177 symptoms of irritable bowel syndrome: Baboş, C. I., Leucuţa, D. C., & Dumitraşcu, D. L. (2022). Meditation and irritable bowel syndrome, a systematic review and meta-analysis. *Journal of Clinical Medicine, 11*(21), 6516. https://doi.org/10.3390/jcm11216516

177 posttraumatic stress disorder: Hilton, L., Maher, A. R., Colaiaco, B., Apaydin, E., Sorbero, M. E., Booth, M., Shanman, R. M., & Hempel, S. (2017). Meditation for posttraumatic stress: Systematic review and meta-analysis. *Psychological Trauma: Theory, Research, Practice and Policy, 9*(4), 453–460. https://doi.org/10.1037/tra0000180

177 fibromyalgia: Aman, M. M., Jason Yong, R., Kaye, A. D., & Urman, R. D. (2018). Evidence-based non-pharmacological therapies for fibromyalgia. *Current Pain and Headache Reports, 22*(5), 33. https://doi.org/10.1007/s11916-018-0688-2

177 help individuals overcome addictions: Garland, E. L., & Howard, M. O. (2018). Mindfulness-based treatment of addiction: Current state of the field and envisioning the next wave of research. *Addiction Science & Clinical Practice, 13*(1), 14. https://doi.org/10.1186/s13722-018-0115-3

177 increase overall brain volume: Luders, E., Cherbuin, N., & Kurth, F. (2015). Forever young(er): Potential age-defying effects of long-term meditation on gray matter atrophy. *Frontiers in Psychology, 5*, 1551. https://doi.org/10.3389/fpsyg.2014.01551

177 the thickness of the lining of the hippocampus: Hölzel, B. K., Carmody, J., Vangel, M., Congleton, C., Yerramsetti, S. M., Gard, T., & Lazar, S. W. (2011). Mindfulness practice leads to increases in regional brain gray matter density. *Psychiatry Research, 191*(1), 36–43. https://doi.org/10.1016/j.pscychresns.2010.08.006

177 emotional reactivity and rumination: ibid.; Brewer, J. A., Worhunsky, P. D., Gray, J. R., Tang, Y. Y., Weber, J., & Kober, H. (2011). Meditation experience is associated with differences in default mode network activity and connectivity. *Proceedings of the National Academy of Sciences of the United States of America*, *108*(50), 20254–20259. https://doi.org/10.1073/pnas.1112029108

177 increasing focus, attention, and memory: Basso, J. C., McHale, A., Ende, V., Oberlin, D. J., & Suzuki, W. A. (2019). Brief, daily meditation enhances attention, memory, mood, and emotional regulation in non-experienced meditators. *Behavioural Brain Research*, *356*, 208–220. https://doi.org/10.1016/j.bbr.2018.08.023; Norris, C. J., Creem, D., Hendler, R., & Kober, H. (2018). Brief mindfulness meditation improves attention in novices: evidence from ERPs and moderation by meuroticism. *Frontiers in Human Neuroscience*, *12*, 315. https://doi.org/10.3389/fnhum.2018.00315; Tsai, S. Y., Jaiswal, S., Chang, C. F., Liang, W. K., Muggleton, N. G., & Juan, C. H. (2018). Meditation effects on the control of involuntary contingent reorienting revealed with electroencephalographic and behavioral evidence. *Frontiers in Integrative Neuroscience*, *12*, 17. https://doi.org/10.3389/fnint.2018.00017; Mrazek, M. D., Franklin, M. S., Phillips, D. T., Baird, B., & Schooler, J. W. (2013). Mindfulness training improves working memory capacity and GRE performance while reducing mind wandering. *Psychological Science*, *24*(5), 776–781. https://doi.org/10.1177/0956797612459659

177 influence the immune system and that regulate levels of glucose and insulin: Khalsa, D. S. (2015). Stress, meditation, and Alzheimer's disease prevention: Where the evidence stands. *Journal of Alzheimer's Disease: JAD*, *48*(1), 1–12. https://doi.org/10.3233/JAD-142766

181 slower rate of cognitive decline: Boyle, P. A., Buchman, A. S., Barnes, L. L., & Bennett, D. A. (2010). Effect of a purpose in life on risk of incident Alzheimer disease and mild cognitive impairment in community-dwelling older persons. *Archives of General Psychiatry*, *67*(3), 304–310. https://doi.org/10.1001/archgenpsychiatry.2009.208

181 associated with larger hippocampal volume: Carlson, M. C., Kuo, J. H., Chuang, Y. F., Varma, V. R., Harris, G., Albert, M. S., Erickson, K. I., Kramer, A. F., Parisi, J. M., Xue, Q. L., Tan, E. J., Tanner, E. K., Gross, A. L., Seeman, T. E., Gruenewald, T. L., McGill, S., Rebok, G. W., & Fried, L. P. (2015). Impact of the Baltimore Experience Corps Trial on cortical and hippocampal volumes. *Alzheimer's & Dementia: The Journal of the Alzheimer's Association*, *11*(11), 1340–1348. https://doi.org/10.1016/j.jalz.2014.12.005; Sakurai, R., Ishii, K., Sakuma, N., Yasunaga, M., Suzuki, H., Murayama, Y., Nishi, M., Uchida, H., Shinkai, S., & Fujiwara, Y. (2018). Preventive effects of an intergenerational program on age-related hippocampal atrophy in older adults: The REPRINTS study. *International Journal of Geriatric Psychiatry*, *33*(2), e264–e272. https://doi.org/10.1002/gps.4785

Chapter 9: Create a Brain-Nourishing Environment

186 the science is mixed: Desai, R. J., Mahesri, M., Lee, S. B., Varma, V. R., Loeffler, T., Schilcher, I., Gerhard, T., Segal, J. B., Ritchey, M. E., Horton, D. B., Kim, S. C.,

Schneeweiss, S., & Thambisetty, M. (2022). No association between initiation of phosphodiesterase-5 inhibitors and risk of incident Alzheimer's disease and related dementia: results from the Drug Repurposing for Effective Alzheimer's Medicines study. *Brain Communications, 4*(5), fcac247. https://doi.org/10.1093/braincomms /fcac247; Fang, J., Zhang, P., Zhou, Y., Chiang, C. W., Tan, J., Hou, Y., Stauffer, S., Li, L., Pieper, A. A., Cummings, J., & Cheng, F. (2021). Endophenotype-based in silico network medicine discovery combined with insurance record data mining identifies sildenafil as a candidate drug for Alzheimer's disease. *Nature Aging, 1*(12), 1175–1188. https://doi.org/10.1038/s43587-021-00138-z

193 it's 80 percent water: Lisa Mosconi. (2022). *The XX Brain* (New York: Avery Publishing), 197.

Chapter 10: Care for the Caregiver (Meaning You)

214 decrease in a general sense of well-being and quality of life: Pinquart, M., & Sörensen, S. (2003). Differences between caregivers and noncaregivers in psychological health and physical health: A meta-analysis. *Psychology and Aging, 18*(2), 250–267. https://doi.org/10.1037/0882-7974.18.2.250

214 significantly lower scores on tests of cognitive function: Falzarano, F., & Siedlecki, K. L. (2021). Differences in cognitive performance between informal caregivers and non-caregivers. *Neuropsychology, Development, and Cognition. Section B, Aging, Neuropsychology and Cognition, 28*(2), 284–307. https://doi.org/10.1080/13825585.2020 .1749228; Dassel, K. B., Carr, D. C., & Vitaliano, P. (2017). Does caring for a spouse with dementia accelerate cognitive decline? Findings from the Health and Retirement Study. *The Gerontologist, 57*(2), 319–328. https://doi.org/10.1093/geront/gnv148

214 Between 50 and 70 percent of dementia caregivers report regular sleep disturbances: Byun, E., Lerdal, A., Gay, C. L., & Lee, K. A. (2016). How adult caregiving impacts sleep: A systematic review. *Current Sleep Medicine Reports, 2*(4), 191–205. https://doi .org/10.1007/s40675-016-0058-8

214 people with dementia experience depression more frequently than the general population: Huang, S. S. (2022). Depression among caregivers of patients with dementia: Associative factors and management approaches. *World Journal of Psychiatry, 12*(1), 59–76. https://doi.org/10.5498/wjp.v12.i1.59

215 a bigger negative impact on well-being than unemployment: Giurge, L., Whillans, A. V., & West, C. (2020). Why time poverty matters for individuals, organisations, and nations. *Nature Human Behaviour, 4*(10), 993–1003. https://www.hks.harvard.edu /centers/mrcbg/programs/growthpolicy/beyond-material-poverty-why-time-poverty -matters-individuals

215 up to a sixfold increase compared to non-caregivers: Norton, M. C., Smith, K. R., Østbye, T., Tschanz, J. T., Corcoran, C., Schwartz, S., Piercy, K. W., Rabins, P. V., Steffens, D. C., Skoog, I., Breitner, J. C., Welsh-Bohmer, K. A., & Cache County Investigators, (2010). Greater risk of dementia when spouse has dementia? The Cache County study. *Journal of the American Geriatrics Society, 58*(5), 895–900. https://doi .org/10.1111/j.1532-5415.2010.02806.x

215 when the sense of caregiving burden is high: Vitaliano, P. P. (2010). An ironic tragedy: are spouses of persons with dementia at higher risk for dementia than spouses of persons without dementia? *Journal of the American Geriatrics Society, 58*(5), 976–978. https://doi.org/10.1111/j.1532-5415.2010.02843.x

215 caregiving actually bestows important gifts: O'Reilly, D., Rosato, M., & Maguire, A. (2015). Caregiving reduces mortality risk for most caregivers: A census-based record linkage study. *International Journal of Epidemiology, 44*(6), 1959–1969. https://doi .org/10.1093/ije/dyv172; Roth, et al.

216 deepened relationships and an increased sense of purpose: Cohen, C. A., Colantonio, A., & Vernich, L. (2002). Positive aspects of caregiving: Rounding out the caregiver experience. *International Journal of Geriatric Psychiatry, 17*(2), 184–188. https://doi .org/10.1002/gps.56

216 experiencing greater overall well-being than non-caregivers: O'Reilly, D., Rosato, M., & Maguire, A. (2015). Caregiving reduces mortality risk for most caregivers: A census-based record linkage study. *International Journal of Epidemiology, 44*(6), 1959–1969. https://doi.org/10.1093/ije/dyv172

216 positive aspects of caregiving help them deal with any negative effects they may experience: Fauziana, R., Sambasivam, R., Vaingankar, J. A., Abdin, E., Ong, H. L., Tan, M. E., Chong, S. A., & Subramaniam, M. (2018). Positive caregiving characteristics as a mediator of caregiving burden and satisfaction with life in caregivers of older adults. *Journal of Geriatric Psychiatry and Neurology, 31*(6), 329–335. https://doi.org/10.1177/0891988718802111

221 shown to reduce the perception of caregiver burden: Lloyd, J., Muers, J., Patterson, T. G., & Marczak, M. (2019). Self-compassion, coping strategies, and caregiver burden in caregivers of people with dementia. *Clinical Gerontologist, 42* (1), 47–59. https://doi .org/10.1080/07317115.2018.1461162

224 enhance a sense of connectedness and life satisfaction: Kerr, S. L., O'Donovan, A., & Pepping, C. A. (2015). Can gratitude and kindness interventions enhance well-being in a clinical sample? *Journal of Happiness Studies: An Interdisciplinary Forum on Subjective Well-Being, 16*(1), 17–36. https://doi.org/10.1007/s10902-013-9492-1; Killen, A., & Macaskill, A. (2015). *Journal of Happiness Studies, 16* (4), 947–964. https://doi/10.1007/s10902-014-9542-3; Kini, P., Wong, J., McInnis, S., Gabana, N., & Brown, J. W. (2016). The effects of gratitude expression on neural activity. *NeuroImage, 128*, 1–10. https://doi.org/10.1016/j.neuroimage.2015.12.040

226 significant relief in symptoms of fibromyalgia and long Covid: Sanabria-Mazo, J. P., Montero-Marin, J., Feliu-Soler, A., Gasión, V., Navarro-Gil, M., Morillo-Sarto, H., Colomer-Carbonell, A., Borràs, X., Tops, M., Luciano, J. V., & García-Campayo, J. (2020). Mindfulness-based program plus amygdala and insula retraining (MAIR) for the treatment of women with fibromyalgia: A pilot randomized controlled trial. *Journal of Clinical Medicine, 9*(10), 3246. https://doi.org/10.3390/jcm9103246

227 dementia caregivers who were assigned regular massages saw a significant reduction in caregiver burden: Szczepańska-Gieracha, J., Jaworska-Burzyńska, L., Boroń-Krupińska, K., & Kowalska, J. (2020). Nonpharmacological forms of therapy to reduce the burden on

caregivers of patients with dementia: A pilot intervention study. *International Journal of Environmental Research and Public Health, 17*(24), 9153. https://doi.org/10.3390/ijerph17249153

Chapter 11: Partner with Your Provider

247 the media reported that as an increase in risk of 26 percent: Dominus, S. (2023). Women have been misled about menopause. *The New York Times*. https://www.nytimes.com/2023/02/01/magazine/menopause-hot-flashes-hormone-therapy.html

247 significantly reduces the risk of all-cause mortality and cardiovascular disease: Hodis, H. N., & Mack, W. J. (2022). Menopausal hormone replacement therapy and reduction of all-cause mortality and cardiovascular disease: It is about time and timing. *Cancer Journal, 28*(3), 208–223. https://doi.org/10.1097/PPO.0000000000000591

248 significant reduction in breast cancer risk compared to the rest of the similarly aged population: Mikkola, T. S., Savolainen-Peltonen, H., Tuomikoski, P., Hoti, F., Vattulainen, P., Gissler, M., & Ylikorkala, O. (2016). Reduced risk of breast cancer mortality in women using postmenopausal hormone therapy: A Finnish nationwide comparative study. *Menopause, 23*(11), 1199–1203. https://doi.org/10.1097/GME.0000000000000698

248 taking hormones reduced the risk of all-cause mortality by 9 percent: Akter, N., Kulinskaya, E., Steel, N., Bakbergenuly, I. (2021). The effect of hormone replacement therapy on the survival of UK women: A retrospective cohort study 1984–2017. *BJOG, 129*, 994–1003. https://doi.org/10.1111/1471-0528.17008

249 "Alzheimer's disease starts earlier in women's brains than men's brains": "Menopause brain" is a real thing. Here's what you can do about it. Ted Radio Hour. (2022). https://www.npr.org/transcripts/973805003

255 when people have enough vitamin D it appears to prevent cognitive decline: Shea, M. K., Barger, K., Dawson-Hughes, B., Leurgans, S. E., Fu, X., James, B. D., Holland, T. M., Agarwal, P., Wang, J., Matuszek, G., Heger, N. E., Schneider, J. A., & Booth, S. L. (2022). Brain vitamin D forms, cognitive decline, and neuropathology in community-dwelling older adults. *Alzheimer's & Dementia: The Journal of the Alzheimer's Association, 19*(6), 2389–2396. https://doi.org/10.1002/alz.12836

255 Higher levels of circulating vitamin K is associated with better cognitive function: Booth, S. L., Shea, M. K., Barger, K., Leurgans, S. E., James, B. D., Holland, T. M., Agarwal, P., Fu, X., Wang, J., Matuszek, G., & Schneider, J. A. (2022). Association of vitamin K with cognitive decline and neuropathology in community-dwelling older persons. *Alzheimer's & Dementia, 8*(1), e12255. https://doi.org/10.1002/trc2.12255

256 Higher levels of omega-3s in the blood are associated with a bigger hippocampus: Satizabal, C. L., Himali, J. J., Beiser, A. S., Ramachandran, V., Melo van Lent, D., Himali, D., Aparicio, H. J., Maillard, P., DeCarli, C. S., Harris, W., & Seshadri, S.

(2022). Association of red blood cell Omega-3 fatty acids with MRI markers and cognitive function in midlife: The Framingham Heart Study. *Neurology*, *99*(23), e2572–e2582. Advance online publication. https://doi.org/10.1212 /WNL.0000000000201296

Chapter 12: A Glimpse into the Near Future

264 raises levels of brain-derived neurotrophic factor (BDNF) and antioxidants: Hamblin, M. R. (2016). Shining light on the head: Photobiomodulation for brain disorders. *BBA Clinical*, *6*, 113–124. https://doi.org/10.1016/j.bbacli.2016.09.002

264 increase in sleep and cognitive function: Chao, L. L. (2019). Effects of home photobiomodulation treatments on cognitive and behavioral function, cerebral perfusion, and resting-state functional connectivity in patients with dementia: A pilot trial. *Photobiomodulation, Photomedicine, and Laser Surgery*, *37*(3), 133–141. https://doi.org/10.1089/photob.2018.4555; Saltmarche, A. E., Naeser, M. A., Ho, K. F., Hamblin, M. R., & Lim, L. (2017). Significant improvement in cognition in mild to moderately severe dementia cases treated with transcranial plus intranasal photobiomodulation: Case series report. *Photomedicine and Laser Surgery*, *35*(8), 432–441. https://doi.org/10.1089/pho.2016.4227

266 even grow new neurons in the hippocampus: Zimmer, C. (2014). Young blood may hold key to reversing aging. *The New York Times*. https://www.nytimes .com/2014/05/05/science/young-blood-may-hold-key-to-reversing-aging.html

266 extended their life spans by 6 to 9 percent: Zhang, B., Lee, D. E., Trapp, A., Tyshkovskiy, A., Lu, A. T., Bareja, A., Kerepesi, C., McKay, L. K., Shindyapina, A. V., Dmitriev, S. E., Baht, G. S., Horvath, S., Gladyshev, V. N., & White, J. P. (2023). Multi-omic rejuvenation and life span extension on exposure to youthful circulation. *Nature Aging*, *3*(8), 948–964. https://doi.org/10.1038/s43587-023-00451-9

266 showed improved cognitive function in patients with mild Alzheimer's: Boada, M., López, O. L., Olazarán, J., Núñez, L., Pfeffer, M., Paricio, M., Lorites, J., Piñol-Ripoll, G., Gámez, J. E., Anaya, F., Kiprov, D., Lima, J., Grifols, C., Torres, M., Costa, M., Bozzo, J., Szczepiorkowski, Z. M., Hendrix, S., & Páez, A. (2020). A randomized, controlled clinical trial of plasma exchange with albumin replacement for Alzheimer's disease: Primary results of the AMBAR study. *Alzheimer's & Dementia: The Journal of the Alzheimer's Association*, *16*(10), 1412–1425. https://doi.org/10.1002/alz.12137; Boada, M., López, O. L., Olazarán, J., Núñez, L., Pfeffer, M., Puente, O., Piñol-Ripoll, G., Gámez, J. E., Anaya, F., Kiprov, D., Alegret, M., Grifols, C., Barceló, M., Bozzo, J., Szczepiorkowski, Z. M., Páez, A., & AMBAR Trial Group (2022). Neuropsychological, neuropsychiatric, and quality-of-life assessments in Alzheimer's disease patients treated with plasma exchange with albumin replacement from the randomized AMBAR study. *Alzheimer's & Dementia: The Journal of the Alzheimer's Association*, *18*(7), 1314–1324. https://doi.org/10.1002 /alz.12477

268   improvement in memory and learning ability after treatment: Qin, C., Wang, K., Zhang, L., & Bai, L. (2022). Stem cell therapy for Alzheimer's disease: An overview of experimental models and reality. *Animal Models and Experimental Medicine, 5*(1), 15–26. https://doi.org/10.1002%2Fame2.12207; Duncan, T., & Valenzuela, M. (2017). Alzheimer's disease, dementia, and stem cell therapy. *Stem Cell Research & Therapy, 8*, 1–9. https://doi.org/10.1186/s13287-017-0567-5

269   promising research on the effectiveness of stem cell treatment for dementia that has been conducted on animals: Qin, C., Wang, K., Zhang, L., & Bai, L. (2022). Stem cell therapy for Alzheimer's disease: An overview of experimental models and reality. *Animal Models and Experimental Medicine, 5*(1), 15–26. https://doi.org /10.1002%2Fame2.12207

270   Cerebrolysin aids in recovery after stroke and traumatic brain injury: Jarosz, K., Kojder, K., Andrzejewska, A., Solek-Pastuszka, J., & Jurczak, A. (2023). Cerebrolysin in patients with TBI: Systematic review and meta-analysis. *Brain Sciences, 13*(3), 507. https://doi.org/10.3390/brainsci13030507; Mureşanu, D. F., Livinţ Popa, L., Chira, D., Dăbală, V., Hapca, E., Vlad, I., Văcăraş, V., Popescu, B. O., Chereches, R., Strilciuc, Ş., & Brainin, M. (2022). Role and impact of Cerebrolysin for ischemic stroke care. *Journal of Clinical Medicine, 11*(5), 1273. https://doi.org/10.3390 /jcm11051273

271   sevenfold more potent than BDNF: Sun, X., Deng, Y., Fu, X., Wang, S., Duan, R., & Zhang, Y. (2021). AngIV-Analog Dihexa rescues cognitive impairment and recovers memory in the APP/PS1 mouse via the PI3K/AKT signaling pathway. *Brain Sciences, 11*(11), 1487. https://doi.org/10.3390/brainsci11111487; McCoy, A. T., Benoist, C. C., Wright, J. W., Kawas, L. H., Bule-Ghogare, J. M., Zhu, M., Appleyard, S. M., Wayman, G. A., & Harding, J. W. (2013). Evaluation of metabolically stabilized angiotensin IV analogs as procognitive/antidementia agents. *The Journal of Pharmacology and Experimental Therapeutics, 344*(1), 141–154. https://doi.org /10.1124/jpet.112.199497

272   looking at the exosomes you have in your body can help diagnose specific types of dementia: Soares Martins, T., Trindade, D., Vaz, M., Campelo, I., Almeida, M., Trigo, G., da Cruz E Silva, O. A. B., & Henriques, A. G. (2021). Diagnostic and therapeutic potential of exosomes in Alzheimer's disease. *Journal of Neurochemistry, 156*(2), 162–181. https://doi.org/10.1111/jnc.15112

273   point to promise as an Alzheimer's therapeutic: Vann Jones, S. A., & O'Kelly, A. (2020). Psychedelics as a treatment for Alzheimer's disease dementia. *Frontiers in Synaptic Neuroscience, 12*(34). https://doi.org/10.3389/fnsyn.2020.00034

273   the FDA issued draft guidance for the study of psychedelics: Siegel, J. S., Daily, J. E., Perry, D. A., & Nicol, G. E. (2023). Psychedelic drug legislative reform and legalization in the US. *JAMA Psychiatry, 80*(1), 77–83. https://doi.org/10.1001 /jamapsychiatry.2022.4101

273   a clinical trial that will evaluate psilocybin as a potential aid for depression in early Alzheimer's disease: Retrieved on November 20, 2023, from https:// hopkinspsychedelic.org/alzheimers

275 shingles vaccine is associated with a 15 percent reduction in risk of developing both Alzheimer's and Parkinson's: Lehrer, S., & Rheinstein, P. H. (2022). Vaccination reduces risk of Alzheimer's disease, Parkinson's disease and other neurodegenerative disorders. *Discovery Medicine, 34*(172), 97–101.

275 from the current 55 million to an estimated 78 million people worldwide by 2030: World Health Organization. (2022). A blueprint for dementia research. https://www.who.int/publications/i/item/9789240058248

INDEX

Page numbers of illustrations appear in italics.

ABOUT THE AUTHOR

DR. HEATHER SANDISON is the founder and medical director of Solcere Health Clinic, a San Diego–based brain optimization clinic, and Marama, the first residential memory-care facility to have the goal of returning its residents to independent living. Her pioneering combination of clinical work, peer-reviewed research, and the development of educational platforms has transformed the lives of patients and caregivers and set new standards in the field of dementia care.